Tired All The Time?"

The Causes, Consequences and Cures

Dr David H. Dighton

MEDICAUSE

First Published 2025

Copyright © David Henry Dighton

David H. Dighton™

Published in the UK by MediCause, 115 High Rd., Loughton, Essex. UK. IG10 4JA

www.daviddighton.com

email: david@daviddighton.com

British Library Cataloguing in Publication Data

A CIP catalogue record for this title is available from the British Library.

ISBN: 978-1-0683597-4-3

Dedication

For all those who spent their energy encouraging me.

I am indebted to Dr. Peter Nixon, cardiologist at Charing Cross Hospital, London, who gave me insight into fatigue, ill-health and cardiovascular disease, and how they might be reversed.

Peter had enough insight to bring new light to the understanding of cardiac illness. He tried to change opinions and remove ignorance, but his colleagues, all of whom were intelligent enough to understand it, were not always predisposed to listen.

About the Author

Formerly,

British Heart Foundation Research Fellow,

St. George's Hospital, London.

Lecturer in Cardiology,

Charing Cross Hospital, London.

Chef de Clinique, Cardiologist, Vrije Universiteit. Amsterdam.

Former Director: Cardiac Centre. Loughton. Essex, UK.

www.daviddighton.com

email:

david@daviddighton.com

Dr. David H. Dighton qualified at the London Hospital Medical College in 1966 with MB and BS (London) degrees. In 1970, after a year or so in NHS general practice, he became a British Heart Foundation Fellow in Cardiology at St. George's Hospital, Hyde Park Corner, London, working with cardiologists Dr. Aubrey

Leatham and Dr. Alan Harris. In 1973, he became a MRCP(UK), and later a Lecturer (London University) in Medicine and Cardiology at Charing Cross Hospital, London.

In 1980, as Chef de Clinique (Assistant Professor) at the Vrije University Hospital, Amsterdam, he helped introduce trans-venous pacing and collaborated in ongoing coronary artery research. After returning to the UK in 1982, he worked both in his own private medical and cardiac practice in Loughton, Essex (The Loughton Clinic, established in 1973), undertaking invasive cardiac investigations at the Wellington Hospital, London. In 2000, he started a private cardiac diagnostic centre, specialising in the early detection and prevention of coronary artery disease (The Cardiac Centre, Loughton). This closed, once the Public Services Authority directed the GMC to withdraw his license to practice in the UK (the political reasons are detailed in his book, 'The NHS. Our Sick Sacred Cow.' 2023). As an independent private cardiologist and general physician, he disagreed with UK medical bureaucracy, and who they thought most qualified to devise, regulate and supervise medical practice; opinions he based on having been a medical student, general physician and cardiologist for sixty years.

In 2003 and 2006, he wrote two books on food and the heart, and between 2022 and 2025, seven books on medical and cardiac subjects. His most recent technical book (2025), explores the possible neurophysiological bases for tiredness, fatigue and exhaustion. This is his eleventh book (see list of works by the author for details). He continues to publish books on cardiac topics, to write haiku and to research cardiac prevention.

His interest in the frontier that lies between art and science in medical practice, led to his magnum opus: *The Art and Science of Medical Practice.* This details not only what he was taught by many experienced physicians, but what he learned from practising both the art and science of medicine in teaching hospitals and in private practice. As medical student, physician and cardiologist, he studied and worked within the fold of the UK medical profession for sixty years.

He has other interests. He is a poor linguist but loves learning languages and communicating in languages other than his mother tongue. He draws and paints in oils on canvas. For his own amusement, he plays the guitar and piano. He likes to compose simple melodies, one of which introduces his YouTube videos for patients on understanding heart problems (Dr. Dighton interviews). Another he played live for a friend on Facebook.

For further information goto: www.daviddighton.com.

To view his artworks – oil on canvas – goto: uniqart4u.co.uk.

Email: david@daviddighton.com.

Other Works by the Author

Eat to Your Heart's Content. The diet and lifestyle for a healthy heart.(2003). HeartShield.

ISBN: 0-9551072-0-2

HeartSense. How to look after your heart.(2006). HeartShield.

ISBN: 0-9551072-1-0

The NHS: Our Sick Sacred Cow: Causes and Cures (2023)

Paperback. ISBN: 978-1-3999-6027-4 (also ebook from: https://stan.store/drdhd001001)

How to Become Heart-Smart. A User's Guide to Heart Health and Heart Disease Prevention. (2023; 1st Ed./**2nd Ed. 2024**. ISBN: 978-1-3999-7461-5 (also ebook from: https://stan.store/drdhd001001)

Who Loses Wins. Winning Weight Loss Battles: A 'Fat Mentality' v A 'Fit Mentality' (2024).

Paperback ISBN: 978-1-7385207-1-8; ebook: 978-1-7385207-2-5. (from: https://stan.store/drdhd001001)

Doctors, Nurses & Patients. How to Survive Medical Practice (2024). ISBN: Paperback: 978-1-7385207-5-6; ebook: 978-1-7385207-6-3 (from: https://stan.store/drdhd001001)

The Art and Science of Medical Practice (2024). ISBN: (hardback: 978-1-7385207-7-0;

Paperback: 978-1-7385207-3-2; ebook: 978-1-7385207-4-9 (from: https://stan.store/drdhd001001)

Poems for Recycling Lives (2024).

ISBN: Paperback: 978-1-7385207-8-7; ebook: 978-1-7385207-9-4

Essential Adult Cardiology. A Textbook for Aspiring Cardiologists.(2025)

ISBN: Hardback 978-0683597-0-5; Paperback 978-0683597-2-9; e-book 978-0683597-1-2

Tiredness, Chronic Fatigue and Exhaustion. Neurophysiology and Cardiovascular Risk. (2025).

Hardback only. ISBN: 978-1-0683597-3-6

www.daviddighton.com   for   more   information.

Contents

Detailed Contents

Introduction

Stresses in Life: Foreground Issues; Background Issues; Subliminal Issues. Traffic Analysis Theory of Tiredness.

PART ONE

The Basics

1. Tiredness, Fatigue and Exhaustion

Definitions of tiredness, fatigue, and exhaustion. The Human Function Curve. 'Healthy' and 'Unhealthy' Tiredness; Sameness, Boredom and its Tiring Effect; Health and Vitality.

2. **Human Energy**

Energy for Life; Forms of Energy; Human Energy Income and Expenditure.

3. Stimulus, Response and Constitution (Stress & Strain)

PART TWO

Spending Energy: Personality Types and the Demands of Life

8. Personalities, Outlooks and Energy Spending

Personal Character and Energy Spending; At-Oneness and Ego; Snobbery; Beauty; Vanity; Sympathy and Antipathy; Delegation and Resignation of Duty; Discipline; Integrity; Talent and Incompetence; The Effect of Upbringing; Choice: Fantasy v Reality; Warrior Virtues; Frustrated Warriors; Neuroticism; Other Energy Spending Traits; Sex and Gender on Mars and Venus; Loners and Followers; Birth Order; Sympathy and Love; Antipathy and Hate; Self-Worth; Incompetence; Key Human Energy Spending Factors.

9. Foreground Stress: Transient Transactions

The Natural Life; Surveillance and Action; Conditioning; Happiness as a Modifier; Reactiveness; Fear; Responses to Stress; Communication; Personal Biases.

10. Background Stresses: Life Problems and their Resolution

Personal Biases; Resolving Conflict, Reducing Stress; Slow Decision Making; Relationships and Mismatched Needs; Three Areas of Need: Affection; Does Love Conquer All?; Control; The Need for Inclusion; Pleasurable and Unpleasurable Relationships; Business Relationships; Pathological Relationships; Assessing Relationships; Life Change; Life Situations; Case Histories: 1 & 2; Constant Competition; Defending Thoughts and Feelings; Attention-Seeking; Limelight and Fame; A Mere Life of Ease; Culture & Relationships; The Family; Baby Bonding; Surviving Parenthood.

11. Subliminal Stresses. The Pool in Which we Swim

Social Factors; Urban or Rural? Environmental Energy Spending; All in Our Genes?

Damocles' Many Swords – Subliminal Threat; Advertising and Subliminal Stress;

The Pleasure Principle; The Wealth Paradox; Past Experience as a Stressor.

PART THREE

Medical Energetics

12. Medical Causes of Fatigue

The Causes of Fatigue; The Sleep Paradox; Myalgic Encephalitis (ME); Chronic Ebstein-Barr Infection (Glandular Fever or Infectious Mononucleosis); Other Infections; Chronic Fatigue Syndrome; Post-Traumatic Stress Disorder (PTSD); Menopause; Other Hormonal Conditions; Heart Failure; Brain Biochemistry and Fatigue; Age; Causative Circumstances; Dietary Influence; Therapeutic Causes; Recognising Fatigue in Others; Rehabilitation.

13. Ill-health, Disease and Medical Catastrophe

Medical Catastrophe; Is Stress Always the Cause of Heart Attacks?; Order and Catastrophe; The Seeds of Catastrophe; The Benefits of Catastrophe.

14. Unlocking Energy: Rest, Sleep. and Traffic Analysis

Sleep and Rest; Perceived Energy Gain; 'All Shook Up'; Energy Saving; The Holiday Effect; The Sleep Paradox; The Sabbath: A

List of Figures & Illustrations

Introduction

"A man who has energy and talent, can be a King amongst men.

A man who has energy alone, with no other particular gift, can be a Prince.

Those who have talent but no gift of energy will be paupers."

Jeffrey Archer. *John Dunn, Radio 2.*
7.6.8

Personal energy is essential for the maintenance of health and to achieve success in life. In this book, I have attempted to explain its absence – all the causes of tiredness, fatigue and exhaustion, most of which are not related to physical illness. Although often trivial in cause and effect, fatigue and exhaustion can be associated with catastrophic, life-threatening sequels, like septicaemia (sepsis), mental breakdown, heart attacks and strokes. As a cardiologist I have seen chronic fatigue ruin lives, and ruin cause fatigue. If doctors took tiredness, fatigue and exhaustion more seriously, they could limit clinical risk, reduce the frequency and severity of symptoms, improve blood pressure, coagulation and immune responses, and even save some lives.

Living a full life needs energy-driven vitality. Energy controls our quality of life and can influence length of life. If we are to achieve what we later regard as worthwhile, we must have energy and the desire to spend it appropriately.

We are all aware of our personal energy balance: the misery of feeling depleted and fatigued, and the exhilaration of boundless vitality. There is a direct financial equivalent – wealth, when money is in excess; poverty, when it is lacking. Some handle both their money and energy with ease; others spend their life worrying about them. One can learn to balance both, but only those with the ability to learn, a willingness to practise, and a mind happy to embrace change, have any chance.

Have you ever wondered why some people suffer from a sudden – 'out-of-the-blue' – medical condition? Many who have lived more than a few decades, will have lost a friend or family member from a sudden heart attack or stroke. They might then have wondered why. Some will have watched a friend or relative slowly deteriorate, without any apparent cause. Others will have seen a friend age rapidly, get tired-out and frightened, for no obvious reason. They may have previously consulted their doctor without being given a diagnosis. Although not all, many such patients will have experienced prolonged tiredness before any sudden event.

Could there be a connection between progressive fatigue and illness? Does the brain have a battery that runs down, to leave us tired and short of energy? Everyone gets tired; something mostly reversed by refreshing sleep. But what about fatigue and long-term (chronic) exhaustion? Why is it not possible to reverse extreme tiredness with one night of refreshing sleep? Might a virus or some hidden disease be the cause? How is it, with all the advances of modern medical science, the causes of tiredness, fatigue, and exhaustion are often a mystery.

It is common for patients to go to their doctor complaining of feeling 'tired all the time' (TATT, some doctors call it) to be investigated for every known medical condition – some treatable – some not. How many patients are told, 'I am pleased to tell you, I have found nothing wrong with you.' Happy not to have a detectable, serious disease, many walk away satisfied. Others might conclude that their tiredness is 'all in their mind'.

In practice, I found only 1.5% of the one thousand fatigued patients I fully investigated, with an organic cause for their fatigue – like diabetes or an under-active thyroid. Many are pigeon-holed by doctors with an unsatisfactory, ill-defined diagnosis, like 'chronic fatigue syndrome' (which explains nothing) or ME (myalgic encephalomyelitis), the cause of which has been long disputed.

From a medical perspective, tiredness is not often serious, unless progressive and prolonged. It can then precede to catastrophes like heart attacks and strokes. It can sometimes explain why high blood pressure is more difficult to control, and why migraine attacks become more frequent. Can it make pneumonia more likely and more difficult to treat? One might ask Hillary Clinton. In 2016, she developed pneumonia after losing the US presidential race to Donald Trump. One might have asked Winston Churchill who in

1943, contracted pneumonia that almost killed him. He became ill soon after a conference in Tehran. He later remarked that he had felt crushed, between a Russian bear (Stalin), and an American elephant (Roosevelt).

What of those dying suddenly? Could tiredness and fatigue have provided a warning? A clue it might be, but one often ignored or downgraded in significance by both patients and doctors alike.

Stress may not be the cause of disease, but it can certainly modify its severity and course. Stress drains our energy, but what qualifies as a biological stress? The problem is, we all define it differently, although for physicists, it couldn't be simpler – it's just an applied force. Some will deny its presence in their life, especially if they cannot do much about it. Stress is not a straightforward concept for doctors or patients. This is because, however we define it, it will impact each of us differently, depending on how much energy we need to spend dealing with it. Energy considerations are more fundamental.

Stress and how we spend our energy on it, will depend on how much it draws our conscious attention; how much it means to us (or to someone else), and how we choose to deal with it.

In three separate chapters (9 to 11), I have classified stressful human transactions as:

- **Foreground Issues:** In the foreground of our lives are many immediate, transient matters to be dealt with. We may not think of them as stresses, but nevertheless, they must be dealt with even if little or no thinking is required. Many are trivial, like whether to buy this or that loaf of bread, or whether to choose coffee or tea to drink. Most involve fast thinking, as opposed to slow thinking (Kahneman, D. 2011).

- **Background Issues:** These consist of the more in-volved, long-term stresses, we find ourselves dealing with on a continuous day-to-day basis. Some hang over us like a cloud, all requiring slow processing. They can be life-shaping: whether to become a doctor or lawyer; whether to move house, marry or separate. They are sub-ject to many influences, especially any personal biases. Some can be modified for the better, allowing us to move on; others seem unalterable; making us feel trapped or not in control.

- **Subliminal Issues:** These are stresses that set the back-drop to our lives – like the scenery of a stage play, they form our living circumstances and environment. Some are of political significance, like the environment, climate change, traffic noise, air pollution and cultural challenges, with only a few having the will or energy to engage in their modification. Most of us give some thought to them, and most of us come to accept them. We have no practical need to think about them, even though they might affect our health.

Even though they can have a considerable effect on patients' lives, and medical conditions, many doctors choose to avoid asking about their personal circumstances. After all, doctors are not social workers or counsellors, and may not see it as their job to make such enquiries. In the UK, they claim to have too little time! This will be a mistake when their patient's progressive fatigue, arises from their personal issues. Some doctors experience heart-sink, when a patient complains of tiredness – many suspect the cause to lie beyond their clinical remit. I wonder if the current trend for doctors to become more specialised, and less interested in the whole person, has led some to become detached and anonymous. I also wonder about the clinical consequences of this in the UK (it is much less common in some nations I have visited).

What part does sleep play in health and illnesses, especially if it is disturbed while dealing with stressful circumstances? What happens during sleep, and why does it refresh some, but not others?

If a virus or some definable disease is not the cause of tiredness, might it arise from a lifestyle issue? Could relationships or job demands be involved? Could diet be responsible? When it comes to avoiding disease or living longer, might taking supplements or a regular diet of bananas liquidised with green vegetable slime, be beneficial?

Is it all in our genes? Are some born to survive, whatever life throws at them, while others – those with a poor constitution – fall at the first hurdle? If our constitution counts, what can we do about it, given that genetic engineering is not yet available?

Modern humans have moved on from natural selection and any equivalent of Darwin's survival of the fittest. By creating safer living conditions, better hygiene and medical intervention, humans have created an advantage over a totally 'natural' life as it was, many millennia ago.

Between 1800 and 2024, the average life expectancy doubled, from approximately 40-years to 80-years, depending on whether one surveys the UK or US data. But why? Have improved public health and nutrition contributed more than medical science?

The deprived now have an improved survival potential, safer procreation, and now live longer, but a large health divide remains. The socially deprived will have shorter lives on average and suffer more medical problems than the wealthy. This disparity in health is so large (the wealthy have 70% to 80% fewer heart attacks than the deprived), it is unlikely to result from food alone. What part do stress, energy spending, and a lack of personal control play? These questions are considered within.

Many choose to ignore survival, living their lives by chance, not by design. The wealthy may not be more intelligent, but they are often self-motivated, persistent, and intolerant of insecurity. How we choose to use our energy, depends not only on our desires and motivations, but on many environmental factors over which the poor and disadvantaged have less control.

While reconnaissance is important, many survive with little more than luck on their side. In the race to reach the South Pole in 1911, Roald Amundsen believed in diligent forethought and preparation. Captain Robert Scott used much less and died as a consequence. Optimism is a wonderful thing, but it works better combined with careful forethought. The experienced and intelligent tend to look before they leap; others simply hope for the best. Science can help, but only when it can reliably predict the future.

Consider some simple predictive examples:

- If we pull hard enough on a piece of elastic, it will snap. That's physics.

- If we mix vinegar with baking soda, carbon dioxide will be released. That's chemistry.

- But what if you are locked into an unhappy relationship? Will that cause you to have a heart attack? That should be medical science!

If you are heading for bankruptcy, might you also be heading for a stroke? Medical science, if predictive enough, should be able to answer these questions. Unfortunately, at the moment, we can only answer them to some extent – and then, only by quoting their statistical probability. Like the elastic of differing strength, all will eventually snap if stretched enough. Likewise, some of us will respond adversely to stress, others will not. But what about for you and me as individuals? For us, the answer most likely depends on our genetic make-up; especially on our liability to 'fur' our arteries (atherosclerosis) or raise our blood pressure (for details read my book *'How to Become HeartSmart'*. 2024). To discover the relationship between stress, spending energy and serious disease, is attempted within.

The reasons for health and ill-health always involve energy – just like every other action and reaction in the universe. When our energy runs out, we die. If we get exhausted and our energy is at a low ebb, many of our bodily processes will change for the worse. Our immunity could fail, and infection might overtake us. Those with angina can deteriorate, getting it more often; some with high blood pressure can become uncontrollable. Among the many background causes are life events – like marriage, divorce, moving house and bankruptcy. Our personal reactions to these situations, like resentment, inescapable servitude, and loss of control, are all important. Where we live, and how we live, are also factors. They can combine with our financial status and education to help predict what will happen to us. Whether our expectations match reality can be of real medical consequence.

There is much to discover. Without getting into too much technical biological detail, the more one understands physical and brain energy – how it becomes available, is stored, and is used – the more we might understand how to balance our personal energy, and how to solve our own life equation. This is better than running short of energy and getting ill. Even though our eventual death remains a certainty (at the moment), the medical challenge is to maximise life's potential by upholding its quality. Money and happiness can help. Although hard to achieve, contentment and composure can both reduce our energy expenditure. Unfortunately, these goals elude many of us, especially those with too little control over their circumstances.

Because I have no wish to overload this text with scientific evidence and references, those interested in them should acquire my previous book: *Tiredness, Fatigue, and Exhaustion. Neurophysiology and Cardiovascular Risk.* 2025.

Initially, I had no wish to use my text as a polemic against the current UK medical establishment, but medical services for patients in general, and those with problems resulting in fatigue are now so deficient, I found it unavoidable.

Energy pervades every thought and action we take, so I have had to consider the psychology, attitudes, and as many life situations as possible, rating them for energy expenditure as causes for non-clinical tiredness, fatigue and exhaustion. In considering every aspect of life today, my views about social structure and the scandal of the health divide, might also be viewed as polemical. Because of the unhealthy way many now live, and how we plan to live in the future – as anonymously as possible, (if an AI-dependent generation has its way) – strong opposition will be needed to counter them. Like life itself, energy needs to be spent overcoming social and medical practice entropy. Without strongly countering the current direction of society and medical practice (a view not yet being expressed sufficiently to put patients first), the diagnosis and relief of many patients complaining of fatigue will defy successful resolution.

To understand fatigue, one needs to know about the biology of energy. From whence it comes, and where it goes. To understand this, you will need to know about what constitutes stress, why our mental and physical constitution matters, and how chronic fatigue arises. I cover these basic topics in PART ONE. In PART TWO, the many ways we spend our energy is considered. Like spending and saving money, it is important to review how our energy comes and goes – not annually with an accountant – but during every minute of every day. In PART THREE, I explore failing energy, ill-health and disease. PART FOUR explores the broader aspects of energy expenditure – how broader social and medical management aspects can affect us. The measures that can help restore our energy, and diminish our tiredness, fatigue and exhaustion, are all described.

These measures draw on my theory of brain traffic blocking neuronal channels during the day, rather like rush-hour traffic blocks roads. During the night and in off-peak periods they open again. I have called this model the Traffic Analysis Theory of Tiredness (See: Chapter 19).

I first contemplated writing this book after working with Dr. Peter Nixon at Charing Cross Hospital, London, in the 1970s. All those years ago, without the decades of experience I now have, I wasn't completely sure of the clinical relevance of what he taught me about fatigue and exhaustion. I am now!

PART ONE

The Basics

CHAPTER ONE

Tiredness, Fatigue and Exhaustion

"Under the look of fatigue,

the attack of migraine and the sigh,

There is always another story,

There is more than meets the eye."

At Last the Secret is Out.

W.H.Auden. April. 1936.

In his last days, Pope Francis portrayed the undeniable face and voice of exhaustion. This was apparent on his last appearance at the Vatican, on the 20th April, Easter 2025. After suffering weeks of energy draining pneumonia, he failed to regain his usual vitality. He died early next day, and was later succeeded by Pope Leo XIV, whose first appearance portrayed a completely different appearance – one of jubilant health and energy.

When someone is fatigued and exhausted, those acquainted with them will usually notice it. It will not be so obvious to those meeting them for the first time. For hospital physicians, nurses and medical students, it can be difficult to appreciate in a stranger. A patient looking exhausted is a reliable sign of illness; especially when prolonged and progressive. The loss of vitality, caused by clinical, psychological or psycho-social distress, should always trigger enquiry and investigation. Friends and family will usually be aware of any stressing factors, and how the patient has for months or years, carried burdens too difficult to bear. Recognising human distress, and offering restorative intervention, is no trivial matter. Recognising it, and helping to overcome it, can save a life.

Every human being comes to know tiredness, with many desiring infinite energy as a superpower. From our first hours of life, the energy we have must be balanced by restorative sleep. Babies grow their brains during sleeping, and wake regularly to feed, and take in their surroundings. Some cry to get attention, quickly tire, then fall asleep again. Restless and uncomfortable babies cry a lot; those who are contented while awake, often sleep peacefully.

New parents have to cope with experiences that are both joyous and tiring. Not all will become exhausted, but many will. Often woken at night, their sleep can get fractionated. The daytime tiredness and increasing irritability that may follow, will not help them cope with a young child. The parents of babies (except those with full-time nannies, attentive aunts, and grandmothers) will nearly all come to know tiredness, fatigue, and even exhaustion. This can quickly lead to an inability to cope – a mental breakdown – or depression, if allowed to continue. For this reason, our personal birthday celebrations should always include honouring our parents – for the stress we might have caused them.

Physical tiredness is centred on muscles. It happens if physical exertion tests our strength and stamina, and when we are pushed to the limits of our endurance. This is easily reversed by adequate rest. Trained for stamina, professional tennis players can play long matches, one day after the other. Interestingly, fitness and physical training builds stamina, and wards off both mental and physical fatigue. Sufficient aerobic exercise, like running, is always accompanied by breathlessness. With weight-training this happens less. It is physical weakness of our muscles that prompts us to rest. Even trained track athletes sometimes lie down on the track after an arduous race or will stand still and bend over to maximise their oxygen grab. While athletes are out running, jumping, swimming and throwing things, the unfit are more likely to be sitting down with their feet up.

Physical tiredness can accompany the satisfaction of achievement – running a marathon or building a wall. Unsatisfying, aimless work, and unwelcome toil, will more often seem tiring. The sleep that follows satisfied achievement is usually more restful, contented, and refreshing. Those who perform unwelcome tasks, harbouring resentment or discontent, often find refreshing sleep more difficult to get.

Mental tiredness limits both our capacity for physical work and mental work. The quality of sleep is most often the determining factor. Occasionally prolonging sleep beyond the usual, can disturb a regular sleep pattern.

I once attended a champion cyclist. Because of Peter's failing performances, his GP and coach thought he might have heart disease. His coach had good reason to think this. His protégé had been suffering from palpitations, shortness of breath, and chest pain on occasions. His accurately timed performance figures had deteriorated to the point where something serious was suspected. Detailed investigation of his bodily systems, including extensive heart, lung, and circulation testing, failed to show anything other than Olympian fitness.

So, what had reduced his performance by 25% on the cycle track? Perhaps he was telling lies about his training schedule. Perhaps his enthusiasm had waned or he was depressed. He initially claimed to have no idea of the cause. The answer, however, emerged from enquiring among his friends and family.

Six months before he came to our hospital, his father had died. He had been the one to encourage him from childhood. His father bought him his first bike and raced with him until their difference in age and skill began to tell. Soon after his father's death, his mother remarried. Peter took an instant dislike to his step-father; a dislike that was mutual. After many acrimonious arguments, Peter decided to leave home. His step-father saw no sense in a young man 'wasting his time' on a bicycle; regularly training in a gymnasium and being fastidious about what he ate and drank. According to him, it was unnatural for a young man to lead a life of restriction and personal discipline. 'Find yourself a girlfriend', he would say. 'Go out and enjoy yourself. Put yourself around a bit - you know what I mean'. Peter knew exactly what he meant, but it wasn't what he wanted. His overriding ambition was to become a top-ranking, competition cyclist.

As the result of conflict, Peter became evermore tired during the day. He was also not sleeping well. His coach gave him regular warnings about his unsatisfactory performance: a trend that could not continue without serious consequences for his sporting career. His symptoms continued to develop so he was referred for heart testing.

The solution to his problem proved simple in the end. His coach, who had seen something similar before, arranged for him to move into a hostel for athletes. Once there, camaraderie encouraged him to flourish as an athlete again. In all, it took Peter one year to get over his father's death, and his mother's untimely remarriage to someone he found incompatible. Once he realised the sporting significance of his failing mental reserve, tiredness, and defective sleep pattern, he changed his strategy. He decided to avoid family members and others who promised nothing but discord. This was not easy for him, but becoming successful among Tour de France cyclists, isn't easy either!

Some people are born with vitality and energy – they can shape the world. Others are born lazy – the world shapes them.

As we progress from babyhood to adulthood, we must all learn to suffer many tribulations brought to us by others: our parents, teachers, workmates, and those who become friends and lovers. Some bring joy, fulfilment and happiness; others bring only tribulation and the loss of contented sleep.

What do I mean by tiredness, fatigue and exhaustion? Here are my definitions:

- Tiredness is that mental state perceived as a mild lack of energy. It is usually overcome by one night of restful sleep. It can be put 'on hold' for a short while by need, necessary motivation or novel stimulation.

- Fatigue is a further state of tiredness, recognised by the inability to perform further when asked to do more; regardless of being stimulated into action.

- Exhaustion is extreme tiredness, characterised by a complete inability to perform, whatever the strength of motivation. If required to perform, performance deteriorates. Exhausted people can be mentally and physically unstable. This risks catastrophe – a road traffic accident for an exhausted driver; a heart attack for someone with narrowed coronary arteries.

For all these reasons, tiredness, fatigue, and especially exhaustion, are not trivial matters. Strangely, learning about them has not featured much in any medical school curriculum, and even now, their recognition is not seen as an important risk factor.

The following diagram (Fig. 1) represents how daily demands cause tiredness and fatigue as demands increase. It will take lots of repeated, tiring activity without sleep, to cause exhaustion. Peter Nixon published our work and called the connection between arousal (motivation) and performance, the human function curve. Normal human performance (completing cognitive tasks, etc.) is usually proportional to arousal, or strength of motivation (Nixon, P.G. 1979).

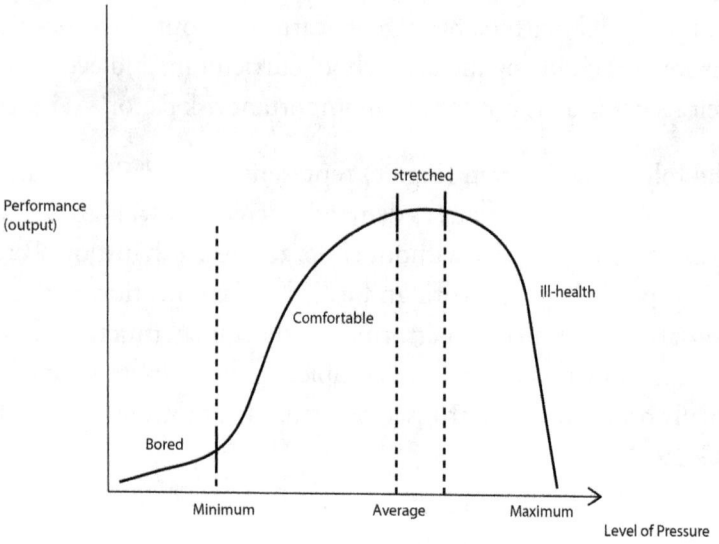

Fig 1. Based on :
(Human Function Curve: Peter Nixon (1979)

What about those who begin their tasks, already tired, fatigued or exhausted? In Fig. 2, I have illustrated their performance. We know that athletes can perform lots of tasks without tiring. Exhausted people are different. Their performance will deteriorate, whatever the motivation. The performances of the tired and fatigued, will lie somewhere in between.

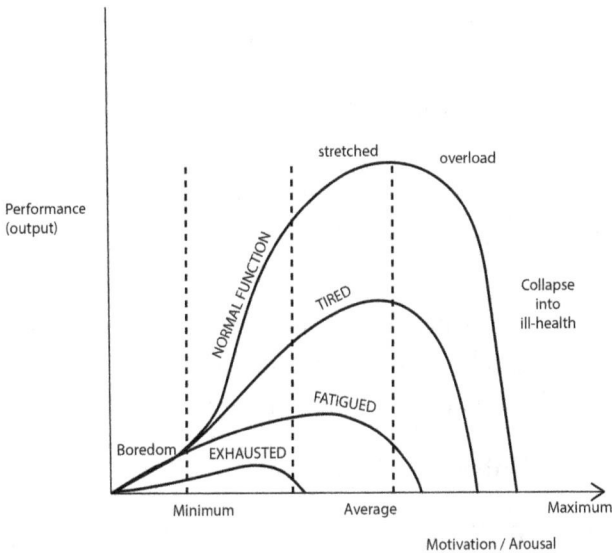

Fig 2.
Human Performance Function in
Normal, Tired, Fatigued, and Exhausted Persons

Fatigue has personal consequences. We will make more mistakes as our energy diminishes. Because some road traffic accidents are caused by fatigue, vehicle tachometers were introduced to stop long-haul drivers driving for too long (1968 in the UK). For young parents at home, mistakes will occur when demands are made of us by our partners and children. Unless a young mother has help, she could become unable to cope with her baby. Here, there is a significant cultural dimension to be considered. The further east one travels from the UK, the more likely help from family members becomes.

> *Jemima Goldsmith had two children with Imran Kahn. When she lived in Pakistan, she hardly saw her children. Many aunties, nieces, and grandparents wanted full involvement.*

The medical consequences of fatigue and exhaustion are serious in relation to mental health and medical events like sepsis, heart attack and stroke. I will discuss these later on.

'Healthy' and 'Unhealthy' Tiredness

It's no fun being tired, although, occasional tiredness is easy to deal with. One night of refreshing sleep usually reverses it. Those who are tired all the time need 'good sleep' but can find it elusive. Some carry on adding to their tiredness, working because they have no option; sometimes because they think they can continue to work regardless of tiredness, and sometimes because they are obsessed by activity and involvement. This being fairly typical of artists, entrepreneurs and the self-employed who are free to work as they wish.

Tired people survive more easily if they perform familiar tasks. Unaccustomed activities, which would otherwise add some spice to life, need more energy. For those who feel trapped or enslaved by work and endeavour, there may be little pleasure or fulfilment in life; their view maybe that life is a never-ending treadmill.

Everyone has experienced tiredness. A fulfilling day's work, an exciting journey abroad; these all cause normal healthy tiredness. A day of aggravation, annoyance, frustration, and disappointment are causes of 'unhealthy' tiredness.

Healthy tiredness is always short-term; unhealthy tiredness can be prolonged (chronic), occurring as it often does, in a setting of continuing dis-ease (discomfort).

Chronic tiredness has many causes. Ten weeks of bereavement, eighteen months of coping with a stroke victim, one year of an intolerable job or marrying the wrong person – all cause unhealthy forms of tiredness. They are unhealthy because they reduce our perceived energy reserve, and because they can cause particular symptoms:

- An inability to sleep,

- Forgetfulness,

- Irritability,

- Poor memory,

- Worsening medical problems – peptic ulcer pain, angina, reduced resistance to infection, higher blood pressure, depression, and even suicide.

- Tiredness can cause misery and depression; misery and depression are causes of tiredness.

Tiredness can be more apparent than real. The tiredness of boredom soon disappears with a pleasant surprise, or when given something exciting to do. This response, separates the bored from the truly tired, fatigued and exhausted who will find little joy in surprise – and just another challenge to cope with. They will not be much fun at a party! Some, not wanting to miss the occasion, will go regardless of their tiredness, trying to find a little pleasure.

Sameness, Boredom and the Tiring Effect

Those brimming with *joie de vivre* may not notice, but boredom can be tiring. Our modern living and working environment are mostly created by large corporations and regulatory bodies; staggering uniformity is cheaper to create than the novel and edifying and will better suit their budget.

Not only are many modern buildings uniform and uninspiring, the design and colour of the clothes most wear can also reflect monotony. Artists like Banksy have come to dispel such boring uniformity; in his case, without wasting years trying to get planning permission.

The uniform shape and colour of bricks and steel girders underpins the shape of modern buildings. Because bricks are the shape they are, most houses will conform to a pattern. Look from the window of any train as towns flash by. Notice the uniformity of the boxes most of us call 'home'. How similar, familiar, and easily predictable they are. One might come to think, after seeing more than one or two, they are all the same. By ignoring important details, we can generalise, with Greek temples, castles, cathedrals, and waste-paper bins, all having strikingly similar aspects! The effect is to create predictability, and predictability can lead to under-stimulation, boredom and fatigue.

As time progresses, uniformity – one aspect of anonymity – is becoming more common. This will remain, while property developers, architects, and town planners, create volume at the expense of individuality. No wonder many long to escape, and take a holiday to a country where the buildings, local dress, and food, are all refreshingly different.

Nature does provide a little more interest, with considerable variation in the detail of plants, grass, and trees, although many can look familiar. In the ancient writings of Plato, Socrates remarks on their similarity. He found he could learn nothing more from being in the countryside (Phaedrus, Plato). What he was looking for was inspiring, novel conversation, and new ideas.

Other examples of planned similarity are to be found in parts of the USA. Many small towns in the non-coastal areas can be amazingly uniform. This has come from the practical utility and fulfilment of public expectation. Many roads in towns form grids, with every highway having its compliment of usual chain eateries and retail outlets. Service utility overrides any need for individuality. Each culture has produced its own form of uniformity, whether it be the temples or cobbled streets of Ancient Rome or Athens, or the grass huts of Polynesia. If not dictated by fashion, the style will be dictated by tradition, the local Chieftain, or local Planning Officer. One benefit of uniformity is that builders can easily and more safely erect the same building each time.

We all live with many subliminal environmental features that influence our everyday life. These features are a potential substrate for discontent, some only perceived after we escape. Even the grandeur of St Peter's in Rome, can seem like a variation on our local church. Familiarity can lead to contempt, although, many are quite content with repetition and variations on the same theme. Many gain reassurance from it, because it reinforces feelings of stability and belonging. Valued feelings of fellowship, ethnic grouping, and patriotism can result.

Any security to be found in our surroundings, lessens our energy expenditure. The challenge of adapting to new environments, consumes energy. One stable island of peace in an otherwise demanding world, should be the place we call 'home'. Those without such an island of peace, will spend more energy adapting to their environment, and are more likely to suffer ill-health. It follows that moving home or changing job, is associated with high energy expenditure, and statistically, an increased likelihood of medical problems.

I well remember both my grandmothers speaking about becoming 'run down'. Both knew what they were talking about, having survived the hardships of London through two world wars. They would have made the diagnosis of an exhausted person from afar. Their prescription for treatment might have been erroneous, however. They would probably have suggested a 'tonic' – a common prescription six decades ago and before. The placebo effect accounts for the improvement of at least 20% of those who took them. Some older tonics contained cocaine, later to be replaced by caffeine to boost energy. Many contained a variety of abstruse herbal compounds. Some contained sulphur and many included iron. A common presumption once was that most fatigued people were anaemic. With the inadequate nutrition of the time, that may have been so in Victorian times. Today, it is a rare cause of fatigue in western countries.

Tonics are still available to 'boost energy and vitality'. Amazon currently (2025) advertises '*Strath Original Liquid Herbal Health Tonic, containing* 61 Vital Nutrients, Vitamins, Minerals & Amino Acids, Swiss Made Natural Supplement Yeast'. Tonics like Metatone, are no longer available ot listed in the drug reference manual used by doctors – the British National Formulary (BNF). Many still buy Sanatogen tonic wine, so the idea of a tonic to relieve fatigue continues.

The advice to, 'take it easy', and 'take time off', has been apt for millennia. However, doctors can be quite disinterested in anyone who complains of being Tired All the Time (TATT) or is 'run down'. Many patients become aware of this and seek advice elsewhere.

Although foods contain locked-in chemical energy, they cannot restore the energy of a tired or fatigued person, unless it comes from some psychological placebo effect, the correction of a low blood sugar (hypoglycaemia), or reverses salt and water depletion. A 'healthy diet' is essential for the preservation of health, but does less to prevent the common, serious diseases of today, like dementia, cancer or heart and lung disease. Vitamins in food are an exception – their absence will each cause a specific disease. A lack of vitamin C causes scurvy, and a lack of vitamin B1 (thiamine) causes Beri Beri. Vitamins, ginseng, herbs and spices contain little or no energy in themselves, and will not directly remove tiredness, unless they are specifically prescribed to treat Beri Beri, scurvy or severe anaemia (due to iron or B12 deficiency). Pernicious anaemia, for instance, is one cause of profound tiredness, cured only by repeated vitamin B12 injections.

Bodily energy is constantly generated – a process that never switches off. In fact, it remains ready to be tapped into, whenever needed. A Combi gas boiler operates in the same way, with lots of gas, awaiting use on demand. Biological energy is locked into one main chemical compound. In the presence of glucose and oxygen, ATP (adenosine triphosphate) is continually produced. It is not to be found in food but manufactured in each of our cells. Life depends on the energy locked into it. Consciousness is also dependent on the brain receiving enough oxygen and glucose (in the absence of too much carbon dioxide), delivered to the brain at a certain blood pressure. If our blood glucose, blood oxygen or blood pressure drop too low, we become unconscious.

Meals rich in fat and sugar can have a soporific effect. Eating too much of the wrong thing, can make some feel unwell. In the same way, metabolism abnormalities and various diseases can cause tiredness, fatigue and exhaustion, by changing our internal chemistry. The high blood glucose of diabetes is brought under control by insulin, and with it renewed vitality. Pneumonia, cured by antibiotics, will restore health once any chemical toxins disappear from our blood stream. These contrast with the more ubiquitous forms of tiredness that are unrelated to illness or disease, and for which solutions will include sleep management and social engineering.

Health and Vitality

For most of us, health is of more immediate importance than any thought of survival. But what is health? It is certainly not just the absence of disease. Any definition must include having sufficient energy for life. That comes from enjoyment, feeling worthwhile, and sleeping well; perhaps also from having a clear conscience, and having sufficient self-esteem.

In the film, Chariots of Fire (All Stars Ltd. 1981), Eric Liddell is woken from a peaceful sleep, by a steward on the overnight train from Scotland to London.

Steward: "Did you sleep well Mr. Liddell?".

Liddell: "Like a log".

Steward: "You must have a clear conscience then, Sir!"

Feeling healthy means we must have sufficient mental and physical energy for our daily needs. A surprising number of people seek extra energy from products sold in health food shops. Apart from a placebo effect, they are mostly wasting their time. There is no extra energy available in a vitamin pill, ginseng or in any of the multitudes of other dubious preparations on sale.

Health is not simply a lack of disease. Until disease draws on our energy, sufficient to cause tiredness, health and disease can easily co-exist. As the energy available to a person wanes, their health will decline, and disease could overtake them.

There are active people, and 'couch-potato' people. There are the energetic and the slothful; the bright and the dull. Such differences are there, from early on in life, and easily observed by kindergarten teachers, college lecturers and sergeant majors. These human characteristics are usually lifelong. The energy possessed by a person, will usually be obvious to anyone who wishes to interact with them.

My father told me one of his many Jewish jokes. A laundry business proprietor needed someone to press and iron clothes. From hundreds of applicants, he chose a strong looking man who claimed to be 'like lightning' when he ironed clothes. After hiring him, and the boss was touring the factory, he noticed the man working very slowly. "I thought you said you were like lightning", enquired the boss. "Ah! Yes!" said the presser, "I am before I get to hold an iron in my hand!"

CHAPTER TWO

Human Energy

There are those who exude energy and vitality; those who would love to have these advantages, and those who never will. We all have periods when we feel energy depleted, unable to work or to lead a normal life. Why does this occur? Might it be an illness or simply a bodily response to our circumstances?

The brain controls how we feel mentally, and variations in its function cause a wide range of thoughts and feelings: from depression to exhilaration; from disinterest to passion. Both exhilaration and passion are fuelled by energy, but where does this energy come from? Knowing that, might allow us to understand why we get tired, fatigued and exhausted. Does our body stop making energy? Does its delivery get blocked? These are some of the questions addressed in this book. Can we identify the source of human energy; improve its delivery, and boost our enjoyment of life, at the same time reducing our disease risk? Understanding these issues in full, should help to reverse and prevent fatigue.

I'm not about to overwhelm you with biological science, but there are some simple principles which put the human condition into perspective. Physics is not much to do with the human condition, but we can borrow some of its concepts to better understand ourselves. To consider energy is to consider how humans, and all plants and creatures work. There is power in knowledge when utilised appropriately.

Energy for Life

It's always our choice – where, and on what, we spend our energy. Those under the control of others may not agree. All tasks can be viewed as pleasant or unpleasant. Unfortunately, we will burn much more energy performing unpleasant or tiresome tasks.

Discussing the nature of energy and its relationship to our existence, will itself spend our energy. We might ask, where does it come from? Since we cannot visualise it, could it be elusively embodied in the strings of subatomic quarks – parts of the electrons, protons and neutrons that together, constitute everything in the universe? Even though it powers life, and the movement of planets, we can neither see energy, handle it directly, nor define it sufficiently. All we can do, is observe what it does for us.

Since nobody fully understands the nature of energy, even a child might ask, 'Is God energy, and is energy God?' The nature of energy would seem to be beyond human understanding, even though it pervades our universe and powers its existence, we cannot know it, except by what it does – manifesting as heat, light, movement, radiation, chemical reactions, etc. Physicists discuss whether it is a particle, a wave, or both, some trying to define it as a subatomic string. Although fascinating, thinking about it, could waste a lot of your time. Even though we may not understand energy, we must all contend with it – how to use it, lose it, or gain it. There would be no life without it, so at least, we must learn to preserve it.

Can sunlight affect our energy? With the occurrence of sun spots, electrically charged sub-atomic particles (plasma) are projected into space. Some hit the earth, and their arrival concentrated at the poles of the earth, results in an *aurora borealis*. These northern lights are either green or red, depending on how they energise the oxygen in our atmosphere. Their arrival, electrically charges water droplets in clouds. This promotes ice formation in cold air, later dropping as rain. Clearing the clouds allows the sun to heat the earth and create warmer weather. There is little doubt that extra light and heat can affect our personal energy levels. Whether the energy from sun storms and plasma can affect us directly, is a matter of conjecture. Sunshine can certainly make us feel happy and energised, whereas winter gloom saddens many of us.

The importance of the sun to human existence was established in ancient times. When Akhnaten (Amenhotep IV), the Egyptian Pharoah, tried to change the religion from worshiping multiple gods to one sun god – the Aten – he sealed his fate. At least, he paid homage to the effect of the sun on crop yields, and its life sustaining effects.

Forms of Energy

All matter in the universe has intrinsic rules of engagement, especially where energy is concerned. It is said that energy cannot be made or destroyed, although it can be stored and transferred. The various types of energy have long been known to science (discovered, not invented). Electrical energy powers our TVs and flows through light bulb filaments to create light. Lifting weights and moving machines takes mechanical energy. Then there is potential energy. When water is pumped up to a mountain reservoir, the energy used is stored for later use. When it later flows downhill and turns a turbine, it can be made to create electrical energy. Energy can also be locked away in chemicals; explosions and fire occur when that energy is released. Petroleum is one of these (chemical energy), but there are many others.

It is chemical energy that powers all living creatures. The chemical energy released by the breakdown of one particular molecule, keeps us alive. This compound is ATP, or adenosine triphosphate.

It is one of the most important, high-energy molecules, synthesised by each of our cells. A fascinating discover was made recently about its manufacture. It is synthesised by a chemical rotor – a molecule (ATPase) that spins around at high speed within our cells (within the mitochondria). It has actually been visualised. Each day, our cells make an amount at least equal to our bodyweight. We need that much energy to power all of our bodily systems. Our lives depend on it, so its production has to be totally dependable and inexhaustible; we would not survive long without it. From an evolutionary point of view, all creatures have a need – to live long enough to breed.

If we stop producing ATP, we will become ill and die. This chemical is ultimately derived from food, but so indirectly, no particular food is needed for its creation. You might think that certain foods help to make more ATP than others. That would be too precarious a requirement for life to continue dependably and is not the case. As long as we have enough carbohydrate, protein, fat, vitamins and specific minerals in our diet, we can produce all the chemical compounds we need to stay alive.

The body works across different scales: from the very small molecular level (within cells), through to the largest holistic scale of organs, like the heart and brain.

At all levels of brain and heart function, both glucose and oxygen are needed. To remain conscious, both must be delivered constantly to our brain cells. The same applies to keeping the heart pumping. In addition, too much carbon dioxide in our blood is not a good thing – it will make us tired, but it will only occur if we have heart or lung disease or have inadequate breathing (sleep apnoea and obesity). You may remember Charles Dickens' Pickwick Papers. Dickens mentions a sleepy, obese boy called Joe, who had breathing problems.

"Sleep!" said the old gentleman, 'he's always asleep. Goes on errands fast asleep, and snores as he waits at table."

"How very odd!" said Mr. Pickwick.

"Ah! Odd indeed," returned the old gentleman; "I'm proud of that boy – wouldn't part with him on any account – he's a natural curiosity!"

Charles Dickens. *Pickwick Papers*, 1837.

Joe probably suffered from what we now call Obesity Hypoventilation Syndrome. Some overweight people have a form of sleep apnoea, caused by obstructed breathing at night (snoring is a symptom). It occurs most in those with a short, thick neck (obstructed sleep apnoea). Breathing can also slow or stop when brain cells fail to provide enough stimulation (central sleep apnoea). The lack of oxygen that results can cause daytime tiredness, and sometimes heart rhythm disturbances, some of which can be fatal.

Human Energy Income and Expenditure

Another Dickensian contributor to the science of human energy (thermodynamics) was Mr. Micawber. You might remember him from David Copperfield. Mr Micawber said of money:

"Annual income twenty pounds, annual expenditure nineteen pounds nineteen and six, result happiness.

Annual income twenty pounds, annual expenditure
twenty pounds nought and six, result misery.'"

Charles Dickens. *David Copperfield.* 1850.

The same rule applies to human energy. If we spend more than we have, it leads to tiredness, fatigue and exhaustion (as well as misery sometimes). We all have kilos of stored energy in fat, muscle and carbohydrate, but that doesn't mean we have energy immediately available. How we tap into enough energy to live and dissolve tiredness, is the subject of this book.

Here are some other thoughts about personal money and energy:

- In human biology, all our energy transactions are strictly accounted for.

- Unlike money, energy cannot be stolen, begged, or borrowed, except from reserves, and then only for a short time.

- Unlike money, energy cannot be spent unless we already have it, waiting in reserve.

- Unlike energy, money can now be spent before we have it, in anticipation of future income.

- Human energy storage capacity is strictly limited, whereas any bank can store as much money as we can find.

It is possible to avoid paying off all your financial debts; debts of personal energy, however, are not allowed. The forfeits are punitive for both – fines and added interest payments for any financial debt; ill-health and disease for those whose personal energy fails.

CHAPTER THREE

Stimulus, Response and Constitution (Stress & Strain)

In the world of school physics, stress is defined as an applied force; strain as the change that results. In biology and medical practice, stressing forces are not so easily defined, and may not be universally accepted as stresses. There is a further complication: any resulting change, will vary from person to person.

Stress can arise within us (feelings of hurt, frustration or indignation) or from our environment (eviction, bankruptcy). Some physiological response (a strain effect) will follow – sometimes innocent and irrelevant; sometimes of serious medical consequence. Our genetic constitution and experience of life can both determine what the response will be – like different types of elastic, our physical and mental characteristics can be weak or strong. We may stretch a lot, or only a little before snapping – a little anxiety at one end of the range – a medical catastrophe, like a heart attack or mental breakdown, at the other.

Because every action leads to a reaction, every stress will cause some change – this is a strain effect. Stress is not limited to unpleasant, negative situations; it is there in every situation. Even the slightest change of circumstances will be responded to, whether coped with well or not, whether consciously or unconsciously.

Can stress be good for us? Since stress is unavoidable, perhaps we should ask if a lot of stress might be good for us? Some are said to thrive on it. This is possibly true for a few, but in over fifty-years of medical practice, I saw hundreds defeated by it. The more exposure we have to it, however, the more likely we are to learn how to cope with it. In 1977, Dr. Robert Sharpe wrote a book entitled, *Thrive on Stress*, for those who wish to explore the concept further.

> *"Life would turn to a stagnant pool, were it not ruffled by the jarring interests, and the unruly passions of men."*
>
> *'On the Pleasures of Hating'*
>
> William Hazlitt.

Stress and our reactions to it, are both important medically (see Fig. 3: two weights on different types of elastic).

In human biological terms, no standard measure of stress exists. Hot and cold environments can be measured accurately, but each of us will perceive them and react to them differently. Some react adversely to crowds, some to solitude. How disturbing we find them, is one measure of our strain response. How we respond individually – with anger, frustration, a fast pulse rate or a higher blood pressure, are important issues for many. Some react emotionally; others physically (blood pressure etc.). Some will react in multiple ways, depending on their inherited constitution and conditioning from life experiences.

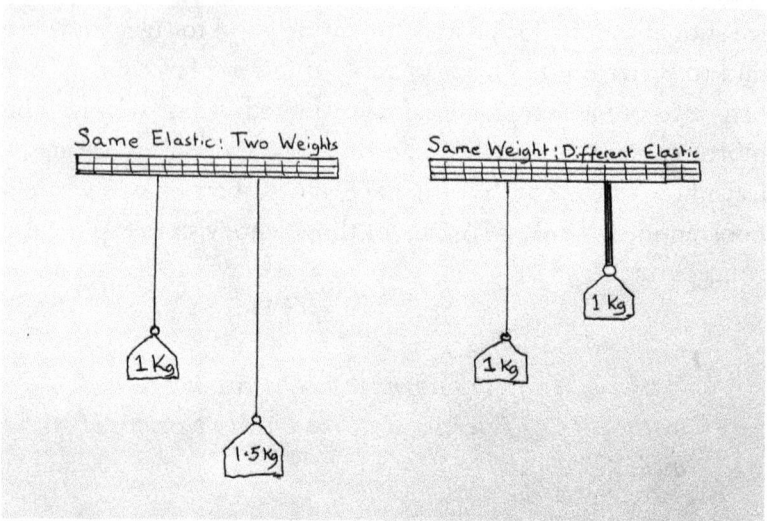

Fig. 3: Elastic & Constitution

On the left. With the same elastic (constitution) and different weights (stress), the stretch (blood pressure, psychological reaction etc.) will be more.

On the right. With the same stress (weight), those with a tougher constitution will stretch less than those with a delicate constitution.

As they hang on to their end of the rope, members of a Tug 'o War team, will know what it is to 'take the strain'. In the same way that each member of the team must resist movement, so change is resisted by our internal body chemistry. The concept of maintaining internal stability was first recognised by Claude Bernard in the mid-nineteenth century. Despite being pulled emotionally by guilt, despondency, love, hate and joy, our bodily systems try their best to keep the internal environment constant. When the pull becomes too great, one tug 'o war team will slip, and is pulled over. When one team is weak and the other strong, the contest soon ends. The same applies to our individual responses to fear, and the sense of losing control. The stress could influence our hormonal, chemical, dynamic, and psychological well-being, up to the point where something gives – and we will all give at our weakest point. At that point, nothing more than a faster pulse might result. For others, a mental breakdown, heart attack or stroke could occur.

For every action there is a reaction, whether it be a piece of elastic, or our heart. What makes the human body complex, are the multiple interactions between different systems, all of which must integrate well if we are to have a healthy mind and body. Those with an equable, composed temperament, will suffer less psychologically from stress, than those who live with anger, frustration, fatigue and exhaustion.

Apart from physical stresses (challenges like heat and cold), there are mental stresses – cognitive challenges: questions to answer, and problems to solve. There are also emotional stresses: bereavement, falling in and out of love, disputes with others, marital separation and divorce. All of these and their consequences, have been known since Adam met Eve.

"Alas, my liege, my wife is dead to-night;

Grief of my son's exile hath stopt her breath:

What further woe conspires against mine age? "

Montague. *Romeo and Juliet V. III.   W. Shake-speare.*

"When sorrows come, they come not as single spies. But in battalions."

Claudius. *Hamlet. Shakespeare.*

"I am ten leagues deep in calamity."

The Mahratta. *Kim. Rudyard Kipling.*

In contrast to weights stretching elastic, understanding the effects of stress on us humans, requires some consideration of our energy costs. Stress arouses us, and we will spend energy on our response: sometimes noticeably, as with fear and aggression, intolerance and anxiety; sometimes subliminally, with increases in blood pressure and cholesterol. These responses to stress are the biological equivalent of stretched elastic. There is one major difference. As we tire, our responses to stress become exaggerated.

Every stress that challenges us, spends our energy. The energy we spend on subliminal stress depends on our lifestyle. Because we get used to it, we can remain unaware of how much energy we are spending. Simply deciding what to eat, whether to turn left or right, or planning our day, all spend some energy. More challenging than the accumulation of small energy-spends, are big shocks to the system: happenings that stop us in our tracks – totally consuming our attention. The sudden news of a close friend dying; the effect of being stopped by the Police for driving too fast or an unpleasant argument, all arrest our attention, and can leave us feeling drained, upset, or aggravated. The stresses most relevant to us, spend the most energy. The most pathological stresses are the prolonged, long-term ones. These arise from situations that need to be pondered at length and will significantly disturb our sleep until an acceptable solution is found.

Constitution

One of my patients was a famous comedian and actor. He always refused my suggestion to have a cardiac screen – one that would detect coronary artery disease (present in his family). He always refused, describing himself as 'strong as a horse'. He succumbed sometime later from a sudden, fatal heart attack. In his case it was the constitution of his heart arteries, not that of his mind and other organs, that decided his fate.

'Constitution', like many popular ideas of merit, is not to be found in medical textbooks. Just as elastic, ships and cars, vary in the way they respond to change, so do we. Never be persuaded by the fantasy of biological equality – that we are all the same – with none of us different from any other.

Take ten people aged eighty-years old. Make a judgement of how old they look. They will not all look the same age. Some might pass for a 65-year old; others might look older, perhaps ninety-two years old. Some will be playing football with their grandchildren, others will be unable to get out of a chair. Each will have a different constitution, one reflection of which is how old they look. Internally, there can be major differences. Some will have furred and narrowed arteries (atherosclerosis), while others have none. Some will be frail, others will show no sign of it.

I once had a receptionist in her 50s who claimed never to have been ill with a virus infection. She certainly never had any days off work in the twenty years I employed her. There were others who took time off every two weeks. Perhaps, their immune systems were different.

Some babies are born robust, others look weak and fragile. This is likely to have consequences – like their liability to illness. When challenged by harsh times, the young and weak can suffer, while the old and tough carry on. This is what an assessment of constitution contributes to a medical appraisal. Constitution remains a clinical judgement, not something definable or easily measured. Using a Clinical Frailty Scale, the elderly can be assessed by those who don't know them. Few doctors will dismiss the reality or significance of such assessments. Nothing, however, beats knowing them and their circumstances personally. Anonymity is not a worthy medical companion. The argument that it will save time and money would never have impressed my patients. Some are now contending that patients will be better off with AI and a computer interface. If the only patient choice is to talk to an inexperienced doctor who knows too little, they could be right.

Constitution is a physical entity, made up of many factors. Bereavement will affect one mourner more than another, affecting an exhausted spouse more than a healthy one. Those bereaved after a short illness, fare better than those who have coped long-term with a protracted illness. To understand the effect of bereavement on those left, requires an understanding of stress, and its individual, variable effects on their energy, immunity, and other bodily systems.

In medical discussions between doctors, stress, constitution and personal energy handling, are mostly ignored or glossed over. Stress is important, but only as a stimulus. It is only one factor helping us understand the lives our patients lead, and only one aspect of what I refer to as the life equation – the income versus the expenditure of our energy – something I always found useful in predicting a patient's medical journey.

Strategy, intelligence, overview, education, the ability to command, self-control, personality, gullibility, rigidity of thought, anxiety, meticulousness, and aggression, are often of a fixed nature, and factors that are constitutional. Can they affect our health and influence our survival? Making costly, incorrect decisions; adopting inefficient strategies; being too obsessive and anxious, can all lead to mental ill-health. Occasionally, those they control, like their immediate family or work force, will also suffer.

Like beauty, constitution may be ill-defined, but will affect our fitness to survive. It should be obvious to every physician, counsellor, and army instructor, how some people deal with life – some without turning a hair – others reacting adversely. To inherit a strong constitution, is to be easily capable of withstanding the tribulations of life. Those with the toughest mental constitution will be resilient, emotionally stable, intelligent, perceptive, self-aware and confident, able to use their energy efficiently. Those with the best, and toughest physical constitution, will be athletically fit, have an immune system that fends off infection, and no tendency to high blood pressure or the 'furring' of their arteries (atherosclerosis).

For early man, a tough physical constitution would have been an advantage. Apart from intelligence, an ability to run fast, stamina, with good sight and hearing, would have headed their list of necessary survival attributes. Nowadays, the ability to withstand hours of unfulfilling, boring work, and the strength to deal with verbal and behavioural abuse, aggression and inequality, are the attributes most needed. We need to be self-aware, and at one with ourselves; congruent with the needs and failings of others. A degree of equanimity will allow us to deal best with all the nonsense, falsity, and data-overload that modern society constantly throws at us.

Subsequent to Darwin's publication of the Origin of the Species, he suffered much indignity – that of widespread rejection of his ideas. Having anticipated this, he held back his publication. At the time, the majority religious view, was that man was the unique creation of God. Darwin's rejection of this idea will have caused him much worry, frustration and perhaps ill-health. He became ill soon after returning on the Beagle to Great Britain in 1836. Some thought his illness was psychosomatic, others have thought it due to Chagas' Disease or lactose intolerance. He made the point that all men and animals are different, and that small differences between them, could affect species survival. The survival I often refer to here, has a different focus – that of only one human lifetime; personal survival within the overcrowded, competitive environment that modern humans have created.

Self-Knowledge and Survival

Personal mind-talk uses energy. The most important relationship we have – is with ourselves. We conduct it through 'mind talk' – the constant conversation we have with ourselves, unless distracted. The content varies, from thoughtful, analytic, and reminiscent, to conjectural, but always influenced by our personal biases. Thoughts may be of the, *'she loves me, she loves me not'* variety, or be prospective – planning and discussing the future. Some occupy their minds entirely with fantasy, vanity and emotional matters; others conduct logical discussions, during which they formulate their future *modus operandi*.

Our mind-talk can be biased by our cynicism, perfection, resentment, jealousy, anger, forgiveness, graciousness, altruism, magnanimity, and a myriad of other ideas, needs and feelings: perceived by others as our attitude and personality. Unfortunately, the time we spend discussing matters with ourselves, can be based too little on fact, and too much on conjecture. If it were not, we would need much less time to mull things over. We could spend much less energy ruminating. When caught on the horns of dilemma, our energy can be consumed easily: even to the point of exhaustion.

If you can't decide what to do . . . do what's right!

To know and accept ourselves for what we are, with all our strengths and limitations, is to approach a state of inner peace – it has been called a state of grace. True self-knowledge requires humility – an almost impossible task for anyone who is overly egotistical, obsessive, arrogant, complacent or vain.

Our Hand of Cards

Experienced card players come to know that the cards they hold, will often predict their chance of winning; although, an expert player can do better with a poor hand than a novice. However, few practiced players will win with a dud hand.

The genetic codes we each carry within our cells, can be likened to a hand of cards. Good genes – good constitution; bad genes – bad constitution. From my experience, those with the best chance of health, are those with characteristics inherited from healthy, long-living parents and grand-parents. Inherit the constitution of a Superman, and you too might shrug off every external force. I have met those who have withstood bereavement, divorce, and bankruptcy, all within one year, without any obvious medical impact (on their internal chemistry, blood pressure or mental health). I saw many others who deteriorated psychologically and faced depression and a failure to cope; others suffered physically with a stroke or heart attack. Doctors need to be aware of each patient's constitutional liability. Many of these can be detected using active medical screening (with challenges including exercise testing) – geared to play devil's advocate, rather than to simply accept the conclusion that nothing is wrong, after not trying hard enough.

As far as personal constitution is concerned, each organ and internal system, has its own predetermined set of responses. Faced with business problems, some people develop chronic anxiety (nervous response) or have repeated migraine (brain arterial response); others get palpitation (heart response), or diarrhoea (bowel response). There are those who get none of these, while others experience several together. You don't have to be worried to get palpitations, but they frequently go together. Those who are subject to palpitation, get more when anxious. Because each system has its own responsiveness, stress will cause palpitation in some, with no response in others.

Taken together, all the characteristic responses of an individual, both physical and mental, define their constitution. They are the biological equivalent of car specifications, or that of a jet fighter, or washing machine. There are fixed physical features, like height, weight, body form, and strength, and dynamic features like decision making, executive functioning and the efficient use of personal power.

It was once traditionally for NASA, only to take those individuals with the best suited constitutional characteristics, to train as astronauts. Once chosen, all protégé astronauts must prove that they can stand up to the physical and mental stresses of space flight and respond favourably to challenges.

A very successful entrepreneur once told me his secret of success. It was to choose only the best people for the jobs he needed done. Selecting the best, more often leads to the best results. The selection of a suitable partner in life; the selection of a suitable profession to match our strengths and abilities, and giving preference to objectivity rather than fantasy, all help to avoid failure.

Chapter Four

Basic Energy Management

Tiredness, or a lack of sufficient energy for living, is the commonest medical complaint of western men and women.

Most people will relish having boundless energy – once they have experienced it. Although a surfeit of energy is common for those in their early years, it gradually tends to wane with age, with the exception of a few. Some are inherently energetic, with others absorbing it from them. Some get invigorated by their surroundings, while others remain untouched. Musicians, actors and public speakers are energised by their audience, while some in the audience get their 'buzz' from 'being there' and enjoying the ambience and occasion.

To sustain biological life requires lots of chemical energy. Well beyond biochemical considerations, our energy powers enthusiasm, drive, ambition, tenacity, and determination. Some use it to control their personal situation; a few will use it to control nations, and to wage wars: Napoleon, the Duke of Wellington, Churchill, Eisenhower, Hitler; Kissinger, Netanyahu, Thatcher, and Elon Musk are examples of past and present high-energy characters. With enough energy to spare, they have made a difference to the world. Others have used their energy to create art, develop theories, write books, think, plan, organise, or build business empires. Not all successful people are delegators, but those who are, have an advantage – they harness the energy of others, and achieve even more.

We rarely hear about those with no obvious energy, or those with no wish to achieve or change the world. Some are content to keep their energy in reserve; to contemplate, secure in the knowledge that very few actually change the world for the better. If at-one with themselves, such people have less need for a strong ego and vanity; their humility and grace can be more endearing and easier to live with than pretentious, powerhouse people. Many are achievers, but they do so quietly, with no desire for fame, wealth or power over others.

Some have energy enough for their own life but will spare too little for relationships or their families. Some with the gift of energy, have lost it dramatically. After losing status or a valued relationship, dramatic medical conditions can result – Elvis Presley after losing Priscilla from his life; Aristotle Onassis after the death of his son Alexander, in a light aircraft crash in 1973; President Richard Nixon who in 1974, resigned the US presidency, rather than be impeached after the Watergate affair; Hillary Clinton after losing the presidency to Donald Trump in 2017. All suffered medical consequences. The less notorious decline, with only their families, friends, and colleagues there to notice any change.

Energy is essential for the enjoyment and fulfilment of life. Energy is the essential ingredient and embodiment of health. Without it, many will experience ill-health.

Since everyone gets tired sometime, tiredness must be regarded as a normal part of life; progressive tiredness leading to fatigue and exhaustion, is not. These can lead to a failure to cope, physical inertia, indecisiveness, irritability, defective judgement and to mental or physical illness – all aspects of personal decline. Not only relationship problems and marital breakdown result from progressive tiredness – heart attacks, strokes, and duodenal ulcer, can also occur to end a period of progressive fatigue. Whereas organic disease in adults is accepted as a legitimate outcome, tiredness and fatigue is often ascribed to laziness, a lack of commitment or the feigning of illness, without respect for any potential risk.

Because of this sense of respectability, we often treat disease with concern, but ill-health with dismay, or irreverence. Mental health, now freely discussed, occupied this distained space for millennia. 'Take it easy', 'Pull yourself together', 'Take a holiday', 'Have a few days off work', or 'Take some Valium', were once typical of the inadequate medical advice dispensed, for those without a physical abnormality. Having a disease is accepted and respectable; ill-health is often thought of differently. All too many patients, better called pre-patients, have been told that there is 'nothing wrong' with them, once their 'objective' blood and other investigations have been returned within 'normal limits'. The test results could be erroneous, or not the best tests to make the diagnosis. Test appropriateness, test relevance, and test accuracy are all relevant technical medical issues. In a similar vein, who would ask: would checking my engine oil, help to diagnose a flat car battery?

To prevent some medical outcomes, we will have to take the forewarning of progressive ill-health seriously. Although many diseases are associated with tiredness, they are not the commonest causes.

Doctors have yet to appreciate the full medical and social significance of fatigue and exhaustion, even though they can forewarn of medical catastrophes, like heart attacks and strokes. There are two problems. First, tiredness is non-specific. On its own, it lacks diagnostic accuracy: there are too many conditions that cause tiredness. Second, not all heart attacks are preceded by tiredness, and not all tired people risk having a heart attack. Also, tiredness as a symptom indicating mental or physical illness, is too sensitive – tiredness is so common, it cannot be relied upon to diagnose disease or the risk of illness; at least, not without further qualification (in-depth enquiry, physical examination and investigation)

The essentials of personal energy management are simple: maximise income; minimise expenditure. We should all know our capacity for energy, and never try to exceed it.

Getting exhausted by a worthwhile endeavour (defined personally), being productive, and pursuing enjoyable pastimes, can be the essence of life – if you have the energy to spare, and are fit enough to sustain the cost. On the other hand, doing nothing can be boring and worthless, but will conserve your energy.

Without energy and its effective management, nobody makes it out into the world in the first place; nobody accomplishes much, achieves self-esteem or enjoys life. It is not easy to make energy management part of life. So many people are unwilling to follow guidance and the sensible rules made by those who have succeeded. Many will suffer before learning what counts. Some remain chronically unwell, and challenge doctors to make them well again, even if they are responsible for their own condition.

Our personal energy management is completely on auto-pilot, and for many of us, never needs to be thought about, let alone managed. For those who get tired or exhausted; those experiencing ill-health or disease, its management is crucial to recovery and preventing fatigue and ill-health in the future. This means managing down-time –sleep and switch-off times, as much as controlling energy expenditure on all the things that engage us in life – some of which spend little energy; some of which will spend lots. We have no battery within us to run down – not like a car with a flat battery that has been left overnight with its headlights on. Instead, we block our brain pathways with thinking and emotional traffic, and like road traffic, these paths will block as we use them during the day and unblock at night – in preparation for the day that follows.

Fortunately, all biological systems have reliable, energy producing biochemical systems, that we never need to think about; systems so reliable, all life has been made possible. These energy-producing mechanisms give up, only as we are dying.

So, what is it that blocks our supply of energy, causing us to feel tired or exhausted? And what unblocks our energy supply, to give us the vitality we need for everyday life? This book attempts to answer these questions, with each chapter that follows, looking into individual aspects of energy management.

Let's look briefly into a few aspects of energy spending, before considering the subject in much more depth.

Perfection

Many spend lots of effort and energy on trying to achieve perfection. Therein lies the Goldilocks principle. For Goldilocks, while roaming the house owned by the three bears, she searched for a bed and some porridge that were 'just right'.

Given some experience, most perfectionists eventually come to realise that imperfection is unavoidable. Wabi Sabi is an old concept of perfection and imperfection. It was an ancient Japanese art to find beauty therein. A villa created by the shogun Ashikaga Yoshimasa (1436 – 1490), was one example. It was converted into a Zen temple after his death. It is considered the icon of Zen-inspired wabi-sabi culture, which flourished in the 15th century.

Energy, Stability and Entropy

Energy is spent everywhere, constructing and maintaining the structures we choose to put in place. Consider the frailty of organisations and physical structures, and the energy involved in maintaining them. Some are stable, others are not. People have similar characteristics, with differences in their ability to withstand stress. How we are designed psychologically and physically, will help predict how we respond.

Entropy is a physical concept biology can borrow. The simple idea is that without maintenance, and energy being spent, every structure in the known universe will steadily disintegrate. A rubbish tip is disorganised; it has no designed structure. Compare this to a finished office building, with rows of carefully placed bricks and panes of glass. To build such a structure, plans are needed, and lots of effort will be required to bring all the separate components together – in the right place and at the right time. Executive organisation is essential. With the building finished, imagine how much effort and energy will have gone into converting piles of steel, wood, electric cable and plastic, into a workable building. The finished structure is said to have high entropy; a pile of rubbish, low entropy.

Entropy is a physical concept; one which reflects the intrinsic energy locked into a structure. To release all that energy in a building, would take lots of time and effort or one massive explosion. Because energy cannot be made or destroyed, the energy quickly released by an explosion, must be equal to all the energy it took to create the building in the first place. Very quickly, any high entropy structure can change into one of low entropy.

Entropy also reflects likelihood. What is the chance of a sugar cube, having dissolved in the sea, being reconstituted back into a similar cube? What is the chance that a chimpanzee will write a poem, while randomly tapping a keyboard? Both are unlikely, because producing order and structured design by chance, very rarely happens. When order is seen in nature – like the formation of basalt columns in the Giant's Causeway, or in the structure of a snowflake, there will be an underlying, predetermining mechanism – in both of these cases, the underlying crystalline structure of the molecules is involved. This is dictated by how atoms and molecules need to be arranged (strict atomic arrangements have to be met). On a larger scale, the pentagon and hexagon shapes seen at the south pole of Jupiter, were completely unexpected, when first seen. They are caused by five or six storm vortices grouping together. So, order (high entropy) can occur naturally. Without an equivalent natural occurrence of structured DNA, none of us would be here today.

Sometimes our minds will construct false order – like seeing the shape of a man on the moon; the outline of body within the shroud of Turin, or the image of a plough among star formations. This is called the pareidolia bias. DNA and blood testing of the stain on the Turin shroud did not find blood of group AB (commoner than others in northern Israel). Also, the figure was rather tall for the region at six feet one inches (185cm.) – so, biased or real, a mystery remains.

Security

To make a safe, dependable life for ourselves, we must make appropriate plans, and consume a lot of energy doing it. Creating a business for instance, takes foresight, time, money and energy, to bring all the right elements together. When COVID-19 came, lockdown quickly destroyed the health of a workforce, and brought an end to many small businesses. The result was financial and social chaos. This has taken lots of money and energy to reconstitute. Public health responses varied from country to country, with corresponding mortality rates related to the uptake of immunisation and how quickly lockdown was introduced. The once high-energy structure of social life was partially disintegrated by a few decisions made by politicians. High-energy, refined structures, are always vulnerable.

The maintenance of business relationships spends a lot of energy. Unfortunately, illness and other changes in circumstances, can quickly bring down an organisation, sometimes permanently. Some structures are inherently insecure.

National security is an international issue; so is personal security. The only way to get it, is to design safe havens. This is one good reason to invest in property. An increasing world population, the slow building of homes, and an ever-greater demand for accommodation, make buying property a secure investment. In many parts of the world, the rich live in enclaves – walled and guarded for their personal safety. Castles have had to be re-invented. Knowing that one is secure at home, relieves worry, tension and reduces energy spending.

Fear is not a listed medical entity, yet it pervades the lives of many, constantly and subliminally spending their energy. Insecurity abounds in modern societies, some capitalist societies choosing to foster it. The drive to achieve security makes us work. If nobody feared prison, not everyone would bother to obey the law. Is fear a substitute for conscience, or is fear the secret that conscience hides? Is it the fear of retribution that keeps us well behaved? Retribution now hangs unseen as a personal threat in all modern societies and cultures. Harnessing fear is good for business. If we fear losing our job, we become more willing slaves, especially if we have a mortgage.

Interviewer: "Spike, do you fear death?"

Spike Milligan: "No. I just don't want to be there when it happens!"

There are so many things to fear, a complete list would fill several large books. There is a point to recognising fear and successfully dealing with it. It is to minimise our energy expenditure, and thus to improve our health. Nothing will induce ill-health quicker than being in constant fear.

In modern society, fear of death, bankruptcy, imprisonment, failure, success, and violence, are all commonplace. In less evolved societies, fear of sickness, or exposure to abuse are ever-present. The unscrupulous have always used fear to motivate others. Doctors use it sometimes, to achieve patient compliance.

Learning

Learning and reconnaissance can save energy spending. As every student knows, the amount of energy spent learning to become a doctor or architect, is considerable. Training our minds to understand new concepts, to think within a framework of reason, experience, and practicality, takes lots of energy. I well remember thinking that my basic exams ('O' Levels, back in the day) were challenging. I then found 'A' levels, even more challenging. Thereafter, learning anatomy, physiology and biochemistry at medical school, surpassed every amount of learning I had experienced. Each subject was equivalent to several 'A' level subjects. Somehow the brain adapts to take on more. We can train ourselves to do it, becoming more efficient as we try. Overcoming all the difficulties we have with understanding and memory, takes lots of energy.

The mind of an educated person becomes highly structured, and far removed from that of an infant whose only quest is to find food. The brain that solved Fermat's last theorem (Andrew Wiles, 1993) was no ordinary one. Some levels of thinking (cognitive functioning) and understanding, can only be appreciated by those who have attempted advanced education. Most people on earth, never need to learn more than is required to run a commercial business. I have often joked that would-be business people need only know one bit of arithmetic – how to subtract two numbers – total expenditure subtracted from the total income – namely, the profit. Following in the steps of Mr. Micawber, happiness results if this subtraction is positive; when negative, misery is not unusual.

Vast amounts of energy are consumed by learning, thinking, feeling and passion. The brain consumes more fuel per minute than any other organ. Memory, reasoning, solving problems, generating new ideas and questioning, all take energy. Processing emotional issues, and dealing with feelings and passion, often require more. We can only guess which consumes most, although it is now possible to measure this using an EEG or brain scanning (to measure oxygen consumption).

"Desires, emotions, passions (you can choose whatever word you will), are the only possible causes of action. Reason is not a cause of action but only a regulator."

David Hume (1711-1776).

The Complex and Complicated

Simple processes like arithmetical addition and subtraction, are straightforward and uncomplicated. The criminal law may be complicated, but at least it is all written down and known. Complex things involve the interaction of several systems, none of which are fully understood. Like the weather, the stock market and human emotions, they are complex and difficult to predict. The sub-systems may be known well enough, but how they react together adds uncertainty. Simple problem solving consumes a minimal amount of energy; solving complex problems consumes a lot more.

Both we and our universe are elegant puzzles. The universe was there, well before we tried to make sense of it, and before we became puzzled by it. It will be there after we are gone. Although less of a puzzle now, it remains puzzling. Some things are difficult to understand and appear complicated. When a system is complex, nobody knows how its separate, complicated and simple parts, interact together. Like the weather, this is a complex system that is quite unpredictable.

The human brain may have complex functioning, but many will benefit from 'keeping things simple'.

Occam's proposition provides some clarity – if it isn't simple, it won't often be correct. Only with full understanding do concepts and ideas appear simple. Thinking, however, is not easily kept simple. As a result, many get confused or retreat into thinking in a binary fashion – coming up with only a black or white conclusion – assuming that there are only two possible answers to any question. They may come to think only in terms of good and bad, strong and weak, high and low, right or wrong. But to understand something more complex, like the weather, consciousness or the stock market, something extra is required.

Sometimes, there is just too much data to comprehend at any one time. We may need to withdraw to a distant point to review the problem in overview. When complex issues are involved, those capable of dealing with them, are often thought to possess a magic art. There is, for instance, an art to medical diagnosis. Proficient doctors, faced with a complicated case, will focus only on the relevant issues and data, and come to a conclusion using their experience to weigh the relevance of each piece of information. This is often done sub-consciously, in the same way an artist will choose the most appropriate form and colour for their work. Since the process does not conform to any rule-based algorithm, we must regard it as an art-form. I have elsewhere referred to this human ability to solve complex issues as nebula thinking. Think of making the best fruit pie ever. One must choose only the best fruits from a large orchard of fruit trees and bushes (equivalent to vast amounts of data), to make the best fruit pie. In the same way, based on anec-dotal experience, many game-changing scientific hypotheses have been put together by those with insight (Dighton. D.H. (2024) The Art and Science of Medical Practice).

Although the aim of science is to understand those fundamental principles that allow the prediction of future events, it is not alone. The descriptive art of a poet, philosopher, or water-colour artist can also be predictive. They too can predict the flow of water in a babbling brook and make sense of it while adding context of human relevance.

Science has long used microscopes and telescopes, but deciding the relevance of what we see remains an art. Science dissects, art creates. Both disciplines can lean on the same skills, while having some sensibility and knowledge of the other. Few other than Leonardo da Vinci have ever succeeded in employing both together.

Collective Energy

Is there such a thing? Does collective power exist in human groups? Collective power seems to exist, especially when groups of like-minded people cooperate to form a football team or build a rocket. Coming together can also achieve intellectual objectives; some sparking new ideas in others. In 1989, the Berlin Wall fell because people power overwhelmed political power. In contrast to dictatorships, democratic governments fall when the majority of people go against them. It would seem that collective power does exist, even if as individuals, we are not much aware of it.

In collective grief and bereavement, a large number of people can consume energy together. The day President John F. Kennedy was assassinated (November, 1963), and the day Diana, Princess of Wales died (August, 1997), group feelings of loss occurred. The whole world seemed to become introspective, quiet and reflective, for a significant length of time. Many people seemed 'in sync' with one another. This is not just a human phenomenon. The death of one elephant will affect the behaviour of the whole family group.

Personal Power

Power is the amount of energy we can bring to bear in unit time. To maintain effective personal power, will consume a lot of energy.

The exercise of power in the UK, once owed something to dress and accent. We were once in awe of pin-striped suits and half-rimmed spectacles; and impressed by a cultured, educated voice. These are now anachronistic and so old-fashioned, they have become the stuff of comedy.

Many are still in awe of certain surroundings – hospitals and courts of law, for instance. For others it can take a beautiful face, outward expressions of wealth, or an impressive uniform, to create a feeling of awe. With the aid of such props, those who possess them know they can bring their power to bear on some others, with very little effort. Those affected by the Halo bias, will more easily succumb.

Most beautiful people are aware of their power over others. The wearers of a military, legal, medical or academic uniform, are usually aware of its effect on the minds of others. Minds can be moved to form opinions and be biased, without the use of words. Those without these power attributes, can spend enormous amounts of energy, trying to achieve the same ends. An ugly man can attract a beautiful woman for a time, using his other desirable attributes, but keeping her will not prove easy. The world is full of attractive men whose power to attract women, requires no more effort than one glance or a smile. Men, on the other hand, are strongly biased by female form and beauty; they are easily swayed by looks, they will readily forget the more important elements of personality, background and behaviour, crucial to maintaining a long-term relationship. Although a weakness, all of this fosters procreation, with few escaping this fundamental evolutionary drive.

Those women who want a relationship with a man, may have the biological drive to be attracted to those who can offer power, money and security, or might soon be able to. To be so discriminating, is a biological strength. Biologically, reproductive females need a secure environment and some privacy to raise their offspring, but men are not always the ones to provide it. Biology and evolution may be subliminal, but they are ever-present to motivate the human psyche.

To function calmly, every civilised society needs citizens who respect its structure and 'objects of power'. A certain type of respectful behaviour is required of us. Respect for the power of the Law when attending Courts; respect for the power of religious faith when visiting places of worship; respect for the power some doctors have over life and death. The white coat and stethoscope, the wigs of judges, the sacred statues and alters, the sacred scrolls kept in the *aron hakodesh* (the Torah Ark), and other vestments of religion, can all influence us. The number of guards and ante-chambers a President or Prime Minister occupies, form the trappings of power, there to trigger respect.

> If respect is deemed missing, discord can result. When President Zalensky of Ukraine, entered the Oval Office of the White House, USA, in February 2025, he was wearing a black sweatshirt featuring an embroidered Ukrainian trident, black slacks and boots. His dress was deemed disrespectful to the office of President Trump. The meeting ended unpleasantly. He was dismissed, and lunch and a press conference together was cancelled.

The personal boundaries of power we each have, may be drawn with a narrow or broad region around our existence. Broad-based personal power over the environment, is often vested only in those who command respect. They will usually dress well, have robes or a uniform; will usually speak well, and behave as if in control. Narrow-based power may apply only to our immediate partners, children, and friends. The only difference is the number of people subjugated.

Some are aware of their power boundaries, others are not. Politicians and judges have their lines of power drawn up for them by legal instrument; they need to be aware of these boundaries. Most beautiful, intelligent, famous, and imposing people are aware of the power they exert over others. There is a simple measure of this power – they only need count the number of people falling in awe at their feet.

Interpersonal power, some of which is embodied in charisma, is a valuable gift. Many are attracted, controlled, or rejected by it.

While it varies with ego, its possession can donate either gratification or disappointment to others. Submissive subjects can be happy in their role, or suffer some loss of self-esteem, caused by agreeing to domination. With freedom as the priority, submission to any form of external power can prove unacceptable. In order to maintain a secure and safe environment, western freedom is never unconditional. It has to include the duty to bend to social pressure and power. In many similar ways, we spend our energy subliminally.

Large ships can make waves which profoundly endanger smaller ships and boats in the vicinity. Similarly, those in the orbit of powerful humans, can be constantly influenced. Large and daunting warships, and imposing powerful people, can bring disruption or protect and bring peace to an area, simply by their presence. Winston Churchill, Adolf Hitler, Napoleon, and Margaret Thatcher, all possessed this rare quality. Few with power these days, other than Donald Trump and Elon Musk, have any comparable charisma.

Human Functionality

Any human energy spending overview must consider the chosen course we each take through life. At the risk of being facile, we can use ships at sea as a metaphor for everyday human functionality.

Ships, like humans, are built to perform different functions. Whereas ships are made fit for travel on the high seas and will mostly perform the job they were designed for, few humans are aware of their design features – in particular, where their talents lie – unless obvious, like outward beauty. Unlike a ship, built for a specific purpose – for war, or container carrying, few of us know what course through life might suit us best; hopefully matching our foremost talents with our chosen vocation. One might think that those who stick to what they are good at, will always be happy. Unfortunately, that is not the case. Many have interests in a vocation or a subject, for which they have little talent. It is common to find a brilliant linguist whose only wish is to become a farmer; or a gifted musician, who only wants to be a car mechanic. Although these vocations could be considered consecutively in life, they are only rarely achieved simultaneously.

One major difference between biological and physical machines, is that machines can be switched off. Our brains are never switched off, even during deep sleep. The human body is always working, converting food into usable fuel and at the same time spending energy, if only on maintenance, while processing information at a subconscious level. Ships need to carry lots of stored energy (coal, oil, wood, or electrical energy in batteries). The body does have its long-term stores – fat and protein, but we store very little energy as carbohydrate, except for glycogen. Like Combi-boilers used for home heating, we can produce power, as and when we need it. On a long-term, reduced calorie diet, we can burn our stored fat as fuel and lose weight. Under extreme famine conditions, we will become emaciated, burning our muscle protein for fuel.

Navigators on board ship, plot their course in order to arrive at their destination on time. This they can do by knowing the power of the engines, by computing the distance to be travelled, and the speed of any headwinds. The safe course of a ship must take account of all possible obstacles – other ships and intervening islands and icebergs. By contrast, only a few people take enough time to plan their route through life, and safeguard against the likely problems ahead. When we are young, we cannot fully appreciate future problems. This value can be learned, however, but only from history, from literature, or from older more experienced friends, family members and acquaintances. We vary much in the amount of forethought we each bring to bear. Without it, our route can be questionable, and our final destination uncertain.

Ella Wheeler Wilcox referred to this determination as 'the set of a soul'. One of Margaret Thatcher's much-loved quotes was hers:

"One ship drives east and another drives west

With the selfsame winds that blow.

'Tis the set of the sails

And not the gales

Which tells us the way to go.

Like the winds of the seas are the ways of fate,

As we voyage along through life:

'Tis the set of a soul

That decides its goal,

And not the calm or the strife."

The Winds of Fate.

Ella Wheeler Wilcox.

Poems of Optimism (1915).

Detours can make us miss our destination and our destiny (after being led astray in youth), but possibly rewarding, when charming, uncharted islands are discovered. Throughout life, detours will become necessary with updated information. Flexibility is a valuable trait, so is dedication to continual reconnaissance and an ability to adjust opinion and attitude. Arriving on time may have to be sacrificed when danger lurks, although the calculation of risks, wise strategic planning with options analysis, are not abilities all possess.

A ship's captain acting on impulse, rather than keeping to a set course, can waste energy. A good plan can be made better or worse by impulsive action, depending on whether the action is guided by experience or ignorance. If good comes of the action, and a good time is had by all, no energy will have been wasted. Every decision involves a gamble. Reliably estimating risk is an art.

With a ship ahead of schedule, additional ports of call might be visited. By working hard, one can get ahead of a schedule and use the spare time for other accomplishments. Working intensely (like an accelerating car) is energy expensive, but then, more time might be made available for rest.

Bad weather can make the unaccustomed sailor sea-sick. With experience, some will learn to avoid doing anything they might find upsetting. Despite a liability to travel sickness (internal stress), some will choose, or be made to choose, cruising holidays in order to satisfy others. Bad weather (an external stress) will cause the ship to waste time and energy. Resilience will be needed to ride out the storm; spending time, keeping all the systems running, and deciding what to do. Occasionally, a storm-force wind will bring ships more quickly to their destination, saving time and energy.

There are those who always fall on their feet – they benefit, even from adversity! This element of chance always needs to be considered.

Taking on more passengers (friends and family) in life, will necessitate greater energy consumption. Further likening our life situation to a ship, we would then sit lower in the water, weighed down by extra responsibilities. This will increase friction through the water; all tasks might become more difficult, with inevitable friction occurring between people. Human friction or conflict, is a common cause of high energy consumption and tiredness. A point could arise, when a heavily laden ship, could be in danger of capsizing. It may not be able to leave port. In human terms – taking on too much responsibility can lead to either inertia or instability.

The captain of every ship knows how to measure his loading limits; he has a Plimsoll Line to guide him. Human beings have no such overload indicator, except for feelings of frustration or the perception of tiredness, fatigue and exhaustion. Sooner or later, a decision might need to be made to off-load cargo. In human terms, it might be those excessive insurance premiums, bank loans, and payments for the third car that need to go. Some of our passengers might need to be offloaded. This might necessitate leaving the 'other' woman or man in your life, or friends who demand more than they give. Similarly, a business can have too many employees, and may need to downsize to remain profitable.

Having arrived in good time at the desired destination, the captain and crew of a ship, could congratulate themselves on a job well done (gaining personal and collective esteem). The passengers will be grateful to have arrived safely, and on schedule. To achieve self-esteem is what many of us work for, from our schooldays onwards.

Despite success, not everyone will be pleased. Mae West once said,

"You can't please all the people, all of the time.

To try, is unrealistic and a waste of energy."

CHAPTER FIVE

Heart and Brain Power

A normal heart and circulation can deliver all the ingredients necessary for the healthy functioning of all our organs and cells. The essential ingredients are delivered by the blood in arteries, while all the by-products of cellular metabolism, one of which is carbon dioxide, are transported away through our veins. Chief among the chemicals necessary for brain function, are oxygen and glucose.

Oxygen is absorbed from the air we breathe and carried around the body attached to red blood cells. Without it, we would only live for a few minutes. If the oxygen in the air we breathe was to run short progressively, we would first become breathless, then tired, then slowly slip into unconsciousness. Nitrous oxide anaesthesia works by displacing the oxygen in the air we breathe, effectively reducing the oxygen supply to the brain. The brain also needs glucose – a basic sugar, derived from the breakdown of carbohydrate (starch and sugars) in the food we eat. Blood glucose level is regulated mainly by insulin and glucagon from the pancreas gland, but also by cortisol and growth hormone. A diabetic who accidentally injects themselves with too much insulin, will drop their blood glucose to a low level, causing them to slip gradually from tiredness, through fatigue to unconsciousness.

Although both oxygen and glucose are essential for our vitality, the reduction of either is an uncommon cause of tiredness. During a healthy life, both are maintained within narrow limits. Their delivery can become diminished for anyone with serious lung or heart disease. The result will be fatigue and shortness of breath in heart failure, or angina for those with coronary artery disease. The build-up of carbon dioxide in the blood also causes somnolence and fatigue. Insufficient or obstructed breathing and lung disease can cause drowsiness.

The brain consumes 20% of all the oxygen absorbed from the lungs. Since brain function depends on a constant supply of oxygen, it has developed a back-up delivery system – a circular artery at its base – the only circular artery in the body (although some arteries in the heart and elsewhere, can connect together in a circular way). At the base of the brain four arteries feed this circular artery – the circle of Willis. Even with three blocked, some blood will get to the brain.

A similar, so called collateral circulation, provides cross-flow between the three main coronary artery branches. If one artery blocks, these extra arteries provide an alternative blood to flow to meet the demand. At the time of a sudden, major artery blockage, their presence can determine life or death. Unfortunately, not everyone has them. In their absence, complete blockage of an artery will usually cause a heart attack (death of heart tissue).

In a healthy heart, the cardiac muscle of the ventricles (right and left pumping chambers) perform the pumping of blood. Within heart muscle (and the brain), the energy needed for contraction comes from chemical breakdown (of ATP synthesised within each cell). The chemical breakdown of ATP provides the energy needed for both heart muscle and brain function.

Both heart and brain tissues need activating. Waves of activation are usually thought due to electric charges flowing from one point to another. In fact, it is the flow of protons, not electrons (electricity), that is involved. Both carry energy. These waves of activation occurring at the cellular level (depolarisation), travel from one point to another, through a specialised conduction network – through the conduction system of the heart, and through neurone cells in the brain.

The wave of activation begins at the top of the heart (from the pacemaker in the right atrium). It then travels to the pumping chambers where it activates contraction. With each beat, an electrocardiogram (ECG) represents the summation of all the activation waves in the heart. Its failure necessitates the implanting of an electronic pacemaker – to provide electrical pulses from a battery, to stimulate heart contraction.

A brain tracing (EEG or Electro-Encephalo-Gram) represents the summation of similar activation waves spreading from one brain cell (neurone) to another, throughout networks of brain cells.There are billions of neurones in an adult brain, connected through trillions of possible pathways. The result of each transmitted wave can be a specific event – a limb movement; a thought or feeling. The exact pathways, and their function are now being studied in detail (connectomics), but from what we know already, specifically activated pathways can give rise to memories, thoughts or feelings. The activated transmission in the brain sometimes fails. With a stroke, certain pathways get damaged, so memory, thinking, speech and movement can falter. Also, when the chemicals involved in nerve transmission (neurotransmitters) become disturbed, dementia and fatigue can occur.

Changing Scale or Dimension

If we change focus from the organisation of the brain as a whole, to what happens at a cellular (neuronal) level, we find completely different activities. Cells are engaged in the manufacture of energy – that which we use to sustain life. They are able to do this unerringly, as long as they are supplied with enough glucose, oxygen, and various nutrients, brought to them by the blood in arteries. The blood also brings along cells that help with maintenance and fight infection. As much as possible, each cell actively maintains its chemical status quo (homeostasis). As one example, the acidity or alkalinity of its internal environment is kept constant, in order for it to function normally. By exchanging oxygen, carbon dioxide and other chemicals, our kidneys and lungs contribute critically to this life sustaining process.

Each cell maintains a negative voltage inside, made possible by cells actively pumping out sodium ions, at the same time causing potassium, calcium and chloride ions to enter. This makes possible all, so-called 'electrical', brain and heart activity. Whereas it is electricity that drives computers (involving the flow of negatively charged electrons), neuronal (brain cells) and heart conduction fibres, engage positively charged protons to create their flow of activity. It is positively charged sodium ions that do the communication and activation work (depolarisation) for neurones and heart cells.

Waves of activity flow from one brain cell to another, following specific pathways, producing distinct thoughts, memories and feelings. The structure of these pathways can be compared to a tree trunk that divides into many branches. Within each branch, there are channels which lead to specific leaves. The complicated combination of leaves available for activation, provides the potential for many separate thoughts, feelings, and actions. After each brain wave excitation, each cell membrane voltage has to be restored, although in the brain, some pathways will remain blocked and inactive, until restored by sleep. It is all this activity at the cellular scale, that consumes lots of ATP, oxygen, glucose, and glycogen (a storage complex of linked glucose molecules) as fuel.

As the wave of activation (depolarisation) progresses through brain tissue, it has to cross multiple gaps called synapses. Brain cells only become connected chemically, once the gaps are crossed. This is accomplished by chemicals called neurotransmitters. Produced on the nearside of the gap (the pre-synapse), they must diffuse across to the far side of the gap (the post-synapse), causing it to activate (depolarising it). These gaps are subject to many controls, one of which is blocking. You may have heard of dopamine and serotonin in relation to happiness, activity and depression. These are just two of many neurotransmitters active in the brain, some of which are involved in the perception of vitality and fatigue. Each part of the brain has its own particular neurotransmitters, although, some like acetylcholine and glutamate are universal.

At first sight, these gaps or synapses, would seem to be unnecessary. It is at these one-way points, however, that control can be exerted – acting like customs officials and passport controllers working at frontiers between countries – they can block entry or hasten your passage. It is at synapses that further activity, to and from the brain, can be boosted or blocked. The causes of tiredness, fatigue and exhaustion involve many molecules and several special synaptic processes.

Brain activity at this molecular level is beyond the scope of this book, but for those interested, I have detailed the relevant facts in my book on neurophysiology and cardiovascular risk (Tiredness, Chronic Fatigue, and Exhaustion. Neurophysiology and Cardio-vascular Risk. 2025).

Energy Flow and Control

Only so much water per minute can flow through a pipe or flow down the plughole in a bath. Only so much traffic can flow through the streets of a city, although over the whole area, lots of traffic movements are taking place. The brain functions similarly. Some believe that too much mental traffic can block neuronal pathways, with inhibiting mechanisms protecting them from overload. Road traffic blocks and backlogs develop quickly, when road traffic volume increases, or three lanes of vehicles try to merge into one. The brain works best when its owner is composed – the equivalent of being in control of traffic flow. At night when there is less traffic, both the brain and the roads in every town gradually unblock, ready for next-day activity.

The Whitehall studies, undertaken by Michael Marmot (1997), which investigated how Whitehall civil servants were functioning in the UK, showed that those who suffer illness most occurred among those with little control of the work they do. The senior civil servants with complete control over their workload, only rarely became over-burdened or suffered illness.

Brain Power

Power is defined as the amount of energy used over time. An accelerating car consumes more power (gas or petrol) than one cruising at a constant speed. Fuel consumption is one way to measure how much power is being used by a machine.

Although not mechanical, the brain also uses power to function. Powered brain activity results in the generation of brain waves. They can be recorded as an EEG (electroencephalogram) from electrodes placed on the scalp. Brain power can be calculated by multiplying the voltage (amplitude) of the EEG waves, with their frequency of oscillation. When we are awake and thinking, our brain waves are full and frequent; when we are deeply asleep (slow-wave, non-dreaming sleep), our brain waves are slower and of lower voltage (thus on a low-power setting). When dreaming, a phase of sleep accompanied by rapid eye movement (REM), we can produce daytime voltage and frequency levels (a normal power setting).

Some human beings, using the power of their personality and position, can induce others to feel energetic. Others can strip others of their power and energy, demoralising them and making them feel diminished, tired or sick. With one stroke of a pen, an anonymous bank manager can ruin the future prospects of a business. By withdrawing overdraft facilities, or asking for the immediate repayment of loans, some families are forced to make a short journey – from wealth and health, to sickness and deprivation. Banks are in business to make a profit and remain solvent; they must enforce strictly defined fiscal policies to protect themselves. When causing harm to others, it will always be politically expedient to remain anonymous.

Real Intelligence & Artificial Intelligence

Intelligent people are better able to connect different facts, ideas, and theories. In this way, they more easily see solutions to questions and find answers to problems. Intelligence is most likely related to the number of brain inter-connections – the greater number of interconnected thought processing neurones, the greater the intelligence. Consciousness and awareness, as well as creativity, must also arise out of this complexity. An interesting question follows. Can a solid-state computer, without a comparable number of interconnections, ever hope to reproduce human consciousness and intelligence? Before that, of course, one needs to ask an even more fundamental question – why do computers need to reproduce human thinking?

A popular outlook at present is that computers are more valuable than human brains, and that AI will make them even more so; they are even said to hold the promise of being able to further humanity. Great marketing, don't you think? Everyone loves a romantic story – like slaves becoming masters or those in rags gaining riches. Here's another one – computers will become human, but only after every science fiction scenario becomes real.

It is true – solid-state computers can calculate faster than any human (one basis for AI is their fast calculation of probability), and can search and organise data, faster than any brain. Human brains, however, can create anew (not just a re-hash of old ideas – from the data uploaded to them). Computers will never use thinking, emotion or personal experience to make wise judgements (those which suit each individual best), unless their data-sets are complete and replete with individual context. Understanding and wise judgement are human functions, which even at best, computers can only mimic.

Alan Türing, who invented the first test to judge whether a computer could ever think like a human being, declared the question to be "too meaningless". He thought computers could only play an imitation game (Türing, A. 1950). In the same vein of thought, the philosopher, J. Searle, proposed an experiment – the Chinese room. He demonstrated that a computer program does not need to 'understand' or 'think' (as we do), in order to appear capable of understanding and thought.

Not everyone aspires to novel thought or invention, so what can computers do for the person in the street. AI will undoubtedly help those of us who don't wish to think much or spend ages getting answers to questions. It might also replace the jobs people love doing the best – especially those that involve creativity. In the past, many had to ask others for answers. With AI, we can find out more for ourselves. The average man in the street may be capable of it, but he has little need for original thought. I disagree with those who think computers will someday generate the original thinking and judgment of Alan Türing, Einstein, Florence Nightingale, Linda Lovelace, Claude Bernard, Isaac Newton, and Richard Feynman. For IT advertisers, this idea will create a lot of false interest.

Some computer experts claim they can build a machine that will program and think for itself, without anyone pulling any strings. Remember the promise of a 'paperless office'? Although it failed that test, we have continued to invest millions of dollars into computer technology, with even more now being invested in AI. Used appropriately, it will undoubted save time for the routine, programmable functions, used by the majority. Plug several AI modules together, and you can have your own AI agent, instead of a human personal assistant. Although these will sell and make untold profits, some lifestyle questions might arise. For instance. What are we going to do with any 'free' time we create, and what will those made redundant, do with themselves?

In what have become the most admired results of human brain activity, speed was never a feature. Passion, conviction and hard graft, were. It took Albert Einstein half his lifetime to formulate the theory of relativity, and Nikola Tesla's conception of AC current took rather longer than a day! Michelangelo's creations suffered nothing from the length of time he took to create them (although his sponsors might have disagreed). Contrast these achievements with the speed of computer processing. Computers allow almost instantaneous calculation, now essential for navigation when using GPS or Forex trading. Creating video from text and text from video is now easy. Like apples and pears, however, brains and computers only need to be complimentary. Obviously, no matter how much a pear aspires to be an apple, or vice versa, only delusion will make it possible.

Although all brains are similar, and computer design is based on similar architecture, computers and brains have little in common other than some functional connectivity. Brains function with diversely connected brain cell networks, creating thinking, emotion, and wise decision-making. Uniqueness lies hidden within the unfathomable number of neuronal connections for which we have only a crude blueprint. Even if we knew the detailed anatomy, brain connections change all the time – something neuroscientists call plasticity. Computers are made to a fixed blueprint, whether their hardware connections and software are written by a human programmer or are self-generated. Brains work on loosely formed assumptions and can have multiple biases; they are not programmed to follow hard and fast rules like computers – differences, fundamental to how each works.

Brains need rest, computers do not (as long as their cooling devices and power supply remain functional and connected). Airports and hospitals, however, are occasionally brought to a complete standstill, when a power failure renders their computer systems useless. Their physical components can fail, with systems that have built-in obsolescence. The complicated wiring and programming of computers must bedazzle those who think them capable of anything – even able to self-diagnose and self-repair – able to create anew, and offer wise judgement as real, rather than artificial. Will they be able to repair one another (outside of science fiction dream states) and will they ever be reliable enough to take charge of a human life? That they can be made more reliable than the average human makes them viable entities.

The brain is an organised physical system and has similarities to some electronic circuitry. Brains came first, of course, and from their work, electronic circuits were born. In electronic circuits, wires, switches, resistors, capacitors, and inductors must be connected to a power source. All the components have a physical form. In the brain there is no single power source, and no equivalent of a battery that will run short of power. Instead, each cell has its own power source, constantly producing a supply of energy derived from the chemical breakdown of high-energy ATP molecules.

In electronic circuits, it is the flow of electrons that activates them. In neurones, it is the flow of protons (positively charged atoms) that powers the brain. Sodium ions ($Na+$), passing into brain cells

(Na+ ion influx) initiates all brain wave activity (waves of depolarisation called action potentials, flowing through neurones). These
waves travel in many directions, throughout a definable network of
multiple neurones, arriving at specific regions of the brain. Like the
brain, electronic circuits can also collect and emit light and sound,
deliver chemicals, and make measurements of heat and acidity
(pH). Unlike electronic circuits, brain functioning releases specific chemicals (neurotransmitters) like acetylcholine (ACh), serotonin, and dopamine, that each affect our consciousness, thinking,
emotion, mood, and attention.

Computer scientists and neurophysiologists argue about consciousness. The question is, will hardware circuitry ever achieve it?
Computer hardware may seem complicated but is no match for
the complexity of brain cell configuration and interconnectivity.
Equally unmatched, is their functioning and output. Since human
consciousness arises from the complexity of an unmapped system,
no electronic device can copy it. It can, however, be simulated
using robots able to create anthropomorphic illusions.

Any semblance of consciousness achieved by a machine, would
have separate features, like ultra-fast processing (sorting, selecting according to given criteria, matching, and calculation), all
inescapably locked into an engineered design, with a need for
prescribed software (even if it is self-generating and correcting).
Unlike the brain, it might have decision pathways, dictated by
calculated probability (as used by AI). Machine 'consciousness'
would be distinguishable from the human sort, by acting as a
complementary alternative.

Computers have one big advantage over brains (while their power
supplies, batteries, circuitry and soldered connections hold up) –
they never tire. Our brains are imperfect, slowing down, making
errors and malfunctioning with the onset of tiredness, fatigue and
exhaustion. Yet a human brain created the Mona Lisa, invented

the microscope, and has come to understand much of the physical universe. The idea that computers can do better is based on
inductive thinking, not on the strict logic that defines everything
computers do.

In all physical systems, order of magnitude or scale is important.
Galaxies exist at a very large scale, yet each is small within the
universe as a whole. Atoms exist at a very small scale. In between
these scales of magnitude lie the solar systems, planets, people,
anatomical features, cells and the biochemistry within. Within
the molecules are atoms, and within them, electrons, protons and
neutrons. Rules applicable to one scale, rarely apply to another.
The behaviour of sub-atomic particles, for instance, cannot yet
be used to predict the movement of any large-scale system, like a
human being or a planet (and vice versa). The cellular actions of
ions (charged atoms) and molecules in brain cells and their connections (neurones, axons and synapses), do not help us understand thoughts and feelings. To understand them, we must consider the integrated actions and interactions of neurones and how
they function on a global scale. It is global brain functioning that
enables our consciousness, perception, thinking, feeling, and life
as we perceive it. This level of functioning is far removed from the
small-scale movements of neurotransmitters and neuronal connections.

Engineered machines also function at different scales, but are only
complicated, not complex. They are all self-limited (even with new
versions available to buy each year), with in-built obsolescence.
It is software that controls all computer functioning, however
clever the outward appearances. It actually makes their functioning completely predictable (at least to programmers). While they
may draw our attention by creating surprising combinations and
insights from data analysis, it would be wrong to think them capable of *de novo* conception.

Those interested to review this subject further, might want to read my more technical book on tiredness, chronic fatigue and neuro-physiology (see under books by the same author and references – Dighton, D.H. 2025). They might also want to refer to the research work of Citri and Malenka, 2008 (see bibliography).

Infinite Brain Power?

When I started to re-research the subject of tiredness, fatigue and exhaustion in 2024, having given it little thought since the 1970s and 80s, I found that neuroscience had moved on. A lot more was known about neurotransmitters and high-energy, chemical ener-gy (ATP) production. My quest remained, to explain tiredness and to reveal its relevance to serious medical problems like heart attacks and strokes.

Could tiredness be caused by a lack of power generation in cells – producing the equivalent of a flat battery? I came to believe that the labels attached to fatigue – a 'flat battery' and 'burnout' were false; more importantly, they have given rise to a misleading conception.

It is possible that ATP, oxygen, glucose and glycogen might run short, but that would require the presence of some disease. I was left to explain how fatigue and exhaustion happened in normal people. I had to explore another possibility: neurotransmitter production failure (known to occur in dementia), causing blocked pathways. As a cardiologist, I was outside of my field of expertise, except that my focus had always been the 'electrics' of the heart.

What I found, came as a surprise. It seems that the normal pro-duction of cellular fuel – high-energy ATP – is completely reliable. Without it being constant and unerring, life beyond a few minutes would be impossible. The other surprise was how much ATP is produced – everyday, it is made in bodyweight amounts.

The biochemical factory within each of our cells (in sub-cellular organelles called mitochondria) does the job. The mechanism never switches off, although, it can alter a little with changing energy demands. Without a mechanism this reliable, life would have been precarious, short, or impossible from the start. Life that has continued for millions of years, first needed something more reliable than any battery or plugged-in power supply. It needed something akin to a nuclear reactor – a totally reliable source of energy, that works irrespective of the weather or the food we eat. Because cellular energy bound in ATP is so much in abundance, tiredness and chronic fatigue are unlikely to be related to its reduced supply in healthy beings; not unless some brain disease or narrowed arteries exist. Since most people who complain of fatigue (98.5% at least) have nothing of the sort, the mechanism of fatigue requires another explanation.

What about neurotransmitter production? Perhaps some deficiency might account for tiredness in otherwise normal people? Neurotransmitters also seem to be produced by near-to-infallible chemical processes; ones that rely on fairly simple chemical elements being brought together. In dementia, acetylcholine production (one of the commonest transmitters in the brain) can be defective (the enzyme acetylcholine synthetase produces it); in the brains of those with dementia, reduced amounts of it are known to occur. Dementia can sometimes be improved by boosting the amount of acetylcholine persisting in the brain. This can be done by switching off its destruction – by inhibiting the enzyme acetylcholinesterase. With this enzyme inhibited, acetylcholine stays around for longer and improves dementia.

Cholinesterase is important in all nervous system functions. It is active in the heart conducting system, where it is involved in the activation of heart pacemakers. Studying this, was one of my early research projects. Unfortunately, I ran out of time and money to pursue it. In the 1970s, I visited Dr. Ann Silver (1929-2023) at her laboratory in Babraham (Cambridge University), to learn more about it. She was then the world authority on the subject and published her landmark textbook on cholinesterases in 1974. In the end, I chose to leave its further study to others. Cardiac researchers have yet to take much interest.

Because the cessation of respiration and heart pacemaker function are incompatible with life, only death will switch off high-energy chemical and neurotransmitter production in the brain stem (that part of the lower brain that automatically controls breathing and heart rate). For this reason, running short of high-energy chemicals or neurotransmitters cannot occur in healthy people.

Stress and the Brain

I mentioned before, in Chapter Three, some of the physical principles that provide useful analogies for understanding brain functioning. For instance, in the same way that elastic lengthens (strain effect) after attaching a weight to it (a stressor), humans experiencing stress might somehow get stretched also (as a form of response). These responses can be straightforward, like an increase in pulse rate, blood pressure or blood cholesterol, and sometimes complicated, like changes in our resistance to infection or blood coagulability. One problem is, we can all react to the same stress in different ways. The way we respond is dependent on our inherited constitution, and our learning and experience (weak or strong elastic provides a useful analogy)(See Fig. 3).

Stretched enough, all elastic snaps, regardless of its constitution. Some situations present the same danger as a cliff edge – they are bi-stable phenomena, equivalent to the sudden snapping of stretched elastic. When standing close to a high cliff edge, all it takes to end up in pieces at the bottom of the cliff, is to take one small step forward (depending on the height of the cliff). The sudden occurrence of heart attacks, strokes, immune problems leading to infection, acute psychosis, and other sudden mental illnesses, might all represent bi-stable, catastrophic medical phenomena.

In a physics laboratory, entities like energy, power, stress, and strain can all be measured. In human beings, the effects of cognitive and emotional stress are not all measurable, although, we can generalise about what stress can lead to. Our internal responses are mostly individual, because inherited human constitution varies so much. Our external, behavioural responses will relate to the type of person we are; to our physical and mental strength, our adaptability, and our capacity to function efficiently under duress.

Clinicians might accept that a stress-strain relationship exists in principle, but patients who have experience of dealing with problems, may come to have a different view. Some accept their significance. Others who live with stress-strain situations can become used to them, many thinking them irrelevant to their medical condition.

Bereavement, bankruptcy, and divorce are social stresses that affect some more than others. Although all such incidents (as applied forces) have to be coped with or ignored, the amount of emotion and cognitive concern they raise (their strain effects), will differ between individuals. In different people, stressful situations can affect one physiological system, more than another. In this way, a stressed patient can become hypertensive or resistant to treatment, if they already have high blood pressure. Blood pressure can become uncontrollable, during acrimonious divorces and legal bankruptcy proceedings. Encouraging relaxation and sleep can then become more effective than escalating the doses of their blood pressure medications. Many others will exhibit no change in their blood pressure, whatever their circumstances.

Unlike weights tied to pieces of elastic, biological systems are more complicated. They are dynamic, changing with time, and needing variable amounts of energy spent on their maintenance. In the brain, different reactions are involved. Different areas of the brain, release varying amounts of energy, causing some distinct waves of activation seen on EEGs (varying frequencies and amplitudes are seen).

The Brain and Electronic Equivalents

Those unfamiliar or uninterested in electric circuits and electronics, might want to skip the next paragraph, describing how waves seen on EEGs might reflect electronic circuitry.

In simple electronic terms, LCR circuits can be used to create pulses. A circuit containing a resistor (R), a capacitor (C), and an induction coil (L), will produce voltage waves similar to those seen on an EEG (electronic ringing circuits). When the circuit current is off, or between voltage pulses, electrons reverberate between the two energy components – the capacitor, and the induction coil. This produces a sinusoidal voltage/current wave. As with the AC current we use every day, these waves represent different levels of power generation.

Hormones and the Brain

A lot of brain chemistry goes on during sleep. Release of the 'stress hormone' cortisol, oxytocin and endorphins, and the female hormones oestrogen and progesterone, can all combine with the effects of the neurotransmitters. Cortisol levels slowly increase as sleep progresses, with growth hormone peaking during the first half of sleep. Another hormone, prolactin, peaks in the middle of the sleep period, decreasing with awakening. Thyroid stimulating hormone increases during sleep, but the secretion of thyroid hormones (triiodothyronine and thyroxine) often decreases.

Most hormones are controlled from an area at the base of the brain called the hypothalamus. It is suggested that growth hormone-release hormone (GHRH) promotes sleep, while corticotropin-releasing hormone, promotes awakening and wakefulness. We now know that the hormones insulin, leptin and ghrelin, influence hunger and satiation (see my book about weight reduction, 'Who Loses Wins' , 2024). When sleep is restricted, leptin and ghrelin activity changes.

In conclusion, every organ is dependent on cellular energy and neurotransmitter synthesis, but the heart and brain are particularly involved in the evolution of fatigue. The theory I prefer is that daytime tiredness is caused by the progressive blocking of synaptic gaps, sometimes blocking whole pathways and networks of activity. They become unblocked and functional again, only during deep, slow-wave sleep, although something similar occurs during meditation, relaxation and exercise.

> *It follows that, sleep does not recharge us, it unblocks our neuronal transmissions.*

I once made an intellectual leap as a young doctor. I moved from two years in general practice, to become a research fellow in cardiology. Initially, my brain seemed to struggle with the challenge. My scientific colleagues were highly intelligent, very knowledgeable and fast thinking. Initially, I felt slow, and struggled to keep up. It took me three months to get 'up to speed'. Did this involve growing new neuronal connections or did some blocked brain pathways – left idle and unused – re-open? Perhaps both happened? This mystery and many others, remain.

Chapter Six

Using Time

"Tempus edax rerum."

(Time, the devourer of everything)

Ovid. *Metamorphoses. xv. 234.*

After length, breadth and height, time is the fourth dimension. Einstein linked mass and energy, creating the best known of all equations: e = mc2. In this equation e = energy, m = mass, and c = the speed of light (with speed comes a time measurement). He also showed that (relatively), time is affected by gravity and speed, but even though his discovery was astonishing, it cannot help with our human predicament – the limited time we have on this earth.

The time, money, and health we have are important. The young mostly have time and health, but no money; the middle-aged have money and health, but much less time. The old may have money, but also failing health and little time.

Change and time are inescapably bound together. Even this moment – 'now' – is constantly passing. 'Now' is a frontier – the point at which past time meets future time.

> *"The trick is to live here and now in the timeless moment.*
>
> *To act as if that's all there is. No beginning, no end."*
>
> *A Season in Hell.* (2012).
>
> Jack Higgins. Hyperfiction.

We all have an unknown lifespan. Both an awareness of time and its measure, distinguish us from most creatures, although whales can migrate to arrive at their feeding grounds on time, and birds can traverse continents to arrive at a certain place at a certain time. Some humans are obsessed with time; others have no sense of it whatsoever. Although the present moment is all we have, it is natural to be concerned about the past, and what the future might hold. The past is gone and cannot be altered. The future is unknown, and cannot be predicted reliably, despite many media gurus proclaiming they know the future.

The older we get, the more likely is the past to become our focus. The young, with too few events in their past, have only the present and future to occupy them. For the young, the passage of time can seem slow, especially when they are bored. It passes fast, however, when they are having fun. At a young age, many dream of being older, secure adults, while older people spend time dreaming of being young again.

The future is always insecure, given the many uncertainties of complex world functioning. Many predict the future based on the past, but that can prove unreliable. This can create a level of anxiety for some who will spend their energy unnecessarily – possibly affecting their health and chances of survival. Since most factors we live with can change on a daily basis, realists plan for their future, written only in pencil. Dreamers are free to plan their castles in the air, while others see no point to any speculation – they happily take each day as it comes.

Those we call efficient, are people who use their time productively, achieving lots in little time. The inefficient take forever – doing whatever they choose to do at their own pace. They can resent or admire those who put time to productive use. Imagine how well one might speak a foreign language, if one spent only thirty minutes every day learning new words.

Time is a precious resource, but it is unidirectional. It only marches forward. The achievements of every industrialised society have depended on its effective use. Personal success and survival can depend on how well we handle time.

Some try to do more and more in less and less time. In 1959, Meyer Friedman and Ray Rosenman first gave a name to such people – Type-A personalities. They were thought to have twice as many heart attacks as their more time-relaxed counterparts; they called them Type-B characters. The faster we accelerate a car, the more fuel we burn. The harder we accelerate through life, the more energy we will use. Burning too much, too quickly, risks fatigue and exhaustion. Fatigue and exhaustion risk heart attacks and strokes in those predisposed to either 'furred' coronary arteries or high blood pressure. Becoming energised is important – without it, those with any ambition will go nowhere and achieve nothing!

The effective use of time means controlling it, whether at work or at play. For busy people, a structured timetable will help to manage their activities. In this way, we might gain hubris, and a feeling of worthiness and self-esteem from achievement.

Many dislike unstructured time; they may find it boring. The Romans made an artform of unstructured time – they called it *otium*. It requires one to be happy with solitude, and content with oneself. An over-structured, busy life can be exhausting.

It may not seem it, but time passes at a constant rate. Although we refer to 'saving time', that is impossible. It can neither be saved or wasted, just managed better.

> *Paul and I drove separately from London to Lyon, in France. It took all day, but he travelled much faster than me, arriving two hours earlier. When I asked him what he did with the two hours, he said, 'I was waiting for you!' What did he achieve by travelling so fast? Did he save time, given that he had nothing better to do than wait for me?*

After Jean Liedloff had rushed to get to the Yakuana settlement in Venezuala, and apologised to the tribal chief for being late. 'Which time is most valuable', he asked, 'that before you arrived, or that after?' (Jean Liedloff, *The Continuum Concept*).

As Bob Hope once said: "Timing is everything", but you don't have to be a comedian to employ good timing. 'Timing' is often crucial to success, whether you trade currencies on Forex or boil eggs. Get it wrong, and your joke could fall flat, or your egg might be too soft. Money traders can lose money, and egg-connoisseurs can get angered by eggs not boiled to perfection.

"There is a tide in the affairs of men
Which, taken at the flood, leads on to fortune;□
Omitted, all the voyage of their life□
Is bound in shallows and in miseries.
On such a full sea are we now afloat;
And we must take the current when it serves,□
Or lose our ventures."

Shakespeare, *Julius Caesar*

Time, like wine bottles, is better filled.

The Time of Your Life is Now

Now is 'when'.

The past and future

Both remain eternal.

"Sed fugit interea, fugit

inreparabile tempus."

(But meanwhile it is flying, irretrievable time is flying).

Virgil

"For what is your life?

It is a vapour,

that appeareth for a little time,

and then vanisheth away."

The Bible

James, 4:14.

These solemn thoughts might induce despair in those who fear death, and those troubled by the ephemeral nature of life. Life is all too short, and a little Yiddish humour can help to lessen its gravity:

Hymie Bard ran a smoked salmon factory in the East End of London. Whenever his employees complained about their long and arduous hours of work, he would say: " I don't know why you're complaining. You're only here for a lifetime, you're not here forever!"

As the fourth dimension, time affects everything in the universe, with nothing exempt. The succession of day and night; the seasons in non-tropical regions; the annual succession of birthdays and anniversaries, Christmas, Yom Kippur, and Ramadan – all serve to make us time aware. On a longer timeframe, our changing bodies mark the passage of decades. Teething, and losing teeth; mumps and measles mark childhood time. Unexpected and unwanted hair growth; menstruation for girls, voice change for boys, mark puberty time. Growing taller, getting spotty, and noticing the 'other' sex – all mark adolescence.

For adults, time is event oriented. Marriage, births, jobs, bereavements, retirement, holidays, changes of house. When older, the middle-aged often ask: "Where did the time go? What have I done with my time?"

Later life is usually marked by the slowing of vital functions: devolving responsibilities, relative immobility, and the need for care. With age, many realise that a youthful mind can still inhabit a worn out and older shell, although the young usually believe that youthfulness belongs to them alone. Some older people will carry on regardless:

> *At 98-years of age, Wally Latimer, a Kansas farmer, decided to take it easy. He decided to slow down. Instead of getting up at dawn, he decided to rise at 6 a.m. Instead of working a 14-hour day on his 40-acre farm, he decided to cut his hours down to 12!*

When asked for the secret of his longevity, he said: "I don't worry, and I don't get mad."

Using time well can be a source of pride.

Time and Perception

A ticking clock marks the progress of time, always moving on-
ward. Our perception of time, however, is never that it passes at
a constant pace. The human mind is incapable of holding any
measure of time for long. We have to be prompted by something
– the movement of the sun; the ticking of a clock or metronome.
Equal amounts of physically measured time can seem long or short
depending on where our mind is focussed.

We tend to measure time in relation to our expectation: a given
journey, a holiday, our life:

> *Jane Port lived her later life fearing that her money
> would soon run out. When she died at 89-years of age
> she left 2.8 million pounds to the National Trust, and
> half a million to the Royal Lifeboat Institution!*

Sometimes a moment can seem like an hour, and an hour like a
moment.

> *"Oh aching time!*
>
> *'Oh moments big as years!"*

> John Keats
> (1795–1821).
>
> *Hyperion, bk.i, 1.64.*

Sometimes, there isn't enough time:

> *"But at my back*
>
> *I always hear*

Time's winged chariot

hurrying near."

Andrew Marvell
(1621-1678).

To His Coy Mistress.

Enjoy yourself and time will seem to fly. Immerse yourself in an enjoyable pastime or job, and hours can seem like minutes. Become discontented or bored, and time will pass with leaden feet.

Contentment is an important aspect of health. To some extent, it relates to losing some awareness of time. In his article on living to 100-years of age (Sunday Times Magazine 20.11.83), Dr. Desmond Morris made the point, that in order to have any chance of living that long, adults should remain vivacious, keep their enthusiasm for future achievement, and remain calm and contented.

When 99-year old, Catherine Booth (grand-daughter of General Booth, founder of the Salvation Army) was asked on TV. "If your grandfather had been alive, would he have come with you?" She replied: "No, he would have been doing something much more important!"

A Time for Everything

"To every thing there is a season, and a time to every purpose under the heaven:

A time to be born, and a time to die; a time to plant, and a time to pluck up that which is planted;

A time to kill, and a time to heal; a time to break down, and a time to build up;

A time to weep, and a time to laugh; a time to mourn, and a time to dance;

A time to cast away stones, and a time to gather stones together; a time to embrace, and a time to refrain from embracing;

A time to get, and a time to lose; a time to keep, and a time to cast away;

A time to rend, and a time to sew; a time to keep silence, and a time to speak;

A time to love, and a time to hate; a time of war, and a time of peace."

The Bible. Ecclesiastes 3:1

Timing is Everything

Would Elvis Presley, the Beatles, Churchill, Picasso, Pasteur, George Washington, or John Wayne, have been so successful had they been born fifty years earlier or later?

If in the right place at the right time, with the appropriate abilities, anything is possible. Even for those with an undoubted ability, there are times when they might achieve nothing, if the time and place are wrong. Survival (or success) often depends on timing.

Timing can rule our destiny. It can be out of phase by centuries, not just minutes, hours, days, months or years. We have all met those who, by virtue of their attitudes, outlook, and personal standards, would have been far less conflicted being born a Victorian, Georgian or Roman.

Effective delivery of the spoken and written word also depends on timing. Knowing what to say, and what not to say at a particular time, can make the difference between being effective or not being heeded.

Life is made so much easier, and less energy expensive, for those with good 'timing'. One should try to get it right by the second, by the minute, hour, day and year.

Alan Wicker was once a well-known TV reporter. He was known for interviewing eccentrics. On one occasion, he interviewed a wealthy passenger on-board the QE2. He was travelling alone and for the whole voyage, stayed cocooned in his large expensive suite. He only rarely ventured outside, taking only one walk around the deck each day. He was content to do nothing. When

Alan Wicker asked what he did with his time, he said: "I do nothing, and I've no time left for doing anything else!"

Time and Culture

We can immerse ourselves in different cultures, by travelling just a few hours by airplane. One obvious difference easily observed, is how different cultures use time. The general pace of life and need to rush, is soon apparent. Tranquillity or frenzy are immediately obvious. Western behaviour is different from that in eastern countries; Latin behaviour is different from the Teutonic. Typical Caucasian behaviour is quite different from that seen in the West-Indies. These are all generalisations, obvious to any observant traveller. Sometimes the differences are stark.

Edward Hall, Emeritus Professor of Anthropology at North-Western University, Illinois, has said that unlike peoples of Europe and North America, the Hispanic cultures of Latin America, put people before schedules.

The time it takes for a track and field athlete to run their preferred distance, is a measure of their athletic prowess. The time they take will rank them in world order.

Attitudes to time and how it is perceived, vary between cultures. Culturally laid-back attitudes can be embodied in the words used for tomorrow: 'Domani', 'Mañana', 'Bukara'. All mean tomorrow – a time when things *might* get done. There use can cause upset among Type-A characters – those with time-urgent personalities, anxious not to waste time.

I wonder if this time-urgent characteristic is of genetic origin or is installed in us during early life. After all, many parents expect their children to achieve, in order to meet their own expectations, based on a given timetable. An age to start school, an age to go to University, and get a job. For a long time, in many cultures, there has been an acceptable time to 'settle down', get married, and have children.

As children, our need for parental approval (complying with many rules and regulations), can create anxiety. Western society requires us not to waste our time and energy on fruitless activity; to be dedicated to productivity, and to keep the capitalist machine revolving. Many societies drive their citizens to achieve self-esteem, while keeping them enslaved (with job insecurity and mortgages). This applies more in particular cultures.

The few Chinese, Japanese (where family honour also pertains), Jewish and professional Indian families I have known, seem to be more driven than most. These are features less obvious in Mediterranean and West-Indian cultures.

Time Overload and Under-load

> *A patient of mine, Joan, was a PhD graduate. After marrying a wealthy land-owner, she soon became pregnant. The family were rich enough to employ housekeepers, kitchen staff, and gardeners. She found herself with time on her hands. Once her child was born, her husband insisted on employing full-time nannies. Her husband, who was much older than her, had lived his life as a country gentleman. He had full-time personal staff and was disinclined to change.*

She found it difficult to do anything other than lead an unaccustomed, under-structured life of luxury. Her underloaded existence inhibited her, and she had become tired, bored and depressed as a result.

As a cause of tiredness, being under-structured is an infrequent finding, found mostly in wealthy patients. Over-structuring is much more common. The majority of tired people have too much to do, and not enough time to do it. Some have enough time but lack the ability to use it efficiently. The effect is to make them feel overburdened.

There are two dependent entities here – volume overload, and time overload. Both can be real or imagined. That depends on how situations are perceived, the motivation available, and the ability to complete tasks through effective organisation.

Many of us have subjected ourselves and our children, to time overload. Remember those exam's?

PHYSICS

ADVANCED LEVEL EXAMINATION

Paper 1

Time Allowed: 3 Hours

(Answer FIVE questions, selecting no more than
TWO from each section.)

Many will remember the syllabus for such exams; getting the books
and guessing just how much they had to learn. The prospect of
learning lots of information could be daunting, and overloading.
Once one made a start, it didn't seem so bad. Clearly, experience
alters perception. Looking back, the work accomplished can seem
much easier than when we first faced it. Memory, intelligence, and
ability can respond to being stretched – at least for the able. For
those genuinely overloaded with information, examination failure
is almost inevitable.

Being overloaded with information and a need for decision
making, can fractionate activity. One can lose direction, with
half-hearted attempts being made to accomplish objectives, none
of which get done well. Some give up and fail; achievers quieten
down, formulate a plan, and act in a determined, structured way.
The energy we bring to any situation will depend on our motivation. Even a fatigued person can stand and walk away, especially if
they have flames licking at their heels.

Time for Survival

The survival of animals in the wild is critically dependant on time,
and timing. Breeding, migration, and feeding, mostly depend for
their success on exact timing. Both the time of year, and the time
of day, can be critical. If an animal attempts to feed at a time when
predators are roaming around, it may get eaten instead. Mating
only works at the right time. This can be conveyed by behaviour
and pheromones.

If someone starts a business at the same time as a nearby, larger
organisation, he risks being overshadowed, eaten up, or taken-over.

Where survival and prosperity are concerned, animals, men, and businesses, all have an opportune ecological time slot.

To have the best chance of success or survival, learning to use time well is essential. This means allocating enough time for work, rest and play. Without a timetable that includes sufficient sleep and relaxation, fatigue is likely. Fatigue can result in ineffectiveness, indecision and inefficiency. More serious fatigue (nearing exhaustion) can lead to the jettisoning of strategies, loss of discipline and the abandonment of an agreed timetable. The ineffective use of time often leads to disappointment and failure. We humans cannot work continuously, so time for unblocking our brain overused neuronal channels (equivalent to, but not the same as, battery recharge) needs to be fitted into every work and play schedule.

Only by conserving time for neuronal restoration can we remain healthy and enjoy the fruits of personal success. Many people are hooked on the wrong strategy. They try:

- work - work - work . . . collapse

The intelligent and successful, adopt another strategy:

- work - rest - work - rest . . . success

Successful people are usually adaptable and will have tried many things to achieve their accomplishments. They might try:

-   work – work – rest - work – work -work

— rest - rest

Future Time

The possible inventions, thought to belong to tomorrow, are always those of to-day. We know nothing about tomorrow. Science fiction dreams belong to to-day, with only some achieving reality tomorrow. When dreams of tomorrow are scientifically feasible, they might become a guiding influence.

The future of science, business and technology, depends on the lateral and creative thinking of a few inspired people. It is their knight's move ideas that change the course of history. Such progress has been a matter of philosophical controversy. Carl Popper suggested that it was progressive: one advance, leading to another. Kühn suggested that progress depends on those who make new, previously unforeseeable jumps. Such conceptual jumps, like coming to understand the revolution of the planets around the sun (Galileo); quantum theory and relativity (Feyneman and Einstein), are intellectual examples; the inception of the light bulb, radio, television, powered flight and the telephone, are practical examples.

When hoping for a better life, many people rely entirely on future possibilities. Some forsake their life to-day, by investing their resources (time, knowledge, money) for a better tomorrow. Many gamble with the time they have. Some dump their spare cash into a pension fund or endowment policy. They should know that while two-thirds of non-smokers live beyond the pension age (66-years in the UK), only one third of smokers will. Not all will live long enough to gain from their investment. Those who don't make it, will have sacrificed their to-day, for the promise of a better tomorrow.

In 1773, Samuel Johnson and James Boswell undertook a tour of Scotland. On their tour of Mull, Dr. Johnson observed:

> *"Plantation (of trees) is naturally the employment of a mind unburdened with care, and vacant of futurity, saturated with present good, and at leisure to derive gratification from the prospect of posterity. He that pines with hunger, is in little care how others shall be fed. The poor man is seldom studious to make his grandson rich. It may be soon discovered, why in a place, which hardly supplies the cravings of necessity, there has been little attention to the delights of fancy, and why distant convenience is unregarded, where the thoughts are turned with incessant solicitude upon every possibility of immediate advantage."*

Samuel Johnson and James Boswell. *A Journey to the Western Islands.*

The contented allow the future to take care of itself; the neurotic live with projections of their future, with all its possible catastrophes and discomforts to worry about. Many wealthy people want to leave a legacy for their grand-children. Others think it wrong to spoil them, removing as it might, their motivation and need for endeavour. The poor often accede to instant self-gratification, since today is all many can rely on. Although impossible to prove over geological time, I doubt that human nature has changed much.

Shipwrecks, Time and Ageing

Stress forces us to spend our energy; each time ageing us a little. The energy we need for body maintenance will be temporarily usurped by our response to stress. If we spend most of our energy on stress, perhaps there will be less available to halt the ageing process.

John de Lorean (inventor of the car in 'Back to the Future') was acquitted from a charge of conspiring to distribute cocaine. When asked how he felt at his acquittal he said: "I've aged 600-years in the last two!"

Premature ageing, noticed by relatives and friends, is commonly observed before a medical catastrophe. If fatigue from stress progresses to the point of exhaustion (before any collapse), the potential victim may look haggard and assume a shambling gait. Their attitude might shift from optimistic to pessimistic, and they can adopt a *'fait accompli'* attitude to life. Even the young can take on a more aged look and geriatric demeanour.

'Wearing well' for one's age, is probably genetic. I have seen it in some families. This conclusion will come to any physician who has served several generations of the same family. Many variations occur, but are they related in any way to how their energy is spent on stress? I suspect the way we each spend energy, like wearing well with time, also has a genetic basis.

Time Clocks & Circadian Rhythm

High and low tides follow a cyclical pattern, in keeping with night and day. Both are related to the movement of the sun, earth, and moon. The earth itself rotates, wobbles and travels around the sun in a cyclical manner that spans thousands of years. Global warming and cooling can be explained by such oscillations. In the human body several biological cycles overlap – temperature, hormones, sleepiness and wakefulness, wax and wane with predictable regularity. There are, however, daily cycles, monthly cycles, and possibly cycles of much longer periodicity. Why should this be? And what functions might they serve?

Everything in the universe is cyclical – it has a waxing and waning nature, be it the heat of the sun, the size of the ozone layer, global warming, the experience of good and bad luck, our liability to infection and fertility and health – all are affected.

The sleep / wakefulness cycle is crucial to normal human functioning. Whatever else sleep does, it helps us regain our mental and physical energy. If by chance, we must remain awake both day and night (sleep deprivation), our ability to concentrate, and our mental and physical coordination will start to fail.

Sleep has its own pattern, dependent partly on melatonin production produced by the pineal gland. Light reaching the eyes, traverses the skull and brain in daylight, switches off melatonin production and promotes wakefulness.

Dreaming occurs during REM sleep. It starts in the first ten minutes of sleep and gets more frequent as sleep progresses. Active dreaming sleep (rapid eye movement sleep or REM), is interspersed with slow-wave, relaxing (resetting) sleep. With daytime stress, the amount of REM sleep increases, and the amount of slow-wave sleep diminishes. The effect is to reduce the restorative effect of sleep.

Because night and day, hormones, temperature and temperament all follow a daily rhythmic pattern, there is an optimum time for sleeping and waking. In animals there are more complex, long-term timing issues which will influence mating, procreation, and survival. Animal survival is critically dependent on innate timing: feeding and sleeping at specific times, can ensure that each animal keeps within its ecological niche, being most awake when its food is available at low risk. Sexual activity in non-tropical climes can also be timed, basing it on the cycle of seasons, so that the offspring have the optimum climatic conditions for growth, life and survival at the time of their birth.

If polar bears did not mate at the right time, their cubs would be unable to survive extreme cold. Food for rapid growth would not be available when they needed it. Survival of migratory animals depends on navigation, and on the time of year. Annual cycles are also exhibited as whales return to feed each year in specific parts of the ocean. Birds sleep, but not all reptiles do. Some animals can sleep with only half their brain alert (dolphins and orca).

Heart attacks and stroke occurrences seem to peak at certain times of day. Strokes occur most on wakening (6 AM to midday). At this time, wakening and arousal begins, and blood pressure is at its highest – strokes due to brain haemorrhage, are then more likely. Weekly timing can apply to heart attacks – they occur most on Monday mornings. Timing also applies to road traffic accidents. Unsurprisingly, they occur mostly during the evening rush-hour, between 4 and 6 PM.

Our individual daily rhythms vary enough to recognise at least two types of individual – 'morning people', and 'evening people'; 'larks' and 'owls' respectively. This is of some consequence since our alertness (arousal), and ability to think, peak at different times. Conflict arises for night people who work as breakfast TV presenters. Dangers can lurk for patients who get ill at night, when attended by a 'morning' doctor. As a resident doctor for two years, I adapted to getting up five times every night and then working all day long.

Most people concentrate best in the morning; a few think and function best in the evening or at night. One of my 'tired-all-the-time' patients was both good at mental arithmetic and a night owl. I recommended her to a casino pit-boss I had seen some time before. He took her on, and she now works the night shift in a famous Las Vegas casino. She is no longer 'tired-all-the-time'.

J.B. came to my clinic for a routine medical screening examination. One of the topics we discussed was his inability to function in the morning. He seemed to be an 'afternoon' person, or perhaps one of those rare birds – a true 'night' person. Luckily, he had netted a fortune after selling his former business, three years before. He was now itching to get back into business. He wasn't looking forward to getting up early every morning. We discussed biorhythms, and what interested him was the fact that most others would be tiring, as he was waking up.He enquired, "Do you mean to say, that if I hold all my important meetings after 4.30 PM, I could more easily get the better of others?"

Since true night people are fairly rare, I told him his chances of gaining an advantage were good. He went on to put this theory into practice. His new business was electrical contracting for major retail outlets. Jobs in that business are often done in the evening and at night – after customers and staff have gone home. He needed night owl staff who could be left without need-ing supervision. J.B. was no longer in conflict with his biorhythms and he then made more money than ever!

Here is a short series of my thoughts (haiku-like senryus) about time:

"Time collapses,

With one sound

Or sight or smell,

Resurrecting the past.

Time expands

As unstructured

Life proceeds:

Immersed in nostalgia.

Time stops

With surprise:

Making love;

Laughter, passion,

And arresting news."

For more, get my little book entitled: *Poems for Recycling Lives* (2024).

If you are in the right place at the right time, with the appropriate abilities and facilities, anything is possible. Nothing, however, may seem possible if the timing and place are inappropriate. Survival (or success) can depend on timing.

The Use of Time. 'Type-A' Behaviour

"If you can wait and not be tired of waiting . . .

Yours is the Earth and everything that's in it,

And – which is more – you'll be a Man, my Son!"

Rudyard Kipling. *'If'*

In their 1974 publication, Meyer Friedman and Ray Rosenman, wrote about the Type-A behaviour trait they had identified earlier (1959). It initially gained recognition as the single most important heart attack risk factor. It was said to double the chance of getting a heart attack. If patients who had suffered a heart attack remained a Type-A character, their chances of another increased fivefold.

Type-A behaviour is easily recognised. These are people who are always rushing, having little time to concentrate on anything. Typically, they have several mobile telephones, and will try to use them all at the same time. They are nearly always late for appointments. As an example. If late for the airport, they might attempt to rush home, feed the cat, deliver flowers to their girlfriend, and post a birthday card to their mother. They find it most difficult to 'do nothing'. On holiday, they will be the one pacing up and down on the beach with a mobile phone in their hand, anxious about something they see as urgent.

Under certain conditions, Type-A behaviour can be induced. Put a person in an overload situation, where urgency matters, and Type-A behaviour can surface. This happened to me once as a casualty (A&E) doctor. On the occasions when I was single-handed, and multiple emergency cases arrived simultaneously, I sensed some time urgency. The same will happen to an understaffed shopkeeper, should a queue of increasingly irritated customers start to form. There are, of course, some people who never feel anxious, time-urgent or rushed by circumstances; these are the laid-back, Type-B personalities.

Kenny Nicholls, a good friend of mine, was an entertainer. He had the most profound Type B personality I ever encountered – often to my annoyance!

One beautiful summer's day we were boating on the upper reaches of the river Thames. We motored gently into a lock, packed to the hilt with boats of all shapes and sizes. There had been a problem ahead, causing a log-jam. Many were loudly expressing their irritation.

All the Type-A boatmen were looking at their watches; getting more irritated by the minute. As the murmur of complaints grew louder, Kenny stood up, introduced himself, and started to sing. Captivated by this unlikely event, his engaging manner, the quality of his singing voice, and his apt sense of timing, caused joy to break free. A few unhurried bars of his song diffused the discontent. By the end of his song, a lengthy ovation replaced the previous angst. Few noticed that the lock had filled, and that they were all free to depart. Strange! Nobody seemed in a hurry; some didn't want to leave. For a few magic moments, he relaxed and galvanised his audience with an impromptu musical rendition.

Should they feel they are wasting time, some will get anxious. A sense of urgency can be diffused, by introducing an attractive preoccupation.

Are Type-A characters born, or are they made? My personal observations suggest that even children at play, can display time-urgent behaviour; in fact, the disruptive desire for instant gratification among two-year-olds, can continue for a lifetime.

CHAPTER SEVEN

The Life Equation

Equality & Balance

For the followers of Zarathustra, and the fanciful diviners of 'the Force' in Star Wars films, good, truth, and light, must be balanced against the forces of evil, untruth and darkness; Ahura Mazda against Ahriman; ying against yang. All balances shift with time; some being felt, others weighed.

In all matter's human, stable balance is elusive. Achieving it usually requires constant work and constant energy expenditure – just to maintain the *status quo*. To be human is to cope with change, and to be human requires many balancing acts. We swing in and out of balance as our lives take shape. In the imaginatively controlled, but necessary fixed conditions of every science laboratory, physicists can achieve equilibrium for a specified time only. Instability, which some will define as chaos, can intervene anytime. Neither science experiments nor life, always go to plan. Despite the inevitability of constant change, humans continually strive for stability. Because change can be fascinating, many have employed art and literature to chart their every challenge.

Both health and success in the business of life (and, the life of a business), require effective energy management. Finding energy, keeping it, and knowing how best to spend it, are key issues for health and the management of ill-health.

Sleep and spending energy are scarcely referred to by doctors in relation to health and disease. The public, on the other hand, are focussed more on diet, vitamins and exercise as essential for health. Since the amount of energy we spend on health and disease, can only ever equal the amount we have available, life proceeds critically dependent on a balance that is little appreciated. We have no natural means to make us aware of this balance – of our energy spending and saving. So much of it, like heat loss from the body, is insensible.

All of life and nature is a balancing act between energy spending and energy generation (from the chemical processes that make it available for use). If we are to lead a healthy life, each side of the equation must balance. By coming to understand this energy equation, tiredness, fatigue, exhaustion, and ill-health, could become less likely. If life is to proceed healthily, and if diseases are to be overcome speedily, we must pay attention to our personal life equation.

Medical science has made many advances in understanding health and disease, but has shown little interest in personal energy when expressed as fatigue, whether related to illness, poor recovery, or sleep disturbance. Doctors understand this, but only rarely feel the need to take it into account – it can start to get too personal. One major problem is the variation between individuals – how some are greatly affected by stress (and energy spending) and others are not. Not all have inherited genetically-driven, physiological processes, that will enhance the likelihood of ill-health, disease and premature death. At the moment, many doctors are claiming they have too little time for their discovery.

Issues of personal energy were better understood in the distant past, when the need for rest, sleep and convalescence, were better appreciated. Doctors then, had none of the advantages of modern medicine, but they did recognise the benefits of sleep, exercise and diet. Patients who had pneumonia were told it would take many weeks for them to recover. Today, we expect patients to be back at work in three days (and patients need to be discharged from hospital, to free beds). In the same way that it takes a certain time for seeds to germinate, and flowers to grow, our bodies also have their own periodicity – the time needed to recover from illness or to learn a new skill.

In UK medical practice, the application of scientific testing and an emphasis on money-saving, efficient patient handling – as if it represents the be-all and end-all of good medical practice – has fast replaced the holistic clinical care doctors once practised five decades ago. In UK private practice (I had over 20,000 private patients, accumulated over five decades), and in many countries I have visited, handling patients with machine-like efficiency, rather than with some sensitivity to individual needs remains unacceptable.

My medical thesis is simple. Personal energy spending and saving are potent predictors of health and ill-health, so we need to attend to both in order to benefit patient progress and clinical outcome.

The structure of our society, and the planning of our environment, our education and skills development, the nature of interpersonal relationships, and how we handle them, all cause us to spend and save energy in ways that can either promote, reduce or destroy our health. The popular concept of 'stress' is but one aspect on the spending side of the life energy equation.

The complete solution of the life equation must include every factor that spends and repletes our energy. In this way, we should be able to make better sense of why some have vitality and are healthy, and others get tired, fatigue, exhausted, and ill. Using the notion of this equation, should better enable us to predict the outcome of every health and life scenario.

Without energy considerations, we cannot know how bereavement might induce a heart attack in one person but leave another unperturbed. Taken alone, the concept of stress, cannot predict these widely disparate outcomes. Only by taking personal medical characteristics (constitution) and personal energy into account, is it possible to understand why one person is made ill by stress, and another is left unaffected. Some seem to thrive on stress, but that might be a romantic illusion, because the life equation and its demands always take priority.

Those who spend most energy, are usually those with obsessive needs, fears, and wasteful anxieties. Only a few meet the world with calm, composure and dignity. Those who become depleted of energy could be at the mercy of their inherited (constitutional) weaknesses – their tendency to high blood pressure, blood clotting or psychological instability. Stress will expose their vulnerability. A few will succumb to their physical weaknesses and develop angina, migraine, peptic ulceration and the like; others might react emotionally, variously becoming anxious, depressed or preoccupied by their problems. Those with enough inherited strength, will keep calm and carry on.

Do we humans react solely as our genetics might predict, or can our experience and circumstances intervene? Actually, there is good evidence for both. Both are involved in predicting clinical outcome. My 50-year experience of sick human beings has allowed me to form many impressions, especially of those struggling with life circumstances and their medical conditions. I suspect that our environment provides the lessons – helping us to adapt our behaviour and outlook to the many stresses and stimuli that befall us, while our genes alone predict how we will react physiologically (or pathophysiologically) – with raised blood lipids, a speeding heart rate, high blood pressure, increased blood coagulability or diminished immune responses. The study of genetics has yet to reveal all the ways in which genes and circumstances interact. Even if we come to know it all, the act of applying it to any individual, will remain a challenging art for doctors to master (see more in my book, *The Art & Science of Medical Practice*, 2024).

Doctors' Enquiries

To understand individual human outcomes requires us to know the fundamental interchanges of energy, demanded by the life we each lead, within the confines of our cultural and social society. Following the simplest principles of energy conservation and utilisation, it is usually quite obvious clinically who are physically and mentally healthy, and who are unhealthy.

In order to understand any unexpected decline in health, it is insufficient for a doctor to enquire superficially about the social and personal circumstances of their patients. Rather, the patient, his family, friends, and work mates, may have to be 'cross-questioned' to reveal the truth. Through risking loss of face and dignity, many are motivated to withhold the truth of their circumstances, even though their life and death could depend on it. Interrogating patients may sound extreme, but it is sometimes appropriate, when life and death issues are at stake. Only from an in-depth understanding of each patient can a prescription for effective change be made – change that will promote health, lead to healthy fulfilment in life, and an improved quality of life, by maximising prevention. Whether this will lead to effective 'disease' prevention strategies is unknown. In some cases, it may be possible, but is yet to be proven.

Interrogation is not always necessary to understand the plight of an individual. By gaining trust, the sympathetic rapport that results, will usually reveal enough. Created by a genuine desire to help through understanding, cathartic revelation sometimes occurs – for physicians, therapists and patients alike.

Some doctors, concentrating solely on their particular area of interest, may have no desire to employ an in-depth holistic approach. Fewer still will be trained to combat the denial and defiant obstruction that some patients employ to conceal their circumstances and energy spending.

Because many physicians are content to treat physical disease, on face value, many will not want to spend extra time to reveal the patient's psychosocial and behavioural features, even if important to their understanding of their patient's tiredness, fatigue or exhaustion. When I was young, very few doctors put any value on preventative intervention, especially if it pertained to health and ill-health, rather than disease. National policies changed after positive evidence for the value of breast and prostate cancer screening was found. National policies have not yet fully grasped the value of all pre- and early diagnosis – diagnosis before any symptom occurs.

Given the relation of fatigue to cardiovascular disease morbidity, there remains a real need for doctors to expose why so many patients become fatigued and exhausted for no obvious reason. Some will be threatened by ill-health, disease, and death, if they spend more energy than they can afford. From their own point of view, patients also have problems. Many fail to recognise the relationship between personal energy saving and spending strategies and their health. Many factors, like aggravation, anger, indignation, anxiety, obsessionality, and resentment, spend excessive amounts of energy, and when combined with poor sleep, can risk their demise.

For doctors sympathetic to understanding the life equation, many will want to raise questions. Among them, will be how they are to find the time for this more intrusive approach, and which of their patients might need it most? In reality, only a few patients will benefit. Because 'patients first' should be our primary practise guide, the numbers of patients who might benefit (the focus of medical bureaucracy) should be secondary. Work for a bureaucracy-led medical organisation, and risk it becoming secondary. Work for yourself, and it must remain primary, if you are to attract any following.

> *Tennis player, Arthur Ashe, was born in 1943. He became Wimbledon Tennis Champion in 1975. In 1979 he had a heart attack and underwent coronary vein by-pass surgery. In 1983, he underwent further heart surgery. His mother had died aged twenty-seven, with hypertensive heart disease.*

> *"Some argue that the high rates of high blood pressure and heart disease reported in black Americans are in part at least attributable to the inordinate control they struggle to exercise over negative feelings, feelings such as anger, resentment, frustration and rage."*

Anthony Clare
on Arthur Ashe.

*In the Psychiatrist's
Chair*

The Art of Healthy Living

There is an art to living, with no accredited masters. A few people seem to 'get it right', although, I know from the many confidences vested in me, that appearances can be quite mistaken. One would need to be a long-living fly on the walls of others, to glimpse the unexpurgated truth. If someone, sometime, has 'got it right', then perhaps their art and science of life should be studied to discern the relevant principles. The purpose of this knowledge could make the mastery of life accessible to many.

The personal energy we have, and take for granted until we lose it, is our most valuable resource; nothing can be achieved without it. Mastery of life as a fully functioning human being, can only be attained by knowing innately or otherwise, how to manage our energy. If there were recognised masters of healthy living, they would be masters of personal energy management.

Disease induction and disease escalation are other aspects of energy management that need consideration. The unifying principles of how this happens must comply with every physical law, common not only to all humans, but to the whole universe.

A stress to one person may not be the same for another, so the concept of stress – strain reactions, lacks universal medical application. This is not so for energy, where the same physical considerations apply in galaxies, stars, on planets, in countries, and for cars, airplanes, hearts, brains and washing machines. Energy is indivisible and universal. There can be no understanding of any functioning system, mechanical or biological, without considering energy. We worry about the prices of oil, electricity and gas as energy sources, but few give thought to personal energy and how we use it.

Energy Balance

The principles of energy flow and conservation, date back to a time when engineers and physicists tried to understand heat, and energy exchange in steam engines. Certain principles were established that have universal significance. The principle of conserving energy for instance, means that the work done by a human or a machine, can only come from the energy put into it. So where does it come from?

Plants not only get their energy from the soil, but from the sunlight falling on their leaves. For animals and humans alike, food is the primary energy source, not sunlight. After digestion and chemical breakdown into various chemical component parts (sugars, amino acids and fats), our cells make specific high-energy phosphate compounds for powering our muscles, heart, brain and nervous system. Like a boiler that produces heat (as a form of energy) from burning coal, paper, wood and oil, animals can use a variety of foods as their source of energy. Evolution has enabled all creatures to use many food sources. Some environments cannot support life, and intelligent beings will move away from them fast. The multiplicity of species, however, is testament to the unfussy nature of animal food requirements.

Returning to Mr. Micawber, we can find in the idea of balancing income and expenditure, a system too insecure to sustain life. What if Micawber had a bad trading week, with poor income and much increased expenditure? He would indeed experience misery. Unfortunately, Mr Micawber was 'forever floored' by his circumstances, despite his excellent advice to David Copperfield.

> *Why is it that advisors are so often incapable of following their own good advice? The recent sacking of Lord Peter Mandelson as the UK ambassador to the US (September 2025), over his relationship with Jeffrey Epstein, stands as an example. Recognised as a brilliant political advisor, Mandelson chose to defend a friend who was later found guilty of sex-related crimes. He was sacked as a consequence.*

We can use the Micawber Principle as a basis for the life equation, but some variations are needed. It is true that our energy income must balance our energy spending. It is true that one can have reserves, like money in the bank, but it is not true that we need to balance our books on a daily basis. As long as we eat something, we can have a long-term, reliable energy supply that will last months. Our biology makes us the equivalent of every financial system, but with much more resilience built in. We carry on churning out usable energy, even during months of famine. Under normal circumstances, with most people having some food to eat, our lives are protected by having an almost limitless cellular energy production line. A reliably powered brain means we can think our way out of challenging and risky situations – especially those threatening our existence. With our muscles and heart being reliably supplied with energy, we can escape danger.

Every animal and human being has the equivalent of a nuclear generator built into each cell – an inexhaustible, protected supply of energy, that stops only with death. It is so reliable, we can forget it completely. The oil business is equivalent in one way – it can reach an almost inexhaustible supply of liquid energy, so its business operations mostly concern controlling its supply to others. Running a grocery shop is more precarious, relying as it does on multiple goods suppliers, and ever-changing customer preferences. This arrangement as a model, would never do for reliable life maintenance.

> *With an almost infinite supply of energy (on a day to day basis), all practical considerations of the life equation need only be one-sided – accounting for variations in energy expenditure, not energy supply.*

Being able to forget energy supply, means that what we accomplish and the quality of our existence, depends (for all practicable purposes) on:

- How much energy we spend.

- How this energy spending affects our capacity to think and work.

- How well we are able to minimise our energy spending (which is never fully switched-off), even during rest, relaxation and sleep.

- How effectively we are able to restore our perceived energy (unblocking neuronal channels) ready for the wakeful activity that follows.

If we are to remain healthy, we need to examine how our energy spending can be minimised during daily life and during relaxation and sleep, and how to use energy efficiently in order to remain a healthily functioning, actively sentient being – fully alert, and physically and mentally capable.

The maintenance of health is a balancing act: the energy we spend on physical and mental activities, must balance the energy we generate. The billions of people now alive, all have personalities and characters that mark them as individuals. The fundamental personality and behavioural differences that distinguish us from one another, can be characterised by how much personal energy we each have available, and how we choose to spend and save it. There is a style to personal energy management that defines each of us as an individual.

If our energy supply starts to fail or cannot compete with the energy needed to fight off a disease process, illness, then death could ensue. Death occurs only once all our power generation stops. Well before that, once our energy supply starts to fail, or is unable to cope with the increasing demands of disease, fatigue leading to exhaustion will precede a serious state of illness which may be irreversible.

Both diseases, and the need to solve stressful situations, can block the available energy we perceive. By failing to reverse neuronal channels, poor sleep creates the perception of unavailable energy. As the process extends, we will progress through tiredness and fatigue to exhaustion.

One definition of a disease is any condition that reduces this cellular energy generation, or one that demands lots more energy than can be made available. Both cause fatigue. We must make sure that our nutrition is adequate (providing the ingredients of biological energy production), but this is far from being an important consideration when trying to understand how everyday fatigue occurs in western societies.

Disease mechanisms are complicated, and how each disturbs energy production and its restoration, is beyond the remit of this book. Instead, I have focussed here on the mechanisms that cause otherwise healthy people to experience daytime tiredness, fatigue and exhaustion.

Forced Energy Spending

Dr. Peter Nixon's experience as an army officer, dealing with crack troops, allowed his observation of exhaustion and its survival implications. He recalled the best soldiers being sent to his 'top gun' commando unit for further training. Early on, they would load the troops with lots of heavy armoury and provisions. They would then marched them all until they dropped or couldn't take another step. They had to learn their limits. Since they were all hand-picked, as 'the best' in their units, most thought themselves invincible. Exhausted people are not invincible – a lesson they all had to learn before they could be trained further.

Although this example is not taken from everyday life, it has parallels for those running several businesses; for those with sales and banking problems, and personal relationship stresses that cause them not to sleep well. Claudius, in Shakespeare's Hamlet, makes the point that sorrows not often come singularly, but in battalions.

With our cellular energy generation being ceaseless, reliable, and almost inexhaustible, the reason we get tired must depend most on our spending of energy – on our choice of daily physical and mental activity.

Everyday Energy Spending

Our calls to action made each day can be large in number. From avoiding people on crowded pavements, to deciding big issues, we are all the time spending our energy, reacting to our environment and coping with our family, friends, and work associates. We humans operate a full-time, ever active, navigation and decision-making system. There is no respite, even during sleep when we might relive our day, or project our fears onto tomorrow. This ceaseless energy spend, is more than adequately matched by the energy produced within each cell of our body. So, until we develop a disease or get our neuronal channels blocked by our chosen daily activity, we can carry on healthily.

In health, physical tiredness depends a lot on physical fitness. Training the body works to increase our strength and endurance. The unfit become physically tired more easily than the fit, and their recovery takes longer. There is little more to learn about mechanical issues, unless we consider blocked arteries (which can deny our muscles an adequate supply of blood and oxygen) or consider what muscle injuries and joint problems will do to us. Mental energy considerations are complex by comparison and are the focus of this book.

Healthy life requires that the energy equation is balanced on a continuous basis, and that depends most on how we control our energy spend. This has little to do with our diet, or the vitamins, minerals or supplements we take. In the western world, any lack of these is rare, whereas tiredness, fatigue and exhaustion, will affect most of us at some time.

Overcoming Entropy

Maintaining our energy balance requires us to keep the *status quo*, at least for long enough to plan for change. We must all deal with change – as something inevitable, enforced by the nature of our universe – enforced by the universal challenge of entropy.

The second law of thermodynamics is that of entropy. The disintegration of order with time, is one way of looking at it. Dealing with it can contribute a large component to the spending side of the life equation.

Humans organise clay into bricks, bricks into houses, houses into towns, towns into counties, counties into countries, countries into continents and so on. We need energy to create all this structure, organising everything from brick manufacture to architects. Town planners must agree, and builders must build to create our modern structured living environment.

While alive, we all have many options to organise our lives. When we die, the edifices we constructed and the organisations we built, will decay unless someone is interested enough to upkeep them. Without an input of energy, the driving force of entropy (natural disintegration) takes over, threatening disarray. This natural, inexorable process is behind human ageing. To the human eye it can be displeasing, so vanity makes many spend their energy trying to overcome it.

If we give in to self-defeating laziness, entropy will assume control of our fate. Unless we constantly spend our energy on overcoming the entropic process, every organisation, system, relationship, and lifestyle will steadily revert to chaos. Confronting such chaos may require more energy than we have. Better to meet and overcome entropy on a daily basis, so that what confronts us is an easily corrected deviation.

The depression that commonly accompanies disaster, can inhibit the flow of energy necessary for recuperation. If an airplane of ship gets too far off course, extra power is needed to bring it back on course. The same applies to human life.

There is no life without energy; no movement, thought or feeling, without energy expenditure. Entropy lies lurking in the wings, ready to assume control. Power is energy at work and accomplishing anything needs lots of it.

Chakras

Speculative parallels can be drawn between ancient Hindu ideas of energy flow within the human body, and the latest discoveries of neurophysiology and energy production within the mitochondria of all cells.

Neither the idea of spiritual life balance, nor the idea that it relates to spiritual energy, is new. The ancient Indian idea of chakras – an energy system that explains human illnesses – was first mentioned in the Vedas, ancient sacred texts dating from 1500 to 1000 BC. The word 'chakra' in Sanskrit means a wheel, envisioned as wheels spinning to provide energy. At the centre of the Indian flag there is a blue wheel with 24 spokes. This represents the Dharma Chakra ('Wheel of Law') – the wheel of law in the Sarnath Lion Capital. The chakra represents the continuing progress of the nation and justice in life.

If one searches Google for information on 'Chakras', the following emerges:

*They are considered **loci of life spiritual energy** or prana, which is thought to **flow among them in pathways called nadi**. The **function of the chakras is to spin,** draw in this energy, and keep the spiritual, mental, emotional and physical health of the body in balance*

There is an interesting comparison to be made here between the concept of chakras and information from current neurophysiological science. The *'loci'* could perhaps represent brain cells or neurones, and *'nadi'*, the pathways representing neuronal pathways within the brain.

Blocked chakras are said to cause both physical and emotional ill-health. Although tempting to consider further this as inspirational (or even knowledge-based) pre-science, they hold no meaning other than a metaphor for what we now know about brain anatomy, physiology and disease pathology.

The chemical, adenosine triphosphate (ATP), represents biochemical energy locked away. On breakdown it supplies all the energy we need for our mental and physical processes. ATP is manufactured within mitochondria by an enzyme molecule called ATP synthetase. This molecule spins (hence my suggested connection with chakras); a remarkable molecular phenomenon that has now been visualised. (Nakamoto, 2008). Could the idea of chakras spinning, have possibly pre-empted what we now know about ATP synthetase spinning and throwing off high-energy ATP molecules in cells? Although completely fanciful, the basic idea has come from a time when biochemistry and cellular biology were completely unknown. Spiritual minded Hindus will no doubt come to their own conclusions.

There are said to be seven main chakras emerging from the spinal cord. To return from ill-health to health, it is thought necessary for various pathways (nadi) to be unblocked, balanced or realigned. As an ancient medical construct, chakra malfunction is thought to explain our emotional and physical ills. Undoubtedly, some will question whether this knowledge is coincidental, or prophetic, since it mirrors some aspects of modern neurophysiological understanding. Others will believe – in parallel to the building of the Pyramids of Giza, and Machu Pichu – that this knowledge was obtained from alien intelligence.

I cannot comment further on what would seem to be prophetic ancient statements, first mentioned three to four thousand years ago. I leave interested readers to enjoy speculating further

PART TWO

SPENDING ENERGY: PERSONALITY TYPES AND THE
DEMANDS OF LIFE

CHAPTER EIGHT

Energy Spending Transactions.

Five human personality traits were researched by Kelly, E.L. and Fiske, D.W. between 1946 and 1951. They described extraversion, agreeableness, openness, conscientiousness and neuroticism amongst graduate students of Chicago University. Neuroticism can be divided into various types of nervousness – anxiety, depression, phobia, hysteria, obsession (overlapping with conscientiousness), and hypochondria. All spend extra energy except perhaps agreeableness and openness. A new trait has been added recently – that of environmental sensitivity –undue reactivity to the light, noise, and temperature, etc. in the places we find ourselves.

Among human beings of all races and cultures are a multitude of different types of character, formed by different personality traits and outlook to life. Each has their place on the personal energy spending spectrum. Some will conserve their energy with minimal spending. Others are powerhouses of human vigour, who rush around and seem to work day and night. Both can accomplish change, if well organised. Taken as an upbeat cliché – '*it (life) takes all sorts*' – intimates challenges in both diversity and coexistence.

As quiet energy spenders, many neurotics are among the biggest. They are not so much energy spenders as energy wasters. They waste their energy trying to satisfy repetitive, anxious and obsessive traits. Some who feel underestimated, may feel they have something to prove. Others will commit their whole life to gaining self-esteem. Some are born deprived and try to accept their lot; others will fight hard to achieve fame, stardom, power and wealth, to overcome adversity and reverse what others might have once thought of them. This desire is often egotistical and vain, and not a basis for inner contentment.

Personal Character and Energy Spending

Natural, high-energy spending characters exist. Some are calm pragmatists. Some are anxious, obsessive, determined egoists. Others are angry or resentful all the time, always wanting to be proven right. Some are time-urgent, Type-A characters, many of whom are trying to pack two lives into one. Many are non-delegators, always refusing help.

Many situations calling for increased energy expenditure are driven by fear. Fear of losing a relationship, income or lifestyle; fear of losing status and possessions. There are innumerable fear-provoking, energy-spending situations to cope with – moving house; coping with winning or losing money; going to prison or relocating in another country. Worse still for some, is the fear of death or the loss of personal control – becoming a slave of one sort or another – trafficked into prostitution or made to do unrelenting, unrewarding work. Under all these circumstances, refreshing quiet sleep, will most likely be replaced by disturbing dreams, during rapid eye movement (REM) sleep. There is sometimes little respite for those leading a troubled life.

There are some in a relationship, who will drain their partner's energy. They are demanding, but never offer to help or contribute. Many use the strategy of appearing lost and needy – enticing others to help and pay the bills. They will often have forgotten their wallet, or they will be short of money for the moment. Yiddish has a specific word for them – *shnorers*. You will need to be strong, resourceful, and energetic to befriend one. They use a seductive strategy – they are fun to be with, while draining your money and energy. Human beings, like physical objects, can be radiators or absorbers of energy; some changing mode as the need requires.

Many other character types exist – world literature and films are replete with them. It might be wise for us to learn about them at school, before life puts us to the test. To help inexperienced doctors, I wrote a small book of my experiences with other professionals. My guess is that many will be alarmed by the fact that such personalities exist in the medical profession. They may have encountered the same characters in different roles – as traders, renowned for being disingenuous and tricky; as car dealers, estate agents, salespeople or influencers. (See my book: *Doctors, Nurses and Patients*. 2024, under 'other works by the author').

At-Oneness and Ego

One can argue that enduring comfort in life exists only when one is ego-free, with no need for self-gratification or status chasing. Perhaps the only real strength is knowing – there is no need for strength – only resignation. Self-knowledge allows one to be comfortable within relationships, despite knowing that most people demand as much as they can get.

Physical strength has always attracted the powerful. The wealthy will have their champions. Few middle-class people, as a form of class distinction, will take physical prowess into account when arguing. In the more violent, less well-endowed stratum of society, it can be physical strength alone that counts. Pride, ego and self-esteem, become matters of push and shove.

Intellectual prowess will put us all in our own place, from junior school onwards. Only a few will learn to adjust to verbal attack and psychological wounding. Because every university intake will consist of top-performing schoolchildren, they will each have to adjust themselves to a new order – to a new intellectual hierarchy. The trauma of displacement, from a top-notch position to a lower one, can be traumatic and lead to anguish. As with everything, there is an energy price to pay. It may take hard work and reduced sleep to win back self-esteem. This can cause fatigue, ill-health and a failure to cope. Perhaps this is why fatigue and ME are common among undergraduate students.

Maintaining an ego consumes vast amounts of energy. Our ego demands that we think of ourselves and portray ourselves as worthy. To maintain a worthy image consistently, we must either be that person, or engage in role play. One aspect of Buddha's enlightenment was not to accept energy wasted on ego – all it does is cause suffering. Many people spend their whole life pursuing fame and wealth, just to prove their self-worth. Misery can come from the sacrifices made getting there. Once they have arrived at their desired status, many will find themselves respected and revered, but not loved.

When the image we wish to portray is not readily accepted by others, some will indulge in drama. They might behave in reactive mode, acting like a spoilt child, a superior being, or a martyr, in order to get their way. Maintaining an ego can cause anxiety, tension, aggression, frustration, and disappointment. When these all fail, self-esteem can be lost and depression can occur.

Western societies rely on a driving economy. The energy for this drive, comes from our egotistical need to improve our acquisitions and status. Many of us, living in western societies, are little more than self-motivated slaves. We may no longer be slaves to a King, Pharaoh, or plantation owner, but many of us are now self-made economic slaves. Rousseau was right. We are all born free, but everywhere in chains. These chains are now of our own making, since many take on more than they can afford, and think themselves more deserving than they are. It follows that the only path to personal freedom lies in lessening the drive of an overbearing ego. We must understand how pathological it can be, and how it is we can become our own worst enemy.

Buddhism recognises the pain and suffering needed to maintain an ego. It prescribes meditation as one route to diminish energy wasting through neuroticism. It aims to promote harmony, contentment, tranquillity, composure, and inner peace. Living for the moment, without projecting the future, does much to switch-off personal high-energy expenditure.

The Buddhist outlook is easily attacked using western cynicism. Cynics might say, it's easy to meditate beneath a Bodhi tree, having left all of our responsibilities behind (a wife and child in Buddha's case). It's altogether another matter to achieve composure while pursuing a modern business. The rejoinder is – few practising Buddhists are inclined to run businesses. From the viewpoint of western ambition, spiritual enlightenment does not appear to be practicable.

Snobbery

Both snobbery and pride provide biases, strong enough to affect our decision making. Both are based on two common errors of judgement: assumption and generalisation. Many assume that everything can be valued, either by price or exclusivity. Snobbery values exclusivity. Reversed snobbery is as bad – assuming that nothing expensive is worth much, and that the wealthy are all daft and spoilt ('you would have to be mad to spend that much on a . . .')

These biases are often poorly informed at worst and based on subjective belief at best. Anti-snobbery for some, is a source of pride. Once it became known that Princess Diana favoured Mark's and Spencer's for 'value for money' clothes, even the worst of clothes snobs, started to shop there. It's a shame, but wealthy people cannot afford to wear their jewellery in public (insurance companies insist it being kept under lock and key). This has had to be accepted, by money snobs and the poor alike. Wearing copies makes sense.

Snobbery reflects what people think of themselves. No actress has played it better than Dame Patricia Routledge (1929-2025), playing Hyacinth Bucket (pronounced 'Bouquet') in the long-running TV comedy series, 'Keeping up Appearances' (1990-1995). Patricia was knighted (2017), an accomplishment well beyond even Hyacinth's aspirations.

Snobs usually lack humility. Avoid them or waste your time and energy, clashing with their perverse views – unless, of course, you find them amusing.

The need to impress, guarantees most will work hard to obtain street cred. To fulfil this need, some young western women looking for a mate will be attracted by male possessions – like property and income. Many western young men are attracted by 'hot' and available, beautiful women. In Masai tribes, women are attracted to the owners of cattle, and men to wide, child-bearing hips. Everywhere, ego is at work, hoping to raise personal status and security. Without doubt, this has been thought worthy of our energy expenditure, from the beginning of time.

The entitled, and those who feel superior, can despise the less well-endowed. Those inclined to inferiority can be uncomfortable mixing with achievers – reminding them, perhaps, of their deficiencies. With the teaching of Christ, love and humility became aspirational. True humility demands that everyone is respected and loved, regardless of status. Together with meekness – another Christian aspiration – both now risk being classed as weakness.

Beauty

> *"It is amazing how complete is the delusion that beauty is goodness."*

> Leo Tolstoy. *The Kreutzer Sonata*, Chapter 5.

Beauty, vanity, and personal gain often come as a package deal. Beautiful people are rarely unaware of how their attractiveness is valued by others. Some use it to gain easy favour: marrying the leader of the pack; seducing others at will, easily gaining favours and recognition.

Beauty is a given – some would say, a divine gift. It is also a money-making, status procuring entity. It is used unashamedly by advertisers whose message is, 'if you want to be *this* beautiful . . . buy the following products'. To the beautiful are often given un-fought-for accolades. As a divine virtue, it can subsume other more lasting and valuable gifts like intelligence, wise judgement, honesty, reliability, and contentment. Beauty like intelligence, can make life easier; much less energy need be spent achieving goals.

Raphael depicted man as a uniformly handsome, powerful, and noble being; he beautified, even those with no actual claim to beauty. Rembrandt and Caravaggio depicted reality, and that forever changed art. Until a few decades ago, regional accents, were never heard on BBC radio or television. They were thought ugly, despite any beauty that might lie beneath. In adverts, we must tolerate a visual diet of hand-picked, ethnically balanced beauties, to whom few compare. Inner beauty might be thought more desirable, but only seldom by the vain. Beauty is the subliminal influencer that drives many to spend their money on vanity – on anything, in fact, that offers enhanced recognition. The vain, however, do possess an insight worth having. Talent and intelligence can be bought, but not so power and beauty.

Predictably, beautiful people mostly end up with matching, beautiful partners. Some will tolerate ugliness, but only in those with desirable future prospects, or those who are already rich and famous enough for their beauty to gain status. It is usually only the rich and famous who can bask in what lesser mortals, biased and in awe, will see as divine light.

Many have met one person in their life who seems to have everything – awesome good looks, brains, an athletic body, wealth, health, a beautiful spouse and gifted children. Surely, they must be happy? One only has to study the plight of many film stars, or famous titled people like Princess Diana of Wales, to understand the common falsity of such an assumption.

Vanity and Fantasy

The vanity business has a trillion-dollar turnover; many fickle followers of fashion and beauty, spending lots of their money and personal energy, trying their best to be noticed or look different. You name it, someone wants it: a bigger butt, a more expensive house, bigger breasts, a larger yacht or a rare expensive car. Multitudes want to look younger, be thinner, have muscles or become sleek. As a result, a massive industry has grown to fulfil such dreams. The service providers are cosmetic product manufacturers, cosmetic surgeons, personal trainers, beauticians, car salesmen, estate agents, ever-ready to help their customers fulfil their desires.

The inevitable has followed – once vanity became big business, the 'disappointment management industry', had to grow. As realisation dawns that we are not all as wealthy, beautiful or charismatic as we might want to be, upset, depression, and disappointment can manifest to consume our thinking time and energy. The providers of psychological services remain in the ascendant.

There are some, who find little else to do in life other than create a false image. Fantasy can be pleasurable in the short-term. Kept within bounds, fantasy serves as a harmless indulgence. Fairyland can brighten an otherwise humdrum life. Although not so much for the young and vital, the use of a mirror, can quickly dispel fantasy. To calmly accept what we see in a mirror, can take a lifetime of adjustment. The sooner we can achieve this acceptance, the happier many of us will be. Only through self-acceptance, can we acquire contentment. Lower energy expenditure is thus achieved. Maintaining a false image, on the other hand, will consume lots of subliminal energy.

Schooling should benefit us by cultivating objectivity – about oneself – and the world around us. This would lead not only to healthier individuals, but to healthier societies.

Apart from the many negative aspects of fantasy and vanity, fantasy does have an important part to play in our lives. It can embody hope, which nobody should have to live without. There would be much less richness to life, without those who are prepared to step beyond rigid objectivity. Man's first flight and first moon walk had first to be imagined. Thereafter, both depended on calculation, nous and a special aptitude to fly – something not all foresaw.

There may be no limits to fantasy, but for what we are required to do in everyday life, there are strict limits to the use of objectivity. Many have to decide each day, whether or not to jump into the unknown, without much supporting evidence or preparation.

With enough homework and a belief in what we are doing, we can improve our chances, but not with any certainty of outcome.

Work Ethic

The famous and super-rich have to be careful about their media exposure; so much falsity is projected on them. One projected view is that they no longer have to work. Successful people mostly work harder than others – it takes a lot more effort than many realise. I remember an interview, recorded with Elton John's partner in 1995. Elton emerges as a character who contradicts the popular projection of someone rich and famous – someone who can 'take it easy'. The fact is, maintaining his creative talent required constant work. His phenomenal record of success was not achieved by 'taking it easy'.

Most people have to work, so that one day, they too can 'take it easy'. Ideally, they will pursue a fulfilling and rewarding lifestyle at the same time. Self-esteem is one reward – gained from giving pleasure to others or from dutiful service – both more fulfilling than 'taking it easy'.

Sympathy and Antipathy

For those of a passionate nature, vast amounts of energy can be spent on love, hate, sympathy, antipathy, friendship or feud.

> "... pleasure asks a greater effort of the mind to support it than pain; and we turn, after a little idle dalliance, from what we love to what we hate."

> *On the Pleasures of Hating*

> William Hazlitt.

The Penguin Book of *Fights, Feuds and Heartfelt Hatreds* (Viking, 1992), provides numerous examples of how energy can be spent. As with money, spending energy can be pleasurable or distasteful; wasteful or worthwhile. The danger with hatred is that it is often unproductive. It lacks magnanimity, and only boosts the ego once the opponent is scarred. When the level of malevolence is low, apparent hatred can be witty and amusing and the basis of many comedy acts.

"Any man that hates dogs and babies, can't be all bad!"

W.C.Fields.

When the level of malevolence is high, instead of being humorous, it can lead to genocide. Examples in history abound. We need look no further than Hitler's hatred of Jews, and the conflict between Serbs and Croats, Catholics and Protestants. Of Catholics and Protestants in Northern Ireland, Jonathon Swift said:

"We have just enough religion to make us hate, not enough to make us love one another."

As cynicism increases with age and *joie de vivre* recedes, it is possible to find hate more enduring than love:

"Pure good soon grows insipid, wants variety and spirit. Pain is a bitter-sweet which never surfeits. Love turns, with a little indulgence, to indifference or disgust: hatred alone is immortal."

On the Pleasure of Hating. William Hazlitt.

The pleasures of loving and the love of giving, can scarcely be surpassed as a boost to well-being. When love happens, ego is shared selflessly with the loved one; energy spent not just on oneself, but also on the one we love. Little will boost our self-image and self-esteem more than recognising the good we find in ourselves. This will reduce our need to spend energy. Love of oneself, can smother us with pride, requiring us to spend lots of energy its maintenance.

Delegation and Resignation of Duty

It can be difficult to decline friendly requests – to attend another late-night party; to be present at an urgent meeting or take another phone call, especially when duty is involved.

I remember being telephoned at 4AM by a patient who complained she couldn't swallow! I wondered what it was she was trying to swallow, and why she had woken me to impart this vital news. Symptoms can provide key information which needs exploring, but this was unusual at 4AM!

Next day, I found her to be depressed. She was concerned about her son's imminent marriage to an unsuitable girlfriend (her opinion, not his). Her powerlessness was the root cause of her psychosomatic problems, not gullet cancer. Although those with early signs of cancer and heart disease can deny symptoms, those with less urgent psychosomatic symptoms will often want to share them at 4AM!

Discipline

To pursue discipline is to foster energy spending. The same question always lies hanging. Is the energy we spend going to be worthwhile?

In his book, *'The Road Less Travelled'*, M. Scott Peck, dedicates his work 'To my parents Elizabeth and David, whose discipline and love gave me the eyes to see grace'. He makes the point that discipline can fortify us to stand up to life and its problems.

Unlike some children who scream for immediate gratification, disciplined adults must take responsibility for their problems, before resolving them. This is one aspect of adulthood. The disciplined person will have learned from his parents (or their surrogates), that rewards usually have to be worked for, and taking responsibility is not always easy. In achieving gratifying solutions, he will have learned that patience, taking time, and applying deliberate resolve are often essential.

We live in an era of trust-fund kids; those with no need for discipline or wealth-producing activity. For them, self-esteem (other than showing off their wealth) can be hard to come by. They will need enough discipline to achieve worthwhile goals unrelated to wealth.

Some people working in an undisciplined system, will demonstrate random behaviour. This may be acceptable when there is no objective or deadline to meet, but a disaster when success or survival is at risk.

Without the disciplined action of all involved, it would be impossible to co-ordinate the actions of a submarine crew, or an army at war. Without discipline, pilots would fly where they fancied, not where they were needed. Without discipline, surgeons might depart from proven procedures. Without strict scientific method-ology, the work of experimenters would not result in reliable con-clusions. Without self-discipline, a patient who needs to alter his lifestyle from sedentary to active, or from resentful to contented, will usually fail. Without discipline, school kids will not study, learn, and go on to achieve academic success. Without applying discipline, parents will rear feral children – those who remain ig-norant of where acceptable social behaviour begins, and where it ends.

Disciplined behaviour improves the chances of survival. Without much imagination, many will be better off sticking to well tried and tested routines. Those who rigidly follow rules are not usually those capable of inventing or discovering new ones.

Discipline applies not only to individuals; it also applies to groups. It applies as much to the survival of nations and ethnic groups, as it does to individuals. Many have speculated about Jewish survival; for what Mark Twain called 'Jewish immortality'. The previous Chief Rabbi in Britain, Jonathan Sacks, suggested how Judaism sanctifies life:

> "... that Judaism is one of the most remarkable celebra-tions of life. Almost the whole of Jewish ritual consists in taking the simplest pleasures – eating, drinking, home, the family, study, debate, friendship and com-munity – and investing them with sanctity; making a blessing over life."

The Times. p11. 14.9.96.

He also suggested on recent social media, that fruitful argument and discussion, pervades all of Jewish teaching and practice, and allows for individuality as well as togetherness.

He mentions nothing of superior intelligence or intellectual ability; scientific, musical or business prowess, given that among Israeli Jews, there is a greater proportion of engineers, lawyers, doctors, and scientists than in any other nation. Jews have won more Nobel Prizes than any other nation (22% of all prize winners, from a group representing only 0.2% of the world population). Sacks does not mention discipline, yet maintaining Jewish dietary laws and many other rituals, requires it.

A highly disciplined way of life is also common to other religious sects, among them Moslems and Christian monks, nuns, the Amish and Mormons. The daily routine of prayer and observance can bring a nation together; thereafter, keeping them together. Both the oppression and rejection experienced by Jews and others, can motivate collective allegiance, although not always sufficient to guarantee survival.

Discipline can be obsessional. There is a compulsive element to it, that might reject alternatives. Obsessive characters are self-disciplined; they find comfort in their prescribed behaviour by finding something they are sure of. Their attention to detail, and their concern to check and re-check, can bring failure if too absorbed in irrelevant detail. They mostly spend vast amounts of energy achieving goals. The carefree and careless need not compare themselves to others, especially if they are gifted and talented enough to make their endeavours effortless.

The cleverest chap at my medical school had almost no need for routine study. He had a photographic memory, and no need to study a topic twice. He spent most of his time relating to others, playing chess and bridge. The rest of us had to stuff our brains, studying as hard as we could.

Norman Schwarzkopf, when discussing Hannibal on BBC Time-watch (1996-7), put the success of both ancient and modern warfare down to logistics: getting all the equipment and men in place

– all ready for action at the right time. That takes discipline. It also takes a determined, disciplined leader, an efficient organisation and a willing workforce.

An efficient machine produces results, using the smallest amount of energy. To be efficient, an organisation and its behaviour must be energy saving. Undisciplined, poorly thought through manoeuvres, waste time, money, and energy. In survival terms, every bit of energy counts. Discipline allows for the more efficient achievement of objectives. Would the Roman Empire, or the Industrial Revolution, have happened without it? Achieving weight loss, smoking cessation, and getting super-fit are associated with benefits – reduced morbidity and mortality. All take energy and self-discipline – and they are what most of us find difficult.

If one accepts that energy conservation principles are beneficial for individuals and organisations, both parents and schools should encourage disciplined behaviour. A lack of discipline fractionates productive behaviour and reduces the chance of personal success. Success, as we each define it, can lead to self-esteem and happiness. Success in the eyes of others, may not only feed our vanity, but also lead to benefits such as promotion and becoming well-known.

Schools need to review their attitude to what are now long despised, disciplined Victorian principles, like those that once promoted the rôte learning of multiplication tables and poetry. The knowledge itself may be of questionable use, but the ability and discipline required to accomplish them, is invaluable. The once appreciated party-pieces of Victorian and Edwardian society, like playing a piano piece, reciting a poem or a speech, gained them self-esteem and social merit. Soirée chanteuses and diseuses were once much applauded.

A lack of self-discipline lets down nobody but us. 'I'll give up smoking next week', I have heard many say. Next week – like mañana – never comes. By committing ourselves to a decision and sticking to it, we raise our integrity and self-esteem, especially with tough commitments. Surprisingly, small commitments can also be worthwhile and difficult to achieve, like being on time, not drinking alcohol for one week or eating no desserts for a while. Some are too used to replaying the 'poor little me' drama. The script reads: *'I'm a weak person. I have little self-control. I'll try not to eat desserts for a week, but I'll most likely fail. What does it matter anyway? I'm happy the way I am. Besides, if I get depressed, sweets and desserts make me feel happy ... etc, etc'.*

If an overweight person has a 'fat mentality', they will be defeated from the start. They will need to accept the drama and identify the implicit falsehoods and truths within their mind-talk script. They must look to the occasions when they were tough, rather than weak with themselves, yet won through. They may have to realise that it is only their mentality and inner voice that defeats them (see: *Who Loses Wins*, David H. Dighton. 2014).

We are all liable to bias, so in one sense, many of us have the equivalent of an Iago accompanying us throughout life. In Shakespeare's Othello, Iago plots to demean the honour of Othello's faithful wife, Desdemona. He does this by spreading false gossip, and even succeeds in convincing Othello that she is unfaithful. This leads him to murder her. Othello learned too late, the truth of Iago's treachery. For this reason, and before taking any action, we must all examine and cross question our every bias. The inner voice we all have, can be malign and try to defeat our efforts to find the truth. This voice will sometimes try its best to deny us a full understanding of why we behave as we do. The risk is that we will inflict pain on those we respect and love, as well as ourselves.

Integrity

If success and self-esteem, dignity and integrity, underlie our feelings of fulfilment, then a disciplined life that induces self-worth should be an essential feature of our education – a process that should be encouraged throughout life. Disciplined routines, verbal or physical, devotional or mundane, can all serve to make us feel successful and fulfilled. Our success will depend on being true to ourselves, and both honest and reliable with others. Personal integrity is thus easily defined.

The realisation of having little personal integrity, unable to keep even the smallest commitment, to oneself or others, will tarnish any positive self-image we had. The erosion of our integrity could make us feel worth less, and in some instances worthless. The possible outcomes are a loss of self-belief, giving up on our ambitions and struggles, and even suicide. Some will decide that it is just too late to change – to become somebody worth knowing. This process can take until middle-age to develop, so it is often called a mid-life crisis. Like all catastrophes that appear sudden, but take time to develop.

After the Second World War in the UK, some young men (a little older than me at the time), were conscripted to serve in the armed forces. Some went in as immature, unruly teenagers; some as 'teddy-boys' ('undisciplined, aggressive, racist louts', some said in the 1950s). I saw for myself how they appeared on discharge. They were proud of their uniform, proud of their army discipline, proud of a tradition they felt part of, and proud of having done their duty. Their subjugation to a traditional disciplined regime, was the source of their pride; they had become imbued with a dignified presence, in contrast to some of their contemporaries. They had learned respect for themselves and for others; they had learned to share, and to respect commands. They had come to understand *esprit de corps* and had lost their arrogant cynicism. Many years after, someone I questioned said they had not enjoyed the experience but recognised how beneficial it was for their maturation. Almost all agreed – military conscription or military service provided a self-improving influence on young men.

The British Public-school system avows similar principles – duty, discipline, and diligence in work, rest and play. It often succeeds by imbuing its pupils with self-worth.

Oscar Wilde, in ironic mood, made Lady Bracknell disagree.

> ". . . The whole theory of modern education is radically unsound. Fortunately, in England, at any rate, education produces no effect whatsoever. If it did, it would prove a serious danger to the upper classes, and probably lead to acts of violence in Grosvenor Square!"

Lady Bracknell. *The Importance of Being Ernest.*
Oscar Wilde.

The Importance of Being Ernest was first performed at the St James' Theatre, London, on the 14th February 1895. In that era, Lady Bracknell would have assumed adherence to duty, diligence, discipline, and respect for others, as the natural attributes of a gentleman. Since only the sons of gentleman went to public schools, they would have already been exposed to acceptable social behaviour. Hence the idea that public schools had no further influence.

If schooling to-day fails to grow personal discipline and integrity, the system should be changed as a matter of urgency. In 1895, as for to-day, any responsibility for self-discipline and respect for others, starts with parents. Undisciplined parents beget undisciplined children. Undisciplined parents and children can beget an undisciplined society. Undisciplined societies fail when they erode self-worth. The undisciplined behaviour of some football fans and political protestors is evidence enough of an eroding effect.

From my own observations, discipline and integrity now seem antiquated, unfashionable, passé and classist, and much less prevalent among the poor and ill-educated. Could they thus be linked to their higher morbidity and mortality (representing by the health divide).

Talent and Incompetence

Do people really rise within organisations, until they meet their level of incompetence (Peter's Principle)? Those with enough talent can get stuck with an inappropriate self-image or choose to stay put. Others will not enjoy the political cut and thrust needed to rise within an organisation.

There are a few young people perfectly capable of doing top jobs, who may never get the chance. It is a myth to think that top jobs are difficult – they are simply more suited to some than others – regardless of talent. This is not a well-kept secret. How can one possibly justify a six-figure annual salary for what is a part-time executive job! At the top, the workload can be quite small, although the responsibility for success and the consequences of failure are not for everyone.

In any position of authority, considerable help from a supporting team is usual. What leaders need is a clear vision of the mission, with the tenacity to see it through, rather than any of the skills necessary to achieve goals. When performance in high office does depend on accumulated experience, there is no substitute for age. For this reason, there is no logic in retiring people before 75-years-of-age. In the NHS, many of my colleagues were offered retirement at 55-years-of age, in a profession where experience is of paramount importance. I reluctantly retired aged 78-years. The cynical viewpoint, at least of medical bureaucracy, is that experience is just the excuse given for repeating the same old mistakes. Bureaucrats certainly know how to handle nonsense and use it to their advantage.

Talented people are everywhere; it is usually their lack of energy and commitment that prevents them becoming a success. Elton John's music teacher was apparently not amused to learn about his ambition. He saw himself as a future pop star, not as a music degree graduate.

Both need and passion can liberate energy. We all have energy, but only a few feel the need to liberate it. Talent is not essential for success. Many find success with oodles of energy and commitment, rather than talent.

Advertisers, PR consultants, and image builders can make anyone a fleeting star. To become an enduring star takes something more. Many pop bands are now constructed from good looking boys and girls, with little to offer other than a pretty face. With the voice-shaping software now available, even I can be made to have a pleasing voice! When individuality, musical dexterity, charisma, and energy combine, a unique talent is easily recognised.

Incompetence in all areas of life, accounts for inefficient and incorrect action, with costs that may not be accounted for until well after the event.

The historical record shows that incompetent behaviour in military matters can lead to dire consequences. In his book on military incompetence, Norman F. Dixon, points to meekness as a culprit. A commanding officer lacking self-assurance, can lose the lives of thousands of soldiers. In the face of adverse reconnaissance about an enemy, some commanders have sent their men into action with little or no chance of survival. Retrospective enquiry has found personal and political factors to be responsible. The reasons can be banal, like disagreeing with a fellow officer, or safeguarding personal property. Some of the most disastrous outcomes of battle, have been caused by trivial personal bias.

During the Second World War, Field Marshall Montgomery well knew before any action took place, that there were overwhelming numbers of German troops around the bridge at Arnhem. Preparations for Allied action were advanced, and the men well prepared. Unfortunately, Monty may have simply lost the heart to cancel the operation at the last minute. Known for his brilliant battle strategies, Montgomery on this occasion, became a slave to his whimsical feelings. He would have met with the Duke of Wellington's disapproval. To paraphrase him, 'Any fool can stand and be cut to pieces; it takes a great commander to know when to retreat'. 'Monty' was nevertheless, one of the greatest commanders. He later redeemed himself at the Battle of the Bulge in the Ardennes after Eisenhower handed control of the US Ninth and First Armies over to him.

"We are all too proud to surrender

and too humble to take the initiative."

Tessa Ransford. *Pity for Professionals.*

The Effect of Upbringing

Survival and success in life, depend on how efficiently we use our energy. Efficient use of energy depends on discipline. Could this explain the obvious success of British public-school boys, and that of some immigrants to Britain? In schools, the children of many Jewish and Asian families are diligent and disciplined enough to excel at academic work. Their application to school work is noticeable, and a source of their success in both business and the professions. In fact, wherever they have settled in the world, they usually achieve social and financial success. My guess is that their discipline and sense of duty are the major factors. Respect for their elders, and long hours of work, are characteristics these cultures share. Unfortunately, their success can instigate resentment among those who choose not to apply themselves, or those who have been spoiled – those with parents who believe their children deserve an easy life.

Can disciplined study be too rigid?

The wife of a Punjabi colleague of mine imposed rigid study discipline on her children. Every night she would insist they did extra study and would test their knowledge afterwards. Their two girls, already blessed with academic talent, became the top achievers at their private school.

Their proud father, a surgical colleague of mine, told me that his eldest daughter had been given a special commendation to become a medical student at Cambridge University. Both short and sweet, it read: 'She is the best pupil we have ever had!' For a public school, over one hundred years old, that was impressive.

Discipline and talent produced a girl who went on to gain the gold medal in medicine at Cambridge. Her father recently told me that her sister had proved to be cleverer! Worthy of a platinum medal perhaps!

Choice: Fantasy v Reality

Only by attaining that state of grace, born of self-knowledge and self-acceptance, can we face the processes of daily living with equanimity. Some must face relationship conflict, divorce and bereavement, others must face poverty, unattractiveness and poor achievement, and yet try to remain composed. Many use fantasy as a safety blanket, creating a honeymoon period, before reality strikes. Doctors, priests, and counsellors then find they have work to do. As often prescribed long ago by the Oracle at Delphi to those seeking advice – to gain comfort with reality requires self-knowledge and self-acceptance. This provides the only non-tenuous form of security, except perhaps for the rich, who can buy their way out of reality and maintain their fantasies.

Pursuing idealism is also part fantasy. It will remain so until we all evolve enough self-knowledge. Who would dare stop the majority believing that one day, they will be rich, famous, clever, or able to make a unique contribution. Fiction provides all the templates needed for vain hope. These hopes keep lots of us going, preventing us from becoming psychotic, neurotic or giving up on life. Unfortunately, few can cope with un-doctored reality. This assures a healthy financial future for fiction writers, and writers of self-help books. Doctors, priests, psychotherapists, and counsellors try their best to help many gain composure through self-realisation. With insecurity on the rise, few will go out of business.

Only those with pronounced inner security can afford to look on life with humour. To be able to laugh at the absurdity of the human predicament, allows for composure and personal energy efficiency. If only one can laugh at vanity, and the silliness of self-indulgent fantasy, one might view reality objectively. There will then be fewer let-downs, and fewer occasions needing correction. As a result, we will cope better. If we can laugh at our fantasies, enjoy them, live with them, but not take them too seriously, we can avoid their betrayal. Without this insight, many spend fortunes on face creams to help them look younger; buy vitamins to ward off disease, and spend fortunes on clothes to enhance their desirability. With no end to vain hope, a growing list of 'must-haves', drives every capitalist society.

After the death of a child, the futility of a life and its self-indulgence, will usually put reality sharply into view. Those so bereaved will want to know 'why', and how this could have happened. It sometimes takes such an emotive catastrophe, to prompt a quest for self-knowledge, and a better understanding of reality.

Who built Stonehenge and the pyramids? Was it mature adults or children? The building of pre-historic homes, Stonehenge, and the pyramids of Giza and Teotihuacán, must have employed many children. In those days, there would have been few people over the age of thirty-years. Early mortality from TB and other infectious diseases, would have assured a nation mostly composed of children and teenagers. Their living conditions must have created a sense of reality much sharper than ours. Perhaps their fantasies related to insuring their passage into an afterlife.

In the early 19th century, the realities of life and death could be stark and medieval. By the age of thirty, many would have experienced the death of both their parents and some siblings. For many young men, the patriotic hopes and aspirations they had to quickly win the First World War, were soon to be dashed after 1914. Standing in the trenches, going 'over the top', seeing their best friends extinguished while standing beside them, was to be the experience of one whole generation of young men. Shell-shock, now called post-traumatic shock disorder (PTSD), was then commonplace, but unrecognised. Many soldiers, found dazed and wandering away from the front line, were shot as deserters. Modern reality is different, although for the moment (2025), it remains the reality for many in the Middle East, Russia and the Ukraine.

Facing up to reality can be beneficial or detrimental; it depends on the individual. Images of crime, accidents and pornography, are now available to all, including children. Most people have no need to store such images in their brain, even if they are real. For many emergency workers, there is no escape. The average policeman, forensic specialist, and fireman must get used to seeing the details of road traffic accidents and crime scenes; horrors, unimagined by most. Although not generally available in the UK, such pictures are not banned in all countries. We are all 'better-off knowing the truth', is one cherished belief of those insensitive to the frailty of human emotion.

With the desire for open access information, and the cherished right to publish, much is available to impressionable minds. The debate about the advisability of access, will continue as long as free access to all information and common sense remain rivals.

Why frighten people unnecessarily, causing anguish and insomnia, amongst the more delicate. This is now a major source of unavoidable background energy expenditure. We all have the choice, however, never to look at another newspaper, watch television, or go to the cinema. We all have the choice to be an information scavenger, or to learn only on a need-to-know basis. Instead of blindly following the now fashionable access to information (which many label as 'progress'), the mental health of some can depend on how information is edited. Information gathering can be a displacement activity; it avoids us thinking for ourselves and considering our individual plight. There is fun to be had, however, finding out for oneself, thinking for oneself, and enjoying the discovery.

Fantasy staves off reality and can help us escape discomfort for a while. To fool us with fantasy can lead to trouble but can be expedient. It can lead to unrealistic thoughts and wrong judgements, but also provide some welcome relief from tragedy. Unnecessary energy expenditure, ill-health and disease, lie in wait for anyone indulging in misplaced fantasy.

Indulging in fantasy, can help form desirable images at the start of a new relationship. Relationships start with idealisation, and can later founder on the gradual disclosure of reality. This applies both to the amorous and those creating a business. Relationship experts suggest that one must hold back; never be too forward and maintain some mystery. 'Keep 'em wanting', said Mae West. 'Never chase', was James Bond's golden rule for cool dudes, trying to encourage women into his bed. The reason it works is simple. Given time, every interested partner will form a projected image – of the car you drive, your home, and your plans for your future (perhaps, together). All may be fair in love and war, but beware. While fantasy sweetens the carrot of seduction, the stick of disillusion can hurt. Ian Fleming cast his James Bond character never to chase, only to woo and ravish.

I once met someone, I strongly suspected was not as nice as she seemed. My assumption proved completely wrong. She was actually much nicer than I thought initially. Our projections and fantasies can be false and inadequate without evidence!

Fantasy is not limited to individuals; organisations also indulge. Dating, advertising, and estate agencies; jewellers, cosmetic and fashion houses, revel in the profit it produces. Advertising helps to justify fantasy. The more prestigious the organisation, the more prone we are to be biased in its favour. As one form of the halo bias, we may believe them to be altruistic and true, despite no corroborative research information. A top-of-the-range-car is still only a car; a mansion still only a house. Are these the most important possessions of a worthwhile person? My advice: follow the money, and always look beyond the sales pitch.

Delusion and fantasy are not the only domains visited by the man in the street, and those born gullible; they are also visited by the educated, intelligent and sophisticated. Politicians provide a good example. They produce well-meaning manifestos, replete with fantasy and delusion. It helps them win votes and retain power.

There are those who cannot afford the luxury of delusion and fantasy; among them are those living on the streets, with little hope of escape (something we and our politicians allow). In this version of reality, there is no place for illusion, although a little fantasy might help to keep them going. A lack of fantasy could withdraw any hope they might have of health or self-esteem. It could depreciate their resistance to infection and promote their demise from pneumonia or septicaemia.

Just occasionally prisoners escape. Papillon escaped and survived to live another life, despite the insuperable odds against him. A few have made their fantasies come true. Energy spent on survival is never wasted, even if indulgent fantasy is involved.

We need to pursue some interest in life, so why not follow the lead of others while trying to make a name for ourselves. One way is to make ourselves more attractive. Heeding the opinions and criticisms of those we respect, can be enlightening and helpful.

Energy is never wasted on enjoyment, unless it involves the type of delusion and fantasy that leads to trouble.

Many believe that some can predict the future. Being correct in the past, does not load the dice for correctly predicting the future. Those who believe it, have fallen for the 'hot hand' bias. Complicated situations that follow a blueprint, are predictable; complex ones like the stock market and weather, are much less so. To think otherwise is delusional. Delusions based on reputation can also be very costly. Any energy spent retaining and honing personal judgement and objectivity, is always energy well spent.

Scientists fight hard to avoid bias, and to prove their results are not just chance findings. Similar objectivity in choosing our bed-fellows is of no less importance, especially when the wrong choice of partner or business associate, can lead to financial ruin or abandonment. Wise judgement, resulting in the best choices, can lead to wonderment; the wrong decisions and choices, can lead to disaster. So, can we learn to judge wisely? Some say, it can't be taught.

Wise judgement is often a strong characteristic of survivors. Although not easily taught, it can be assimilated as an apprentice, working alongside an experienced, knowledgeable master. It also helps to be blessed with self-knowledge and awareness and be sensitive to self-delusion.

The topic of medical judgement and decision making is considered more in my book for inexperienced doctors, *The Art & Science of Medical Practice* (2024).

Warrior Virtues

Honour, duty, self-sacrifice, loyalty, honest endeavour, and excellence in combat, once marked the Arthurian Knight, fighting for just causes. In our imagination he was educated and wise, capable of moral and intellectual judgement that would outlast the test of time. Shouldn't these legendary chivalric values still inspire us today?

Over the course of my lifetime, these qualities have become steadily eroded, and independent judgement, virtue and honour, have been erased by government approved rules and regulations. Justice is now handled by the police, lawyers and law courts, more interested in group compliance than any cause. Yet individuals remain, who could benefit from the personal help of Sir Galahad, known for his gallantry and purity, acting altruistically in the name of honour, love and respect for others, while adhering to all the rules. One alternative would be to choose his father, and be guided by Sir Lancelot, with his more romantic view of life and disregard for convention.

Everyday opportunities arise for each of us to emulate a knight. Supporting a fellow pupil when bullied or harassed at school. Stepping in when a teacher is seen to be unfair to a fellow pupil. Helping an elderly person across a busy road; stopping to help someone injured in an accident: all minor acts of chivalry. Like the attributes of a true Christian, these knightly virtues belong to only a few. Those who are too busy, mindless, or too selfish to be involved, are focussed on their pursuit of wealth and acquisition. Do they not know what self-esteem they are missing?

Are we slowly becoming willing slaves to greed-driven capitalist desires, instead of having generous, chivalric aspirations? Might knights dispensing magnanimity and philanthropy return? I don't believe they ever disappeared, but they now lie imprisoned, chained up in forgotten castles by capitalist jailers who demand payment before releasing them. Altruism, and doing something for no financial gain, now seems to set a bad example.

There was once a mysterious stranger who offered two brothers a promise.

'Plant these seeds', he said, 'and for each of you, a small tree will grow. After your first good deed, a bank note for a large sum will grow on your tree. With the second good deed, two notes will grow, and so on. Finally, the whole tree will be replete with money.'

The older brother couldn't wait for his tree to grow and couldn't wait to do good deeds. The younger brother completely forgot his tree. As a result, his tree became tall and strong. After twenty or so deeds, the older brother stopped helping others, and started picking the money from his tree. After all, he had a business to run, taxes to pay, a big house to upkeep, and an expensive lifestyle to maintain. Then something unexpected happened. As he was counting the money, it all dissolved before his eyes. He was furious. He had been deceived. He was left with nothing more than his consuming greed and debts.

His younger brother, who did good deeds with no thought of reward, had forgotten his tree. Until, that is, he was asked to donate to charity. He told the charity he had no money but offered his tree instead. They wouldn't accept the tree; they only wanted cash, cheques or bank transfers. So, he kept the tree, and with the money travelled the world distributing his fortune to those in need.

With which brother do you identify?

Nowadays, the fields of battle are company board rooms and playing fields, rather than the jousting arena. Winning and gaining honour, is to be found mostly in sporting arenas or on battlefields. The noble aspirations reflected in the Arthurian legend, are now mostly a dream; remnants of noble characters belonging only to the few whose desire is still to achieve self-worth at no expense to others.

Parents now spoil their children to the point where discipline and self-discipline are disappearing. Achieving anything from hard work and endeavour, with the self-esteem that comes from it, might now seem unnecessary. With worthwhile pride in ourselves gone, only vanity will remain. Many are sadly reduced to having pride only in their possessions – their cars, the clothes they wear, and the houses they possess. Many are proud to be a club member; one among others who have accumulated similar artefacts. The possession of objects and money is now for many the only source of their personal dignity. Far less obvious are acts of chivalry. Those capable of them still exists but meeting one could be a rarity.

Human survival has always depended on selfishness, so those with the drive to survive comfortably, are not always those with noble virtues. Western society thrives on greed and selfishness, so noble virtues might now seem *passé*.

Frustrated Warriors

If abused by an aggressive telephone caller, we cannot smite him with a gauntlet, and challenge him to a dual. Those in business may find it better to be reasonable. In this way they might keep their customer and comply with regulations. Most will try to make the aggressor see sense, rather than directly challenge them. Frustration must be bottled-up or profits put at risk. Withholding verbal or other retribution, can deny us personal satisfaction. Unexpressed aggression can lead to internalised self-disappointment, with much energy used to rationalise it.

In the UK, perhaps the commonest source of frustration and aggression, arises on our roads.

*"The dangerous behaviour of other road users re-
mains a significant worry for UK drivers. A third
(29%) say the poor standard of other people's driving
is a top concern this year."*

*"The ongoing lack of funding for maintenance works
have served only to worsen the dire state of the UK's
local roads. It is no surprise, therefore, that this issue
remains by far the top concern of Britain's drivers.'"*

RAC Report on Motoring 2024

Occasional road rage and feelings of anger sometimes result. The commonest risk taken is reckless speeding, with avoiding capture being part of the thrill. Although such behaviour cannot be condoned, it is probably the result of being a frustrated warrior.

Aggression on the telephone or by text message, can save us from embarrassing personal confrontations, although, the wounds words can inflict will last however delivered. I have known couples whose relationship has broken down, become impersonal, and led to separation by text message. One telephone call or text message can end a relationship and destroy hopes – without compassion. In seconds, the hopes of a family can be destroyed, and might have to suffer without responding physically. Some are quick-witted enough to retaliate rapidly, instantly cleansing themselves of anger and resentment. The problem is, few of us can match the now legendary Groucho Marks or Oscar Wilde, or much heckled stand-up comedians, like Bob Monkhouse or Frank Skinner. For most of us, our thoughts will be *sur les escaliers* – retorts formed after the most opportune moment has passed.

Before the letter, telephone, or telegram, we had to meet our aggressors face-to-face. The outcome depended on the physical strength of the aggressor and the weapons they carried. Aggression can now be metered out anonymously, by corporate bodies using emails and WhatsApp messages. Our feelings, however, are anachronistic and primitive – remaining firmly pre-historic, with a suppressed need for physical aggression. The vestiges we are now left with are all impotent – frustration, anger and resentment – all with the potential to hurt us more than the aggressor.

Frustration and resentment will cause the outpouring of adrenaline, cortisone and energy, none of which is healthy. At times of extreme arousal, some hormones can promote blood clotting, with the potential to cause a heart attack or stroke. Whether or not they do, could depend on another inherited characteristic – whether the victim has 'furred' (atherosclerosis) or thinned arteries (see my book *Heart-Smart* or my textbook of Cardiology – *Essential Adult Cardiology*). If blood pressure becomes too high, brain arteries could burst – the cause of hemorrhagic stroke.

Anonymous communication is no longer limited to fictitious drama. Every day, death can be metered out over the telephone or by email, by those we accept as legitimate agencies, like tax officials and debt collectors. This is the western way of life, and because it is underwritten as socially acceptable, it is also the western way of death.

> *My patient John was involved in a long struggle to convince UK, VAT officials, he did not owe what they were demanding. His blood pressure had become uncontrollable and his angina no longer responded to medication. I wrote a letter, stating that should he die, the responsibility would be theirs. This was quickly followed by a telephone call from the head man at the*

VAT tax office. He asked, whether or not my letter was a joke. I confirmed that it was not and gave him much more detail. He was then gracious enough to drop the case against my patient. He asked whether it might be best for him to telephone my patient. I suggested it might be best for both of us to contact him. One month later, John's blood pressure had normalised on minimal treatment, and he seemed no longer to have angina.

In his book, the Gulag Archipelago, Aleksandr Solzhenitsyn relates how the former KGB in Russia, claimed they could kill anyone, without laying a hand on them! The physically adverse effects of interrogation are the military equivalent of what many suffer in everyday life, through money-grabbing, injustice, and hurtful behaviour. If we dump one lover for another, are we not guilty of a similar emotional crime? If a corporate organisation dispenses with our services, some will go on to commit suicide; some might have a heart attack; others might live their life with lifelong resentment and dejection. Given that anonymity is now acceptable, who will readily accept any moral responsibility after such events happen?

It took decades to find those responsible for the UK Post Office scandal, after many postmaster's lives had been ruined by the corporation. It also took ten years of anguish, to discover that Tom Hayes and Carlo Polombo, did not rig the Libor rates (2025) – that was done by others. The perpetrators were able to remain anonymous for years.

We are fast moving away from humane responsibility. Are we still responsible for one another? Can we get away with emotional crimes, only because in modern western society, only criminal acts are punished? Society allows us plenty of freedom to kill with words, but not once to kill with a knife.

Perhaps we should adapt both ourselves and society. Since our genes control our ability to adapt, our inheritance probably decides how much we can change. We cannot all achieve enlightenment, even with so many 'New Age' psychobabble sirens beckoning us.

A great deal depends on whether change suits our purpose. Some enjoy change and adaptation; others find any change disturbing. Marcus Aurelius, Emperor of Rome (AD 161 – 180), advocated getting used to change, for change he observed, was an essential fact of life and nature. The contemporary thinker M. Scott Peck agrees:

> *"The essence of life is change, a panoply of growth and decay. Elect life and growth, and you elect change and the prospect of death."*
>
> M.Scott Peck.
>
> *The Road Less Travelled. Chapter: The Risk of Loss.*

Neuroticism

Very few human beings are without any neurotic trait. Anxiety, perfectionism (obsessionality), phobia, hypochondriasis, depression and hysteria are those usually considered – all with high energy expenditure. Freud thought that neurotics constantly repeat things, seeming not to remember effectively. He thought them emotionally ineducable.

There is a paradox to be observed. Relaxed people can make others feel anxious.

I well remember waiting to board an airplane on the Greek island of Kephalonia. Having checked-in to the small airport, my friend and I returned to our hotel – conveniently overlooking the airport runway. It was only a few miles away, so we thought to drive back to the airport, only after watching our airplane arrive.

My friend Rod, a very relaxed physician, much enjoyed waiting; sipping his retsina by the pool. Being calm and composed, he decided to start driving back to the airport, only after seeing our fellow passengers snaking out of the departure terminal, walking towards the waiting airplane. Despite the fact that we had a fifteen-minute drive, he remained relaxed and unhurried, despite not allowing for any other exigencies – like a burst tyre, or his car failing to start. His argument: 'They can't depart without us! We've checked in!' The effect on even the calmest of his companions (me), was to induce anxiety – for several others, the reaction could best be described as:

' #### PANIC !!!!! '

Anxiety is a survival factor when it promotes appropriate vigilance and surveillance. It is detrimental when it limits awareness. Many human physiological systems are Goldilocks compliant – everything needs to be 'just right' – for optimum functioning. The rule is – not too much or too little. With no anxiety, we might roam the jungle, absent-mindedly at risk from predators. With the will to survive, a little anxiety could prompt some appropriate precautions.

Sometimes reconnaissance is impossible, and survival will be a matter of luck. The following light-hearted, facetious fable makes the point.

> *A sparrow was happily flying along when it met an icy wind. Its wings froze, and it fell to the ground like a stone. While lying semi-conscious, a cow happened to walk by and defaecated on it. The faecal heat defrosted the bird and brought it back to life. The bird, now happy again, wriggled free, and sang a cheerful song of delight. A local cat, hearing the song, pounced and ate the happy little bird!*

There are at least four morals to be drawn from this tale:

1. First, it is difficult to predict when ill-fate will strike. So, enjoy life while you can.

2. Second, not all those who s**t on you, are an enemy.

3. Third, those who haul you out of the mire, are not always friends, and

4. Fourth, when you are comfortable, even if up to your neck in s**t, keep quiet, and don't tempt providence!

Film: *'Assassins'*, with Sylvester Stallone and
Antonio Banderas.

The tendency to be anxious can be traced back through families and is most likely inherited. Depression and anxiety can result from the action of a brain neurotransmitter like serotonin, which after being released, is taken back into nerve cells. Anti-depressants, like fluoxetine (Prozac), work by inhibiting this re-uptake; a process known to be controlled by two genes on chromosome-17. The presence of one gene, lowers the levels of the protein which transports serotonin. Subjects who have this gene, are more anxious than those without it (Lesch, et al. 1996).

Obsessive people are driven to check and re-check all they do; often seeking perfection. If they could adequately remember, re-checking might not be necessary.

The fearful traveller needs constant reassurance of safety. Even though a passenger may have safely flown ten times before, they will remain anxious, regardless of their past experience. Statistics and logic are of little consequence. Many catastrophise irrationally, displacing knowledge and experience with an emotional response; assuming the worst with each airplane take-off: thanking God for allowing them to survive after landing safely. On any flight, one third of passengers are anxious, and another third are fearful. In 2024, twenty-five million Americans were found to fear flying (aerophobia or aviophobia)(See: Stratos Jets. 2024).

Other Energy Spending Traits

Will-power and persistence may be immeasurable, but we all know something about those who possess them. Those who have it, can overcome goals beyond any expectation; without it, many will give in to their weaknesses. It is critically linked to self-esteem.

When Ray Kroc (1902-1984) was asked how he expanded McDonald's® into a world-wide food outlet, he used one word – 'persistence'!

Aggressiveness and impatience; a sense of time urgency (Type-A personality); frustration, indignation and resentment, all spend energy regardless of need. Comfort in life, belongs only to those who spend the least amount of energy – at all times. Spend too much and we quickly tire; spend too little, and some will feel composed, but others will become withdrawn, apathetic or depressed. With some willingness, discipline, and an ability to change, only regulated energy spending equates to a healthy life. The ability to reduce unacceptable energy expenditure, can lead to the feeling of 'being at one' with life. For those who seem to have mastered it, contentment, self-esteem, and composure in life are common characteristics. They are usually free to do as they wish and only rarely are a slave to others.

> "In death, a free man loses the pleasure of life, a slave loses the pain."

> Film: *Spartacus (1966)*.

Sex and Gender on Mars and Venus

Unprecedented in thousands of years of cultural history, is the projection that men and women should now think and behave in the same way. This implies that the 'Y' chromosome, possessed only by males, has no potency. Only those ignorant of DNA, and its biological significance, can harbour this irrational view. They are perhaps more concerned to promote their assumed image, than their biology. As John Gray explained it, gender behavioural differences are better understood, once we accept the metaphor that 'men are from Mars and women are from Venus'.

> "Men mistakenly expect women to think, communicate, and react the way men do; women mistakenly

DR DAVID H. DIGHTON

expect men to feel, communicate, and respond the way women do. We have forgotten that men and women are supposed to be different. As a result, our relationships are filled with unnecessary friction and conflict.

Clearly recognising and respecting these differences dramatically reduces confusion when dealing with the opposite sex."

John Gray

Men are from Mars, Women are from Venus.

These behavioural differences top the list of major sources of aggravation for adults in relationships. Coexisting is perhaps the commonest cause of adult energy drain. For many men and women living together, considerable energy-consuming compromise is required to achieve any harmony. The different sets of views, values and aspirations, held many men and women, will reliably predict incompatibility. They matter little to the mating process (the biological, evolutionary prerogative) – it is driven more by lust and love than rationality. Among those who elect to live a single life, some will fear loneliness and emotional detachment.

Loners and Followers

Once we have reached adulthood, we are expected to have found our persona; no longer insecure, with others needed to direct us. Such a state of autonomy requires decision making and coping, and a higher energy-spending state. Individuality of purpose characterises loners, mavericks, the self-employed, and the independent-minded.

Working with those more able and energetic than oneself, can motivate learning and achievement. I remember once playing the guitar in an amateur music group. We were once joined by some career professionals. The effect on us was memorable. They raised our playing to new heights. Similarly, an average child at school, will often benefit from having a brighter, more able friend. The bright chap will also benefit from the reiteration of knowledge needed to teach his less able friend.

Henri Charrière wrote his novel 'Papillon' in 1969. It was the memoir of his incarceration on Devil's Island, a penal colony in French Guyana. Although the island was virtually inescapable, he worked relentlessly to keep fit, aiming not to surrender to his circumstances. He designed his escape, while remaining subdued. His fellow inmates were mostly resigned to death, as their only escape. He was different. He had the energy of an innocent. The injustice he felt, spurned him on, and gave him spirit enough to fight for a redress.

By enthusing others, inspiring others, leading and encouraging them to gain self-esteem, there are those capable of energising their compatriots. With every act of kindness, one person donates energy to another. There is no proof for the transfer of 'psychic energy' between people, but little doubt that mutual benefit occurs (probably boosting brain serotonin levels). The effect is real enough.

If mind-reading, telepathy, or extra-sensory perception existed, some form of energy transfer would have to occur between people. Critical proof, like that for the existence of extra-terrestrial aliens is eagerly awaited, but that responsibility must rest with the believers. Few scientists would waste their time on such contentions; a few might treat them with sceptical open-mindedness.

Some Views of Personal Energy

I have learned a lot about personal energy from patients. Here are some of their comments:

"Try being out of work for two years, with no money to spend and nothing much to live for. How energetic would you feel?"

"I don't believe in rushing around. I'm happy with a quiet existence. I own my own house. I'm comfortable. At my age, I deserve to take it easy."

"I think I'm wasting my life if all I do is sit, read or watch TV. There's more to life. I play hard and work hard. I like achieving things – things which give me self-esteem. I'll never be out of work. I'd start another business, mow lawns, or emigrate. I wouldn't care what I did."

"I don't believe in spending energy when I can pay others to spend theirs. Delegation, that's the thing. I owe my success to it. With WhatsApp and e-mail, who needs to go to work?"

Birth Order

We cannot change it, but does birth order matter? In general, first-born children are given the freedom to explore their interests; the second-born, must develop in the shadow of the first, and are sometimes demeaned by the experience. The last-born might become the most capable, devious or rebellious, having had to avoid or withstand the behaviour of their older siblings.

The first-born is often more anxious than the others. Some, fearing displacement, may have to fight to keep their number one spot. The second born, are usually more relaxed and amenable, having long adapted to secondment. The second born can, however, feel the need to seek attention by exhibiting eccentric, rebellious, or irreverent behaviour – especially if they found it difficult to accept subordination.

These considerations while fixed and too general, might help to understand others. The behaviour we each display will mostly depend on our own innate personality, but noting parental and family group dynamics, can source valuable insights.

Family dynamics from early on in life, will often affect the mental health of adults. Many come to portray a mask or projected personality, rather than their genuine nature. I suspect that any face behind a mask, is moulded more than we like to admit, by early family influences.

Love

For those with a passionate nature, vast amounts of energy can be spent on love and hate, sympathy and antipathy, friendship and feud.

There is well-being to be had from the pleasures of loving and the love of giving. Little else can boost self-image and self-esteem more than recognising the good we possess. Unfortunately, if narcissistic, we can drown in pride.

Love happens, once our ego is selflessly shared with another. Our energy will then be spent on two people. The pleasure of giving and receiving is perceived to release our energy.

Once a baby is born, most mothers will bond with them and envelop them in love. Loving mothers accept the dependence. All their baby demands is a nipple or teat to feed on, regardless of time or place. Fatigue and exhaustion are common outcomes for mothers whose sleep gets disturbed and fractionated, diminishing the sleep-refreshing process. The welfare of their helpless infant sustains their sacrifice. The loss of calories in breast milk adds further to their energy loss.

Long ago, it was common for mothers to feed their children until they could walk – they would have teeth by then! This exhausting practice seriously debilitated them and reduced their resistance to infection, sometimes with fatal consequences. Some faced death in the name of unconditional love.

Many mothers are anxious about what to expect with their first child. This often dissipates with the second. Better education and the presence of an attentive, knowledgeable aunt or grandmother, will help to allay their concern. Delegation of the child to the father, a grandmother, nanny or friend, may be essential if the mother is to survive healthily. Organising the necessary support prior to birth, should allay anxiety. (Read Carol Hart's book for more details).

Self-Worth

Self-worth has many sources – after having made a worthy contribution to life or simply from realising one's personal expectations. This does not have to involve paradigm shifting research, winning a Nobel Prize or gaining a knighthood. For most of us, simply helping others, completing an assignment, bringing up a family or walking across the room for the first time after an accident or stroke, will suffice. For those with hard-earned skills, it can come from their efficient and successful use.

Both satisfaction and dissatisfaction can come from earning money. Unfortunately, there is little justice to be had here; those who contribute most to society, often earn least. Some top executives earn more in one year than a fireman will earn in a lifetime. I once paid more for curtains than I was paid for saving a life. What makes such ridiculousness bearable, is that saving lives can never be measured using any monetary currency. Instead, we will have to rely on kudos and improved self-worth. However, such worth has no value at the supermarket check-out!

There is much perversity to human thinking. For instance, the skill to save a life holds infinite value minutes before a life-saving act but is of little value the moment directly after! Since most of us are now too self-centred and disinterested to care, few will spend their energy agitating about social issues.

Western society preferentially rewards entrepreneurs, rather than the skilled and highly educated. For some, these differentials are a source of anger and resentment. Many who take their teachers' advice and pursue higher education, are likely to find eventually, their lives ruled by business people with more money and less education. Teachers meanwhile, are being paid less than both the labourers who build schools, and the many pupils who spurned their advice.

One can only ignore social differentials by turning a blind eye to merit. Western societies mostly remain stable, except for a few political activists and dissidents, with no realistic hope of removing the greed for power many seek over others. For as long as stark capitalist differentials exist, there will be an undercurrent of dissatisfaction among those without the power to change it. The health divide will persist because much less personal energy needs to be spent by the fortunate.

The health divide is not the responsibility of any health service. Doctors and nurses are powerless to deal with it – an inability matched by a general public too busy trying to live and get rich, to think about the actual basis for their discontent and dis-ease. Many will protest, by suggesting that, 'someone should do something about the way things are.' But, who?

Politicians are mostly impotent when trying to tackle the underly-ing structural defects of society – on which all citizens must spend their energy. Politicians are bureaucratic tinkerers; dependent on a public majority to keep them in power. The public must be allowed their greed, and to vote for the party promising them the most – lower taxes, cheaper beer, petrol at low prices and affordable cigarettes.

All empires and economic systems have their day, with political situations swinging between good and bad times; public content and discontent. Caught in a time trap of varying longevity, most will not live long enough to see much change in the quality of their daily life – change is often that slow.

The smart way to cope with modern western society, is to accept it, and make maximum use if it. Otherwise, one might think of moving away from it. As a winner, one could move to an island of peace or retire to the countryside. As a loser, one might be destined for the isolation of a prison cell or the anonymity of a cardboard box on a city street. To stay and work for the system, and battle against it, is to spend more energy on maintaining and improving your situation, than on your health.

When the majority become dissatisfied, either war or revolution can be expected. We risk catastrophe – one small move, leading to sudden change. The fall of the Berlin Wall, and the end of the Russian Communist State, were examples. Being involved, could result in unbeatable camaraderie, honour in victory, or the desolation of defeat. After every storm (during which vast amounts of energy will be discharged), there will usually be calm (necessary for equilibration). What follows socially is also inevitable. There is a need to resurrect comfortable living conditions involving the enthusiastic spending of personal energy.

Some seek a life of peace and solitude in a monastery or academic institution. The pious devotion to prayer, study, and research, is a minority pursuit. For the religious, however, the devotional life is less an escape, than a duty to their God. The mores of society at large are then rejected in favour of a more disciplined set of rules and duties. To some, these would be more onerous than any adherence to common law.

The monastic life is an introspective one, aspiring to strict Christian ideals. They are not the same as freedom from the neurotic ego (nirvana) sought by Buddhists. Such a life is almost totally predictable (being strictly timetabled), is minimally stressed (with few external demands), and requires minimal individual energy expenditure. This is perhaps the healthiest, most energy efficient, state of human existence. It is as far from the western way of life (and death) as one can get.

Several studies available show that monks and nuns live longer than average. I am surprised by this, given that individual genetic predisposition is thought more predictive of medical outcomes, than living circumstances. Could pre-selection be at work, or might it arise from fasting, meditation, or the absence of everyday stress? Could it be ascribed to the possession of a religious faith? These questions have yet to be answered (see Michel Poulain, 2012).

Key Human Energy Spending Factors

In summary, individual energy spending depends most on the following factors:

1. **Personality:** People are either high or low energy spenders from birth, the assumption being that personality is largely inherited and mostly unalterable. The egoist and extravert can spend more energy on any given task, than any unassuming introvert.

2. **Neuroticism.** Anxious and obsessive people spend lots more energy than others; the calm and indolent spends less.

3. **Behaviour**. Although partly inherited, behaviour can be modified by life circumstances. The *modus operandi* of rushing around, taking less and less time to achieve more and more (Type-A behaviour), spends excessive amounts of mental and physical energy.

4. **Circumstances.** Our past regrets and resentments, may never go away. They can steadily eat away at our composure, burning energy while carrying all the heavy burdens of our past. Many conflicts and struggles arise from relationships, our social interactions and environment, often arising between those of different background, social class and education. Life changes must be coped with, adding to the tally of our everyday energy expenditure. Why do people continue to live with conflict? The usual reason is, it can be too disruptive and expensive to change. Marital separation and moving to a new house, can prevent further contact between established friends, in-laws and acquaintances – all too painful to contemplate. As you will read in the next chapter, stresses arising from our immediate circumstances are almost always dealt with using reflex, fast reactions. More sinister, are the long-term problems, hanging over us like a dark cloud. They require slow thinking.

5. **Attitudes, Beliefs and Convictions.** Passion and commitment spend energy, achieving both the worthwhile and the pointless. Much depends on the strength of our attitudes and conviction, and a lot depends on our ability to delegate.

6. **Abilities, Intelligence and Aptitude.** Are you suited to your situation? Are you being over-used or under-used? Are you a good communicator? Are you knowledgeable, able, and intelligent enough to have an easy time at work and in social settings? These will all help to decide how much energy you need to spend on life.

CHAPTER NINE

Foreground Stress: Transient Transactions

Foreground challenges are those we deal with, minute by minute every day. They need no pondering or deliberation and are processed fast. They differ from background issues, which need some deliberation and slow processing.

The Natural Life

The original reason for improved mental activity must have been to enable survival. For six to seven million years, several pre-historic variant species of the genus Homo (man) – Homo Habilis, Erectus, Heidelberg, and Neanderthalensis – learned to negotiate the perils existing in their lives. As they did, their brains (the cerebral cortex) grew larger. Without the ability to learn, imagine and use forethought, they would have quickly perished. They had to learn quickly how to react successfully to danger and potential risk. A heightened sense of awareness would have been essential. Overcoming immediate dangers needed fast responses. The same still applies today – each day we are all required to respond with many fast responses. Alongside these, we have learned to design our living conditions to reduce future risks and danger. So far,

Homo sapiens (the wise or astute man) is succeeding, but with much need for further development.

Surveillance and Action

Awareness is a constant survival requirement, as are the immediate judgements needed to define our safety at any point in time. Those standing on a cliff edge might pull back to safer ground, without any conscious thought. Each day we will all make many instinctive survival moves. With a bus or train moving around a lot, one must quickly find a hand-hold. This differs from having to jump a gap. We must first know our athletic prowess, then estimate the gap, then decide how likely we are to jump safely across. This requires slow, not fast thinking. When walking in a crowd, we must instantaneously navigate other people, avoiding them as much as possible. Most of these judgments and decisions are on auto-pilot; once discovered or pointed out, we can avoid danger, and proceed safely. All these thoughts and moves consume energy, even when automatic.

Travelling to work and working in an office, requires hundreds of small decisions to be made every day. Living quietly in the country, and staying put, will spend less. None of this energy is accountable, yet none is avoidable. Depending on the number of transient reactions we take, and the number and significance of the issues we are pondering, we all get to the end of each day, more or less tired from the summed energy we have spent.

Added to the many automatic responses we make, are many small, almost inconsequential decisions – like choosing food from a menu or choosing which cake to buy. In the early days of car manufacture (specifically the Model T: 1919 – 1925), Henry Ford made the decision-making process easier. He told his customers they could have any colour car they liked – as long as it was black!

Being faced by a large menu in a restaurant can be irksome. The Marx Brothers had a solution. When they arrived at a restaurant as a family group, they simply asked for 'one of everything and a cup of tea'! A notable energy saving stratagem.

I have often found modern saloon car driving to be relaxing. Driving a demanding sports car, on the other hand, can be energy sapping. Keeping within the correct lane; keeping an appropriate distance from other cars, and adhering to speed limits, all demand rapid processing energy. On the long drive from London to the South of France, my son and I took turns to drive my Porsche Carrera 911. Although exhilarating and enjoyable, it took much more energy to drive than a grand tourer. Heightened awareness, and a greater number of fast decisions, will drain a driver's energy. When already tired, concentration will be affected, and driving is made dangerous. Add adverse road conditions, like fog and heavy rain, requires even more focus. The advice to stop frequently for rests, is an essential safety measure.

The more experience of driving or dealing with repetitive tasks one has, the more automatic and energy saving they should become.

The instantaneous responses we might experience throughout any day, range from the enjoyable to the alarming. Glimpsing something beautiful or seeing an unexpected goal scored during a football match are the enjoyable sort; responding to a sudden disagreement or suddenly experiencing dangerous driving, are of the alarming sort. None requiring pondering (although that may follow once we later think more about it); at the time, each will drain a small packet of our energy.

Conditioning

Many of our in-built, automatic responses and reflexes, alter with experience or conditioning. Having once vomited on a cruise, some will later react similarly to the slightest movement on a boat trip. Even the sight of a ship might incite their nausea. Such highly reactive states result from conditioned reflexes. Desensitisation, and freedom from such symptoms, can be achieved by exposing subjects to graded stimuli, culminating in the real thing. Highly adaptive people may only need one adverse exposure for them to change and gain benefit.

Our immediate response to aggression and abuse, and our response to compliments and adoration, have their part to play in our quality of life. They might make one's life a misery or be the source of growth and self-esteem. Learning to deal with them can be taught at an intellectual level, but that may not alter our emotional responses.

Happiness as a Modifier

A normally happy person will react differently if miserable – one of the effects of those dark decision clouds or dilemmas, hanging over a person, causing insecurity, and requiring lots of pondering. Being in a good mood minimises energy expenditure. When in a bad mood many become irritable and overreact unnecessarily. Those who keep their emotions under control, tend to make better decisions (Gu-Seo, Myeong 2008). Those easily swayed by their good or bad mood, may react erratically and be inconsistent decision makers. This can lead to unforeseen stresses in what follows. They could be 'cruising for a bruising' or 'brewing up trouble'. Their immediate reactions can be unpredictable. Those in a good mood are more likely to react calmly.

With training, some may be able to reduce or remove unwanted conditioned reflexes. We cannot much alter our propensity to change – as part of our genetic constitution, but we can modify the degree of change. Unfortunately, such modifications may only be transient. Most people do well initially having read an instruction book on relaxation, but then quickly revert once exposed to trauma. Diets can be maintained, but for many, it may only be temporary. This is because few understand their 'Fat Mentality' (see my book: *Who Loses Wins*). Many people get inspired to 'get fit', but few maintain it for long. Giving up smoking is possible, but how many eventually revert back to the habit? Changing our immediate responses to the sight of food or others smoking, is far from easy.

Reactiveness

Our bodily systems need to react in order to maintain our internal physiological and chemical stability (homeostasis), but sometimes these reactions are harmful. Blood pressure for instance, can change quickly without us knowing it. The frustration of waiting in a queue is enough for some to raise their blood pressure. For others, just the sight of a queue will do it.

Our inheritance should predict how we react and in which direction. This is obvious to any doctor who has seen patients react in different ways to the same life change. Some become irritable and aggressive; some respond with high or low blood pressure (as a cause of fainting). For some it might explain their raised blood cholesterol or erratic pulse. Our personality and conditioning help to determine how we will react.

Reactiveness can be over-the-top, the aim being to keep our ego in place at all costs.

As a result:

"The mass of men lead lives of quiet desperation."

Henry D.Thoreau

Some distinctive differences in response might have impacted evolution. In evolutionary terms, small differences can sometimes determine survival. Some factors are adaptable, like our behaviour; others like gender and age are not. Some are partially adaptable, like our ability to sense danger, intelligence, and our ability to run and jump.

Fear

Fear will commonly incite a spontaneous reaction. Sensing fear and responding to it immediately, are hard-wired into our being, for evolutionary survival reasons.

> *"I'm afraid of being alone. I'm afraid of not being alone. I'm afraid of what I am, and I'm afraid of what I'm not. I'm afraid of what I will become, and I'm afraid of what I might not become."*

This is how Frankie (Michelle Pfeiffer), expresses her fear to Johnny (Al Pacino), in the film 'Frankie and Johnny' (1991). The female character Frankie reveals to Johnny, how she had been abused by a former lover. She can no longer have children. She lost a child after being irrevocably damaged during pregnancy.

Such is the long-term, inhibiting nature of fear. One can lose self-respect, and no longer know what it is we need or want – afraid of being afraid; not knowing what to do for the best. Afraid to do anything, in case abuse returns. Difficult to explain, spontaneous responses can arise.

What many fear most is being judged. If they knew themselves well enough, perhaps they wouldn't fear it.

Immediate Responses to Stress

Depending on the stimulus, we can be suddenly overcome by a wave of fear, aggression, panic or delight. Adrenaline will sometimes flood out of our nerve endings and into our circulation, causing our hands to tremble and our heart to palpitate. In our brains, neurotransmitter can flow instantaneously, inciting in us, a myriad of possible feelings. All this drains energy, and there is not much we can do about it in the short-term.

Although William Harvey (1578-1657) published his discovery of the human circulation of blood (published in his famous treatise, *de Motu Cordis*, 1628), he was left pondering how and why the human heart responds as it does to emotion. He failed to find out. The automatic (autonomic) nervous system that partly controls heart rate, had yet to be discovered. This would have to wait for John Langely (1852-1925) to describe it in 1898, 270-years later.

Harvey wrote: *'the heart of all creatures is the foundation of their life, the Prince of all their parts, that on which all growth depends and from whence all strength and vigour flows.'* Although this sense of 'vigour' comes from the brain, it is the delivery of oxygen and glucose by the heart and circulation that makes vigour possible.

Exercise is a stress, and emotion is a response to a thought, feeling, another person or a situation. Both can raise our pulse rate and blood pressure. There are a number of physiological mechanisms involved, one of which includes the synthesis of hormones like adrenaline and nor-adrenaline in nerve fibres. For those with un-comfortable, fast heart rhythms (tachycardias), avoiding immediate stress can sometimes help. For those prone to high blood pressure, avoiding long-term stress can help with stroke prevention.

While working at Charing Cross Hospital, London in the 1970's, I decided to undertake a simple experiment. I wanted to find out how aroused, anxious, and worried people, responded to an adrenaline-like substance, isoprenaline. I gave it intravenously in very small doses (5 micrograms) (five millionths of a gram) and recorded the heart rate changes that followed.

Some of my patients were subsequently sedated, and I then repeated the experiment. To my surprise, I found their heart rate responses were much less. I concluded that the body has control of responsiveness; one that determines how the heart will respond to adrenaline-like chemicals. Obviously, anxiety or arousal is a factor. But how else might the heart's responsiveness connect to patients' state of mind? This returned me to William Harvey's question.

The heart of an anxious, unrelaxed person speeded to twice the rate seen before, with an acceleration that was five times greater. The same person, when relaxed, composed, and untroubled, was much less sensitive to the adrenaline-like substance I gave them. The automatic (autonomic) sympathetic nervous system which is activated by anxiety is most likely responsible for the phenomenon. It might explain why some anxious people suffer from palpitation, and why palpitations are sporadic – occurring mostly at times when patients are stressed (and adrenaline-sensitive).

These heart responses may run parallel to behavioural ones – how we respond to bad driving or the immediate awe of beauty. The amount of adrenaline and other hormones we produce is likely to be proportional to amount of energy we consume while responding.

Communication

Communicating spontaneously with people requires no previous pondering. Much of the energy we spend on immediate responses, occurs during verbal communication.

You are in a foreign land and are asked a question by a passer-by. Have you ever tried to make yourself understood by someone who cannot speak your language? The frustration of trying to communicate can depend on how serious the need is. An iPhone and translator earpiece can now help, although learning another language has many advantages – there being more to communication than words. Instantaneous translation is with us, except perhaps for speaking to experts and nerds – their speech is often replete with obscure acronyms and jargon.

When translating between languages, there are many problems with meaning. The actual meaning of a phrase in one language and culture, may not be understood similarly in another; there will often be interfering contextual and cultural factors. Take the word 'NO', for instance. In some languages it is an absolute; under no circumstances does it mean 'YES'. In other languages it can mean 'MAYBE' and is used as an opening gambit for further negotiation.

Considerable amounts of energy are spent achieving correct understanding. It is troublesome that one may not be able to verify whether both parties have achieved the same understanding. Resorting to drawings diagrams and pictures, shoulder shrugging, grimacing, anger, frustration, and a little laughter, can all help. Facial gestures, hand movements, and complex behaviour patterns (and the motives behind them), are there to be immediately interpreted, understood or misinterpreted, within their cultural and social context. More subtle, non-verbal aspects of communication – facial micro-behaviour, for instance – can aid understanding. Subtle facial changes in expression and eye-movements, are always important to note.

Those who have tried to learn another language, soon realise that there are important cultural aspects to learn. What to say, what not to say, and when. How to address others acceptably. These are not small matters. No language can be fully assimilated without an understanding of its associated values and attitudes – something of its distinctive essence. Some nationals are more forgiving of mistakes than others. The French are stricter about correctness than Italians, but as the language learning master Michel Thomas once opined, who would want to speak to anyone who is unforgiving about a student's language errors, especially if they are trying their best.

Detecting shyness, embarrassment, anxiety and apprehension, and compensating for it, are major features of communication expertise. They help interpret the responses of others.

The pressure to communicate with gregarious people, can spend lots of energy, especially when arguments arise from misunderstanding and inadequate communication. To communicate effectively, clarity and conciseness are key – saying only what you mean and meaning only what you say. Effective communication relies on choosing words, terms, and concepts, understandable to both parties. Respect for educational level, social status, intelligence, and cultural difference, are all essential.

When any matter is contentious, an understanding of one another's psychological position is invaluable. As Charlie Munger once said: 'know your opponent's arguments better than they do.'

Some find it difficult to step outside their gender, family, and national context, and communicate with others effectively. There was a time when doctors never moderated their language for those with a limited vocabulary. That is no longer acceptable, even though some doctors continue to explain medical conditions to patients in terms that are too technical and unlikely to be understood. I am equally mystified by patients who say they understand, when they don't. There are patients unable to understand, and others who refuse to understand.

Six decades ago, many patients saw no need to understand, simply because they had complete trust in doctors. Poor communication partly persists and contributes to the current state of patient dissatisfaction and distrust of the medical profession.

Personal Biases

Our immediate reactions can be biased, but not always to the same extent as those in play when we have to consider our long term, background situations (next chapter) using slow thinking (see Kahneman. 2011)). Every list of the biases we might be subject to, will be long. I have compiled my own. See Appendix 1.

I have witnessed many reactions to fame. With a famous person in my waiting room, some will react in a predictable way. They might be overcome with awe; stunned, mumbling and unable to speak coherently. Fame can do it – the 'halo bias' at work. Some will go on to demean themselves in the presence of greatness, offering to do anything the hallowed person might desire.

Small, personal and impersonal transactions, all consume our energy. They are all part of life, and mostly unavoidable, but the accumulative effect the can have on our health is unknown. Every human, and every animal must live with them, so whatever effect they have, we must learn to live with them. Reacting less actively and conserving energy is likely to have health benefits, but that probably means we will lead a restrained life, rather than one full of excitement.

CHAPTER TEN

Background Stresses: Life Problems and their Resolution

We all have background stresses, some hanging over us like slow moving clouds. There will always be situations and relationships that need resolution, with no immediate solution in sight. Many problems need to be pondered at length; considered from every angle; researched for what might be best to do. The process of dealing with background stress will often need a lot of slow thinking (see, Kahneman, 2011), with some thoughts easily influenced by our biases.

These are the situations that keep us up at night, disturb our sleep, and cause us to be fatigued the next day. If we get tired enough, our decision-making ability will slowly deteriorate and become defective, sometimes resulting in a state of suspended indecision and ineffectiveness. We may not be able to concentrate and will seem distracted – our mind seeming to be elsewhere. Our executive functioning – getting our self together and being able to co-ordinate our actions – could suffer. Without insight, some will say, 'I don't know what's happening to me. I'm not my usual self.'

In turn, this situation can lead to even more perturbed sleep, and even greater levels of tiredness and daytime fatigue. When the situation is potentially life changing, like losing a job or the break-up of a special relationship, it can lead to exhaustion. Exhaustion can then lead to mental breakdown (unable to cope or think normally) or to physical illness in those old enough and predisposed to suffer them (heart attacks, glandular fever, post-operative infection, strokes, etc.).

If we choose to spend our energy on an exhilarating life, we will need to refresh ourselves constantly. Failure to replenish our energy will lead to tiredness and chronic fatigue. Some have referred to this as 'burning the candle at both ends', risking 'burn-out' or getting a 'flat battery'. Alternatively, we might choose a subdued life, enjoying composure and contentment while spending little energy.

> *Goldie Hawn, a notable film actress, appeared long ago in Rowan and Martin's Laugh-in (1968-1973). She demonstrated her supposed life, by holding up a candle lit at both ends. She then said, "See Mum, I can do it!"*

> *I bumped into her, walking through the same door in a famous London restaurant. I regret not having the courage to tell her how much I enjoyed the scene she once played – given how relevant it had become to my thoughts on energy spending.*

Personal Biases

Long-term considerations using slow thinking are subject to many biases. See Appendix 1 for a list. Arguments which expose these biases, can cause emotional outbursts. If we know our self well enough (and few do) we should be fully aware of our biases, delusions and self-deceptions. Such self-mastery engenders respect from others and can create favourable conditions for the resolution of disagreements. When negative, biases might take the form: 'I'm no good; ugly and useless. Nobody would dream of marrying me, employing me or taking a second look at me.' When positive, our biases can seem boastful, egocentric, selfish and contemptuous. The boxer Mohammed Ali used to say: "I *AM* the greatest!", but he was not exaggerating – as a boxer, he was!

Many accept their biases and self-deceits and feel comfortable with them. This serves to boost their ego and self-esteem. Old soldiers and fisherman all have impressive stories to tell. The powerful, the revered and famous, can bring our biases to the forefront. Many tend to credit them gratuitously with exaggerated attributes – intelligence, knowledge, and charisma, as examples of the halo bias. They might then fantasise and exaggerate their significance. 'What a privilege!' they might say. 'They took time out (of their precious time) just to speak to . . . ME!' The reflected glory coming from the attention, may justify being blinded by the light of a dazzling halo.

Parents can have a crucial effect on the development of biases. Some parents consistently destroy the chance of their children gaining self-esteem. How many young children have been told they are 'useless', 'no good', 'a no-hoper' – in short, a failure. The alternative is to extol their merits and virtues, in a loving and appreciative way. For a practical guide to how parents can preserve, maintain, and boost self-identity and self-esteem in their children, see Adele Faber and Elaine Mazlish's book: *'How to Talk So Kids Will Listen, and Listen So Kids Will Talk'* (Avon, 1980).

Conditioning

Competence in handling situations can relate to how we choose to use our energy. If we are shy and fearful of meeting others or take endless steps to avoid confrontation, we might be spending energy unnecessarily. Some adaptation and conditioning could be of benefit. By exposing ourselves to people from all walks of life, with many and various attitudes, presumptions, and patterns of behaviour, we might better conserve our energy and live more comfortably. The more we protect individuals from society (common among the educated middle and upper socio-economic classes), so they follow a given path of school, university, and a professional existence, the less adapted to everyday life they could become.

The rôle of drama taught at school, of adult acting courses, and rôle-play tuition for those inept with others, could all prove important to their future mental health. Since the academic information learned up to the age of 18-years could be learned quicker by most intelligent people, I suggest that some school time is given to lessons about relationships. Everyone could benefit from such lessons, whereas algebra and history will benefit far fewer. Our health can depend a lot on our relationships – for most of us, a major factor for our energy spending and energy saving.

Resolving Conflict, Reducing Stress

Emotionally charged arguments in a relationship, will usually result from not having fully appreciated the basic psychological needs, character or position of the other person. Since passion is irrational, conflict can continue, despite logical agreement.

Business arguments often proceed in a more orderly manner. Since it may be undermining for emotions to show, arguments can be scripted or subject to an agenda. In all arguments, feelings, pride, security and respect, risk being damaged. Heated battles always leave wounds.

If each party is open-minded enough to say to themselves: 'My position is always to try and fully understand the other person, rather than concentrate on myself', quick resolutions would be achieved more readily. This requires each person to have their say, and for each person to engage fully in what is said.

Re-iteration is a valuable tool. Once an opponent has had their say, each of their statements can be repeated, and offered back to them for confirmation or denial. The aim is to achieve clarity and to remove any misunderstanding. The other person then knows that you know what they think. Next, you can reveal how you are thinking.

It is best when arguing, to be open about the way you feel; especially about the things you really want or could live with comfortably. If either party is uncomfortable with this, yet acquiesces, and says 'Yes', when they should say 'No', arguments will soon restart.

Question: What is so difficult about stating what you really feel and want?

Answer: It may expose your weakness, ignorance, arrogance, greed or vanity, and all that you have yet to admit to yourself.

In any argument, it is essential to expose whether the other party is knowledgeable, and self-aware of their biases. Reaching agreement can be impossible with the arrogant and ignorant. Many are too arrogant to accept their ignorance, and too ignorant to be aware of their arrogance. Best to relate to them through a third party (a counsellor, solicitor or impartial friend) who can point out the facts impartially and not create further sources of conflict.

Because of the pressures upon them, and their need to meet their responsibilities and duties, their attitude and actions can falsely appear greedy, vain or arrogant. By explaining personal needs and stresses, the other party might be more willing to help; others, however, will use this to seek an advantage.

By making personal comments about how you feel, you may encourage sympathy, and even get help. By saying, "It hurts me to know you think I am telling lies", you may be thought naive, but it will underline your humanity, and dispel any thoughts of your insensitivity.

To get full and easy resolution of conflicts, it helps to be happy with yourself; at-one with your weaknesses and strengths, and happy to state them without feeling compromised. You will need respect for others and their right to individuality. It is essential to understand their attitudes and reasons for believing what they do. The conflict between two such people is soon resolved.

Slow Decision Making

Our future welfare will much depend on the decisions we make today.

If the butterfly effect is real, even a seemingly irrelevant decision made today, could affect our situation in twenty-five years' time. From the standpoint of having had a long life, I can testify this to be true. Decision making is a vital issue. We should all study it at home and at school before we embark on adult life.

Dilemmas are often stressful. The degree of stress involved, being dependent on the relevance of the decision. An incorrect choice will affect our life-plan or that of someone else.

I have often seen men separated from their wives, who cannot decide whether to return or to stay with their new-found lover. They may love both women, and in being unable to decide between them, fail to adjust to the stress and energy expenditure of indecision. How are they to end their agony, and preserve the mental health of all involved?

A dilemma will always involve both logic and emotion. One problem is that logic cannot be used to solve an emotional problem, and *vice versa*. In the end, correctness of choice with logical dilemmas can depend on the evidence. How much intellectual intelligence it will take to override any emotional factors is another matter. Having emotional intelligence will be beneficial when feelings are the issue. How comfortable one is with the contemplated decision is a good way to perceive and resolve the matter. This requires personal integrity – knowing oneself well enough to admit to our true emotional needs – what *actually* makes us happy. Achieving that feeling of comfort with a decision, can be thought of as trivial – many have a preference only for logic in their decision making. Where the heart goes, however, the mind soon follows. You may recall my previous, David Hume quote:

> *"Desires, emotions, passions (you can choose whatever word you will), are the only possible causes of action. Reason is not a cause of action but only a regulator."*

David Hume (1711-1776).

In decision making, one must always try to achieve an absence of conflict. By conflict, I mean that feeling of disquiet, unease or discomfort which accompanies one or other choice in a dilemma. It will usually be felt more when the 'wrong' decision is being discussed.

It is critically important to notice one's feelings. In a world so obsessed with gratification from sensory perception – from images, auditory signals, and written material – it's not easy to notice oneself in action. Some people will go to any length to avoid confronting their feelings. They will find it easier to go to bed, turn on the TV, take alcohol or drugs, and talk about something else, rather than engage in some introspection. Solving problems can depend on noticing one's feelings and responding to them. We must be free to feel discomfort; to notice the causes, use them, and value them for what they can tell us about ourselves. If we could all do that, there would be fewer who suffer on the horns of dilemmas.

Indifferent relationships, lacking any excitement, rarely produce discomfort. There will be little need for introspection, and no fear of failure or criticism. There are special, friendship relationships, where one is free to say almost anything without causing upset. These are healthy long-term relationships that work. They satisfy those who seek comfort and want to reject challenge and change. Many seek short-term gratification through satisfying lust, excitement, and the novelty of the new and unconquered. They are best put down to experience.

The impetuous can come to regret their decisions. Aggressive sales techniques persuade them easily. It is easy to be seduced by a need to please others, rather than remain objective. With a growing discomfort about a decision, our ego might reassert itself. Once we can admit our inner feelings of discomfort with decisions, we should make fewer unsustainable ones. It is especially important to be aware of meekness, self-gratification, and people-pleasing, in decision-making. Consider only the strength of the arguments and the truth, and always – be in touch with your discomfort. Even so, only a few have the gumption to cancel a wedding in the days before the ceremony or say 'NO' at the altar. Better to notice feelings of discomfort much earlier and avoid catastrophes that could affect many people.

Setting deadlines pressurises decision making and spends a lot more energy than unrushed deliberation. Pressurised situations, involving time pressure (time overload) and volume overload, can force bad decisions, although they may seem expedient at the time. The real test is how long they will last as appropriate and sensible.

Some of us are driven to achieve specific goals by a certain age. A diminishing number of young people in western society, still want to be married at thirty; have children by thirty-five and have a successful business by forty. Many are forced along this path by the demands of others. The juvenile mind is more likely to be influenced by peer pressure, but at all ages, most feel the need to emulate accepted behaviour; following in the steps of their peer group and complying with the current fashion.

The fear of not fitting-in or being seen as non-conformist, is a sad state of mind. For conformists, this can be a source of pleasure or stress. As time progresses, many will have to cope with any mismatch between their expectations and the realities they face.

As Vladimir Putin wisely said, (with reference to peace negotiations):

"все разочарования происходят от чрезмерных ожиданий."

"All disappointment arises from excessive expectations."

Putin, Vladimir. *Associated Press. 1st August 2025.*

Under stressful circumstances, snap decisions can be made, just to relieve annoyance. A lack of composure, and a lack of concentration and mental agility, will not foster wise decision making. Under such circumstances many become vulnerable – too easily accepting that marriage is right for them; accepting retirement, based on age alone; selling their house or buying a dog – all perhaps, to be later regretted. When signing a contract, at least the law allows for a cooling off period.

Relationships and Mismatched Needs

All relationships start by noticing what each chooses to portray. They might progress to understanding the other person as an individual, with all their personal characteristics. After that, some will progress further to understand the fundamental psychological needs of the other person, and whether any mutual compatibility exists.

In all new relationships, a lot of time will be spent trying to understand the other person as a character. So how many character types are there, and how can one identify them without much experience in life? These challenges must be met within all relationships, whether within families, those with whom we work or those we ask for advice. Some degree of judgment and classification is usual, even though the process may wrongly bias us, through a lack of sufficient information. Being a fly on their wall would save a lot of time, and answer many questions, but that isn't yet possible.

One might study Theophrastus, who centuries ago, wrote about the 30 different types of people he had met. Others might refer to astrological Sun signs, and the characters they are thought to represent. One might study books on psychology, but nothing beats the experiences of dealing with many people. Otherwise, I recommend the exploration of relationships undertaken by Woody Allen in his films. At every level, understanding others is an art, requiring some animal instinct. Some will never acquire it. Among them are many nerds and those on the autistic spectrum.

Grief awaits those who do not appreciate the basic primal needs of others. These pervade and challenge every relationship, and we should all study them from early on in life. They are the commonest source of human conflict, and often the biggest drain on our personal energy resources – potentially health giving or life ruining.

Relationships flounder on mismatches at the interface between three areas of inter-personal contact. According to William Schultz (see references), who studied the relationships between pilots as they were flying in the 1950s, compatibility depends on a primal need for the giving and receiving of affection, control, and inclusion (shared values and interests).

Discord arises when the affection sought by one partner, is not forthcoming from the other. If receiving affection is not their need, discord will arise with those offering it. The same giving and taking applies to the need for being in control and the desire to be controlled. The same also applies to the sharing of interests, opinions, and values (inclusion). Those who dislike being controlled, will naturally feel conflicted with those who want to control them. The need to give and receive affection, control and inclusion, are basic inter-personal compatibility factors.

It would be unusual to find perfectly matched needs between any two people chosen at random. The directly calculated chance of a perfect match (with matched giving and taking in each of the three domains) is 2^6 to one (64 : 1), but that assumes that each domain trait is equally common. That is not so. In my experience, wanting to be controlled and having no need for affection, are rarer than the alternative possibilities.

If we assume that one in ten people will reject affection when it is offered, and one in ten will not mind being controlled by another, the odds of finding a match in a roomful of random strangers becomes more like: 64 x 10 x 10, i.e. 6400 : 1. In my experience, this is the more likely probability figure for finding a perfect relationship. The take home message is this: we either need to use a questionnaire-based dating system or meet many thousands of people. Unfortunately, few lives will be long enough to meet that many, although, the odds will be reduced by our pre-selected social preferences – most of us live among those with a similar background.

A major problem with new relationships, is the time it takes for true traits to become revealed. While some are shy, others have learned to hide their true proclivities, until they get what they want from a relationship. This is a common, dishonest, interpersonal tactic. (See Eric Berne's, *Games People Play*, 1964).

Relationship problems consume a great deal of cognitive and emotional energy. Some require long-term, high-energy expenditure. It is no exaggeration to state, that living in a negative relationship, infused with resentment and anger, can be lethal – either from suicide, murder or illness. Compared to riding a motor cycle, and undertaking extreme sports, the risk of death from an intolerable, inescapable relationship, is no worse.

A common social media trend now, is to question the need for relationships. Some men are now promoting the notion – 'get a wife OR get a life.' Apart from procreation, avoiding relationships might make some biomedical sense.

The value of a loving, supportive, mutually agreeable relationship has untold benefits – benefits unmatched by little else in life. The problem is finding that special one. Unfortunately, the odds are against it unless we change our approach. We can choose to move in matching social circles or be matched by questionnaire. Unless we use some science to find that one perfect relationship, the majority of us will live with the stress of inter-personal conflict. As familiarity grows, so can contempt. Contempt and a lack of respect promote abuse. There are major cultural differences (sets of variously held values) between males and females. In a marriage or partnership, they can either be 'in sync' or 'out-of-phase'. Hence, the dictum: compromise is the *sine qua non* of a bearable relationship.

The bare statistics of relationship breakdown are interesting. Why is relationship breakdown most common among lesbian couples? Why is it less for heterosexual couples, and least of all for male homosexual couples?

Three Areas of Need

When choosing to relate to another person, we all have three fundamental needs to satisfy. These will determine the happiness we feel, both in brief encounters and in longer-term relationships. Affection, control, and inclusion are the key areas of need to consider when trying to understand conflict and compatibility. I refer here to the needs which truly represent us – not those we admire in others or have assimilated from others; none of which are truly our own.

Knowing our true needs can be obscured by the suggestions of those stronger than us. Quite often, I am told that I should have a better car. I ignore them, knowing that acquiring objects is my weakest need. Like ancient sirens, adverts offer us similar charms. But do the products on offer fit our needs? Will we be happy after buying them? How many people strive their whole life for what others wish for, only to find that when they have them, they are no happier? What went wrong? The major reason is failing to recognise our own true needs.

So strongly influential are our basic needs, we have little option but to satisfy them. The conflict of not complying will make us unhappy, and like all other forms of conflict, we might burn lots of our energy. It will seem unacceptably selfish to some, but without our true needs being gratified, many will not understand the true source of their unhappiness or discontent.

Affection

Knowing that one has a need to give affection to others, should prompt us to find a partner whose need is to receive it. In this way, both will find happiness. We might, for instance seek to foster children, where the pre-requisite is to give affection and care for others. Without this need being fulfilled, we may never find fulfilment and contentment. Some people object to being spoiled or being smothered by affection. Many are suspicious of those too ready to offer affection – they may appear too needy. Some of these people will be incompatible with those whose true need is to give affection.

Having broken up with a long-term partner, some will come to fear affection, worried it will again lead to feelings of abandonment and loneliness. Some will try to convince themselves, they have no further need for affection. If only poetically (but more likely, genetically), this attitude may not be what is written on their soul. Only with all our psychological overlays stripped away, can we come to know our true primal needs.

Does Love Conquer All?

"Omnia vincit Amor."

Virgil

In the name of love, volumes of poetry have been written. The Taj Mahal was built for the love of one woman, and cathedrals, mosques and temples for the love of God. Business empires have been grown by providing products and services, but partly for the love of money. Some are successful, but there have been many failures, with no less energy spent, and no fewer sacrifices made.

Aesop had something to say on the matter of love and sacrifice, hence the story of the lion and the woodsman's daughter.

A lion fell in love with a very beautiful young woman – the daughter of a woodsman. The lion approached the woodsman requesting his daughter's hand in marriage. This he refused, disregarding the lion's superior strength.

The woodsman explained his concern. A lion might unknowingly harm his daughter with his great strength, and his sharp claws and teeth. Nevertheless, he said he would think about it overnight and give him an answer next day.

Next day the woodsman respectfully suggested that if he was to allow his daughter to marry him, he must have his claws and teeth removed. Because the lion so loved his daughter, he agreed. When he came back the next day the woodsman simply dismissed him. He now had nothing to fear. For love, the lion had resigned every means he had to dominate others.

Romantic love can be obsessive; an addiction – the dedicated pre-occupation of an infatuated mind. When 'in love', fantasies are created, and all thoughts and duties curtailed, except for those needed for survival. Such feelings have inspired poetry and much prose. They can also inspire uncharacteristic largesse and the spending of large amounts of energy. Love can raise our plane of consciousness. From the point of view of others, a better person may emerge.

"Who needs physics, when you've got chemistry?"

TV Film: *Peggy Sue
Got Married* (1987)

Love is not the only strong, energy spending, motivational factor. Hate, duty, fear, faith, pleasure, greed, vanity, self-gratification, and snobbery are some among the others. The stronger our conviction, the more energy we will spend on their pursuit.

"I am a battleground with greed and vanity fighting."

George
Melee.

*TV Interview with
Michael Aspel. Feb. 1988.*

Control

The same principle applies to the need to give and receive control. If one is not a person who takes kindly to being controlled – being ordered to do things, as a subordinate in an organisation –discontent will ensue. For those who cannot accept control as part of their nature, being self-employed or becoming the chief executive of a company, will suit them better; being a middle manager or shop-floor worker, would not. For those uncomfortable in such career positions, it can lead to ill-health (Marmot, Bosma et al. 1997).

Those with a need to be controlled, should seek a partner who wishes to be in control. Then they both might find happiness.

It requires intelligence and self-confidence to be self-employed, in control of the welfare of employees (and often, their families). If a person with a strong need to control others, doesn't have the ability, he may have fewer opportunities to satisfy his needs. Without considerable inter-personal relationship skills, it might be difficult for him to gain enough respect from others. Those without the appropriate skills, should forget becoming a captain of men. Many, however, will put their failure down to bad luck!

Bureaucratic control is implicit in all western societies. There are many diverse ways to control citizens, using the law and financial pressures. Many find this degree of control, not to their liking, and a subliminal source of their discontent – the subject of the next chapter.

The Need for Inclusion

Some people are gregarious, freely sharing pastimes, hobbies, values, attitudes and beliefs; others are loners. Not everybody wants to belong to a political party, play football for their school, become a faithful follower of a sect or sporting team, or feel needed by a group. Those who have this need must seek like-minded people: those with whom they can share their interests and desires.

Others who are solitary rather than group types by nature, will be more comfortable playing golf, singles tennis or snooker; being self-employed, a writer or a lone explorer. This might be because they are shy, not because they desire isolation from others. Again, I refer to what is our natural trait, not that which has become acquired.

Because they are most likely inherited, such traits lie close to the surface, being obvious from observed behaviour, even at an early age. The loners stand aside while the groupies club together. The assumption that all humans are gregarious is an obvious oversimplification. There is an element of delusion in the idea that there is safety in numbers. There are a few who pursue solitude, while for some, it may be inescapable: being lonely in a crowd is what some architects of modern cities have inadvertently engineered. Every lonely Londoner or New Yorker can feel some consolation as part of a large anonymous group. For the truly desolate and lonely, every group will offer some potential for contact; to find someone out there who may come to care for us – if only . .! For those seeking companionship, city living rather than a rural existence, will better serve their needs.

There are many who feel unhappy but know not why. It could be necessary for them to acknowledge their own behaviour, and to examine their natural leanings in the most selfless way possible. As with the desires for affection and control over others, self-acknowledgement of a natural loner status might prevent us making the mistake of trying to be a family person.

When relating to others, we each have a different need to give, and receive affection, control, and inclusion. The presumed, but rarely occurring 'Darby and Joan' relationship, is one in which Darby loves to love and be loved by Joan; Joan, being a romantic, loves to love and be loved by Darby. Darby wants to be in control, while Joan honouring his judgement and skill, is happy leaving him to make all the decisions. While enjoying the same activities, they might never disagree about what to do with their lives. What purgatory some will think. Yet for the few who have it, their perfect compatibility can be ideal. It is also ideal biologically, because the energy expenditure needed to maintain such harmony is minimal.

The absence of discord (on which some sharpen their acumen), can be a perverse source of unhappiness. Not having true insights into our needs and hopes – as alluded to by the Buddha – can lead us to pursue the false aims of our ego, and cause insecurity or unhappiness.

Are relationships worth it? And if so, which ones? This is a question all teenagers should be asked to consider at school. The problem is, pre-coital humans are driven mostly by physical attractiveness, and procreation without a secure relationship. For those past middle-age, with such biological imperatives lost, the need for relationships must lie elsewhere. Will another person provide help or companionship? Perhaps affection, shared coping and control. Perhaps a shared outlook and interests might fill the need.

Although slow to gain any scientific credibility, death from a broken heart, due to emotional rejection or bereavement, can occur. Such was the said fate of *Elaine of Astolat*, who died of a broken heart because Sir Lancelot at King Arthur's Court, did not return her love and affection. Many statistics support the idea. (see my book: *Tiredness, Chronic Fatigue and Exhaustion*, 2025).

"Death ends life, but it does not end a relationship."

Cruse for Widows Organisation.

Robert Anderson.

When he was three years old, Roald Dahl's sister
Astri, aged seven, died of appendicitis. His father
died of a 'broken heart' two months later.

'Boy: Tales of Childhood'
Roald Dahl

From a physical point of view, the energy spent on a relationship can be great. This might encourage health or become an important proponent of ill-health and disease. This energy can help to reduce or maintain illness, and affect the rate of recovery. With reduced energy available, we will be less able to fight off any adverse consequences.

For the sake of perspective, it is appropriate to think of relationship problems as major factors influencing morbidity and mortality. Money spent on teaching relationship skills, could be more important to many than teaching algebra.

From the biological point of view, relationships are irrelevant. The ultimate aim of attraction is procreation. The aim of sex is to ensure the survival of a species. Knowing this, as a matter of biological science, is of no use whatsoever when negotiating a relationship. Feelings, biases, and the need for love and companionship, are the strong driving forces in play. Managing them is an art, not a science.

As relationships move forward, neuroticisms may surface: anxiety, depressiveness, phobias, perfectionism, emotionality, and hypochondria, can all strain a relationship if found difficult to handle. For some, finding anxiety in another can hasten intimacy; especially for those capable of pacifying and calming others. For some, intolerant of anxiety, encountering it will quickly bring the relationship to an end. Not all have the capacity to cope with dependent people.

It might take a lot of exposure and some intimacy, to appreciate the fundamental character of another person – some would say – to find out what is truly 'written on their soul'. What needs to be discovered are their true needs, motivations and drives. Some relationships never get this far; they falter once dissimilar attitudes to sex, money, education, lifestyle, religious conviction, status, class, and background, come to light. Most of us want an answer to a key question. How are we to know when we have found that rare, one-in-a-lifetime relationship – one that will afford us relief from energy spending, and provide us with contentment, spiritual nourishment and fulfilment?

We all have a tendency towards an open or closed nature. This has been crystallised in the model of interpersonal relations devised by Luft and Ingham at UCLA – the Johari Window. They consider people of four types:

- Known Self: known to self and others,

- Blind Self: known to others but unknown to self;

- Hidden Self: Known only to self;

- Unknown Self: unknown to others or self.

When you are free and open, others will easily get to know you. You may not, however, fully know yourself (the blind self). This feature was given to the fictional character Dorothy, played by Judy Garland, in the film, *The Wizard of Oz*. What she really wanted and needed, she already had, but didn't know it. She falsely believed that only the Wizard of Oz could put things right. Unfortunately, he proved to be a charlatan. How often does this reflect life?

One product of a good relationship when it occurs, is that a closed person (with a hidden or unknown self) opens up and is discovered. The prerequisite is that they feel comfortable enough to do so. Eventually, one of Dorothy's companions, the lion, whose character appears to be that of a coward, finds his courage – something he was previously blind to. His unknown self provided him protection. An individual with no insight into themselves, might give nothing away for others to warm to. As a result, most will avoid them.

Pleasurable and Unpleasant Relationships

The most pleasurable relationships are those which require no effort to maintain; with no energy spent on conflict, discord or feelings of discomfort. Mutual respect, trust, understanding and benevolent sympathy are the important elements. Openness, and a willingness to be seen as we really are, sharing all one's thoughts and feelings, defines a loving relationship. It requires the mutual loss of ego boundaries.

Human behaviour can seem unpredictable, because we are all guided by two conflicting aspects of brain activity – logic and emotion. In speaking to ourselves, feelings can clash with logic, and *vice versa*. Both generate mind-talk, each side freely advising the other. Unfortunately, neither is a good listener.

In matters of affection, 'being sensible' or taking a logical approach, rarely has much impact. Even though a certain course of action seems logical, sensible, and straightforward, many who feel uncomfortable will forget the logic and 'go with their feelings'. In so doing, they may decide to fulfil a transient desire, rather than a core need. We may decide to associate with an attractive friend, rather than a more intelligent one. Many badly matched relationships begin simply by 'fancying' someone attractive (but perhaps incompatible). The application of science is hardly romantic, but every moment spent in assessing compatibility could pay dividends.

We all have unfortunate, inbuilt biases. They favour the strong, wealthy, and beautiful, when a timider, quietly successful, less attractive companion, might be the more compatible. Some relationships can be fun for a while, but unwise in the long term. When feelings and logic conflict, beware of martyring; accepting the drama – 'I deserve to have some fun for once; my life up to now has been so tough!'

One-sided Relationships

One-sided relationships are especially unfortunate, and unfortunately common. The set-up is friend and lover, not lover with lover. One partner – acting as a friend – might provide some sex, companionship, and friendly help, but not love. At the same time, the other could exude unconditional love. Once the loving partner realises they are spending their unconditional love (and energy) on friendship, resentment and retribution can grow. Dejection and humiliation become likely. I have seen unmatched passion lead to much anger, hatred, and even suicide.

Some friend-zoned lovers will spend considerable amounts of energy, trying to make mutual love happen. It never will, of course, but their vain hope sustains them. The friendly partner has it easy. All they have to do, is turn up and tolerate a little discontent and guilt. With no alternative partner on the horizon, some will use the situation to their advantage. Only rarely do users suffer. Parasitism comes with its own book of rational justifications. To glimpse the truth, the friend-zoned lover must examine who it is that is making all the plans, initiating meetings, making the telephone calls, and paying all the bills. Even then, their love can blind them to the truth. One unfortunate characteristic of many humans, is their propensity to use others; they benefit, but the one being used pays the emotional price.

Imperfect relationships usually require some change of attitude and some re-orientation of strategy, to make them work. When love is unequal in a relationship, the situation is unstable. Lasting mutual satisfaction is rarely achieved, but many persist in trying to make it work. Two people can learn to live with unequal love, but the amount of adaptation and rationalisation needed to keep the relationship afloat, can be exhausting. The golden rule is – avoid all such unbalanced relationships. Life is too short and our energy too valuable.

Being 'in love' can so consume a person, they could seem to have a medical problem. They can become anorexic (love-sick), sleep fitfully, and spend their mental energy ruminating on the one they love. In the early stages of a relationship, before love has been declared or at least, only declared by one partner, the energy expenditure can be so excessive, they lose weight. Their behaviour becomes noticeably different: pre-occupied, depressed, irritable, and disinterested in anything other than the object of their affection. All this can disappear with the joy of togetherness. For Romeo and Juliet, being in love meant that 'parting was such sweet sorrow'. Although not regarded as psychiatric, the obsessionality, desperation, and craving on display, are only rarely regarded as normal human behaviour.

Lucy Goodison did extensive field work on the 'in love' experience. She says,

> "... falling in love does not go away. We all do it. It is gripping, exciting. We long for it. It makes other more politically 'correct' areas of our life pale by comparison. It keeps cropping up. Its power is unquestionable."

The power she refers to can accomplish both creation and destruction. Such strength of feeling can impart both self-confidence and meaning to life. She quotes two of her interviewees:

*"The experience . . . gives us a glimpse of the exuberance
and energy which might be set free when our relations
with one another are liberated from the system that
perverts them . . . Being in love shatters constraints."*

*"I have a feeling, a strange feeling: she seems to poten-
tiate me. I am expanding: will I burst like a star on the
world?"*

Genuine love involves extending one's own ego boundary to include another person, engulfing their wishes, needs and desires,
as if our own. Love this strong, is mostly obvious, but for those
who are shy and retiring, it can remain well hidden. Sometimes,
their heartache can last a lifetime; with longing for what might
have been. Love that escapes notice, might be a wonderful opportunity missed. Unfortunately, one-side and half-hearted affection,
is much more common than the instant mutual love of Romeo
and Juliet. Mutual love of this sort is rare enough to be regarded as
a once-in-a- lifetime experience. Love can grow to be mutual, but
this not quite the same thing.

An important question for the young, is how long should they
wait to find a perfect partner? While waiting we might ask ourselves, would *we* make a wonderful partner, and are *we* selfishly
looking for a partner to keep with our other favoured possessions?

My boss, Dr. Peter Nixon at Charing Cross Hospital, London,
used to say: 'one can find someone to love on any street corner, but
to find someone you love to hate, is much more difficult!' He was
referring to acrimonious couples who still love one another, but
who have developed dismissive behaviours, because their partner
is no longer acting as they would want. These partnerships are

strongly bound. The death of one can quickly lead to their partner's demise.

Relationships most often start with physical attraction, and most often flounder on the hard facts of conflicting needs. Nothing is more seductive than being liked, admired or just plain 'fancied'. In James Redfield's, Celestine Prophecy, he fancifully makes notice of the energy passing between people and the Universe. He poetically says of meeting others:

> *"by seeing the beauty in every face we lift others into their wisest self and increase the chances of hearing a synchronistic message."*

Relationships that survive beyond the opening gambits, will often develop amoebically – constantly probing and testing in different directions. Eventually, one partner will proffer a remark loaded with attitude. The other will either find this attractive or immediately unacceptable. Mapping attitudes and outlook takes place through questioning. The aim is to reach comfortable territory. Sometimes only non-verbal behaviour can be relied on to detect discord. Relationships with a poor prognosis, continually meet the rejection of ideas and attitudes. Parting will then be a joy, not a sorrow.

Two people can find one another acceptable, after just a few moments. Their acceptance of one another, will be obvious from the start – verbally and non-verbally. A relaxed, empathetical closeness; smiling, long eye contact – all non-verbal evidence of instant attraction. Once the territories explored verbally confirm compatibility, great joy can follow, as the prospects of this relationship come into view. Because of the shyness and reserve some have, the process can be slow, much time and energy being spent without progress.

Each culture dictates the acceptable time for progressing intimacy. Even 'love at first sight' (I was yours after the first 'Hello') will take time to mature into 'the real thing'. What better use of energy than finding a perfect partner (one who will surely save your energy in the long run)?

These initial meetings are a time for honesty, not fantasy. Honesty at this stage will shortcut any unnecessary energy expenditure later on. Get your feelings, needs, and attitudes out into the open. If your potential partner is going to run, let it be sooner not later. If it's only sex you're after, attractiveness and erotic fantasy will suffice. The biological imperative to procreate will justify any energy expenditure.

Lives can be made or lost because of relationships. But what exactly do I mean by a life 'being made'. There is an energetic definition. Life is 'made' when it is deemed worthwhile; a joy worth preserving; a constant pleasure to experience, with self-esteem and worthiness gained as a result. In biological terms, contentment will make one's life least wasteful of energy, and make survival more likely when any call on extra energy needs to be met. By 'likely', I mean that the odds are in its favour, but not guaranteed.

The whole universe of worthwhile experience, shared by two people, will be bounded by their egos. This means that nothing or nobody can interfere. Many lovers are quite happy with this; indeed, it will define their state of happiness. For some, it will last until death. Following the death of such a partner, love will often be re-expressed in ritual, constant nostalgic memory recall, and memorials. Constructing the Albert Hall was just one of Queen Victoria's testaments to her love for Prince Albert; the Taj Mahal is the enduring testament of Mughal Shah Jahan's love for his third wife. She was his soul-mate – Mumtaz Mahal – a Persian princess.

People change only a little with age. If relationship partners develop at the same rate, in the same direction, and to the same degree, a basis for their enduring relationship exists. If both lead separate lives, and expose themselves to different influences, they risk parting unless their love is strong enough to withstand external influences. Some age-related, change of outlook is inevitable: the young look to the future, the old look to reminiscence. No two people have the same innate rate of development, so working together and sharing life's pleasures, will hedge against any disparity. With love and respect in place, each partner can learn from the other.

Although the ages of partners may differ, their level of maturity can be similar. Some difference in maturity can be attractive. The less mature partner might help the older one to re-visit their youth, adding zest and fun to their life. The older one can supply the wisdom of experience. Because the older partner may have learned the knack of energy efficiency, and have more nous about life, a younger partner can benefit.

Most people behave like their contemporaries – they are largely bound to comply with an acceptable image – one befitting their age. From a health point of view, is this advisable? Why should a sixty-year old man be happy doing no exercise, except that it better befits his body image? Why should he not consider trekking overland to Machu Pichu? More might, if it were not for imposed expectations. Sadly, in the western world, a well-earned retirement (from life), and a life of ease till death, is what most have come to expect.

While youth is being wasted on the young, money is being wasted on the old.

Trust between people comes with exposure and an understanding of their circumstances. Mutual trust features in most fulfilling relationships.

Once one party seeks an outside relationship, no amount of trying to keep together will work without a sufficient need. The need to 'try' in a relationship, signals one that is defective.

The only tactic worth trying to get a separated partner to return, is to completely ignore them. Freedom means freedom of choice, and if they have found somebody more suitable, then let it be – separation could be for the best. If they return to try again, hope of success requires an understanding of their true motivations for leaving.

Partners who find another relationship, should be left to see how that new relationship plays out. Maybe they were mistaken about suitability. It is common among breaking relationships for one partner to claim that the other has 'made a big mistake.' The way to handle it, albeit superhuman, is to send them off to be with their new-found lover – full time. Instead of hanging on to them, let them go as an irreproachable act of love and consideration. Who will match such generosity of spirit? This allows the quickest (energy saving) resolution.

By restricting sexual freedom, Islam restricts the energy wasted on changing partners. While the Christian Church has always advocated the same, it does not enforce any code of behaviour that guarantees it.

Uncertainty and procrastination can both cause personal damage in relationships. Both can be cruel; both can be expedient. Acting precipitously saves energy. Prolonged and dragged out relationship conflict, costs vast amounts of energy, with serious consequences for the health of all involved. The ensuing tiredness, accompanied by indecision, can prolong the state of affairs, wasting further energy.

The fallout from a broken partnership will often spread to involve parents and grandparents, many of whom may want to retain their relationships with children and grandchildren. I have seen grandparents, separated from their grandchildren by marital breakdown, suffer pneumonia as a consequence.

Business Relationships

In business, one may have no choice, but to get on with associates and clients. The more secure the business and one's role within it, the less need for duplicity. If the business is desperate for profit, the employees might start to feel insecure. Now, personal politics can surface. To be profitably duplicitous is a useful political and business gambit.

Pathological Relationships

In all physical systems, energy is spent overcoming resistance. In human terms, we spend lots of energy overcoming any resistance to our will. By collaborating with others, energy can be pooled, to achieve mutual objectives more efficiently. We can 'pull together' and more easily overcome resistance, with a lower energy cost to each individual. This is the fundamental justification for delegation and associating with others – a biological reason in fact, for forming relationships. All other reasons, apart from the evolutionary drive for procreation, are either vain or romantic.

Where others are concerned, one should try to respect them, try to understand them, feel for them, and help them if possible, but never become dependent on them, even if in-love with them or in business with them. In short, never become controlled by others unless you cannot help it or desire it.

In a rather old Beatles cartoon film, The Yellow Submarine, Blue Meanies are portrayed. Their like, actually exist in reality, not just in cartoons. Acting as demanding, angry, aggressive, obsessive, self-possessed, mean users of others, they can be as lethal as any poison. They can suck others dry of energy, causing their mental breakdown or inducing a stroke or heart attack (depending on any predisposition).

> *When 16-year old Pauline Reade was abducted and murdered by the Moors Murderers, Paul Brady and Myra Hindley in 1963, her mother suffered mental anguish for 37-years until her death, aged 72-years. In 2000, she was recorded saying she never stopped thinking about it, and never slept properly again. She suffered a mental breakdown as a consequence.*

Duncan Staff. *The Moors Murders. BBC TWO. Longtail. 2025.*

Beware of becoming obliged to mean and nasty people. Neither trust them, nor tolerate them. Be cautious when thinking you have mis-judged them and want to change them. One of their techniques is to make you feel obliged and indebted. They will know what to say when the time is right, like – 'you will be promoted in due course; you will soon be in charge and adopt the position you deserve'. Forget such promises, they are fantasy not fact. Such offers are usually made by self-interested people with hidden interests. They will always profit in energy terms, getting others to do work for them. Their profit, your loss.

Michael Marmot's Whitehall study showed that middle management (caught between the demands of executives and office staff) have the worst of health outcomes. Those not in control, are pressured both by those in charge and those whose work they need to encourage.

Those who think that the significance of control is exaggerated, are at risk. Those unable to sense this as a danger risk unnecessary trouble.

If there is interpersonal evil in the world, one of its manifestations exists in controlling others. High risk organisations, like aviation and the armed forces, need control to contain risk; some others impose more control than necessary. Few organisations now allow free thinking, even though it is the only source of useful progress.

Many exist who care too little for the plight of others and think it appropriate to be as they are. They are guided by simple mores – 'survival of the fittest'; 'who dares wins'; 'dog eat dog', 'kill or be killed'. Forget worrying about the food you eat as a cause of heart attacks and cancer and start worrying about who you are eating with. Metaphorically, you might be their next meal!

There are people who are good and generous, loving and kind, genuine and true, but since they are often quiet and unassuming, you may fail to identify them. With them, lunch can be free, simply because they respect you. Respect is the only basis for a fruitful relationship. Never compromise its value.

Remember that all 'Meanies' are practised in making use of others. They are always presentable, but capable of doing you harm. They are what guerrilla fighters are to regular forces: stealthy, secretive, hidden in plain sight and deadly. My advice is to end all relationships with them, before getting trapped in their web of false promises. Recognising them, and dispensing with them, is one prerequisite for happy survival.

Assessing Relationships

As long as trust and respect last, mutual testing is continuous within all relationships. The value and security of the relationship will be frequently tested and questioned, and often continues for life. Once respect and trust have departed a relationship, neither counselling nor cognitive therapy are likely to help it survive happily.

Early on in any relationship, the appropriateness, value and stability of the relationship, will be in question; sometimes subliminally, sometimes during discussions or what can resemble interrogation. There is truth in the observation that what most people dread in any relationship, is a partner saying, 'we need to talk'. Many men will immediately conclude that their behaviour and commitment are under scrutiny; not in a casual, helpful or supportive way, but in a manner reminiscent of the Spanish Inquisition. Many men will anticipate a declaration of intolerance; of dissatisfaction, or of impending break-up. They will prepare for an oncoming threat, a warning or at least an ultimatum. Men can feel ill-prepared, having to address emotionally-laden female issues; women must counter male pragmatism.

Western men know that if they didn't work such long hours, and were at home more, they might provide more assistance with family matters. This is far less the expectation in eastern cultures. Men are aware of one female definition of male failure – not having enough money to spend all day at home, helping with the children (whose growing up milestones are easily missed), and the household chores. Separate, biologically driven roles might have to be discussed. Gender equality issues will need an airing. Men might see a female question hanging in the air. Perhaps she made a mistake and should have committed herself to another – a more successful alpha male – one who could have provided her with more security and made her happier and richer. Just a minute. Isn't this a partnership? Is it the prime duty of every person to make their partner happy?

When the time comes for 'the talk', many will have wrongly thought the worst. To his relief, all she may have wanted to discuss, was a new washer/dryer!

The best tests of relationship security are to be found in human action, not words. The degree of friendship, affiliation or love, is easily judged by observing behaviour and responses to situations. Although more reliable than words, there are confounders. Laziness and a lack of organisational ability can affect impressions as much as the degree of affection. Look for birthdays and anniversaries being remembered. Is the suggestion of spending time together grabbed or ignored? How much unprompted mutual affectionate behaviour occurs or are there growing signs of distancing?

People reveal their true selves in the small, inconsequential things they do. What they say and do, when they are the centre of attention, could be politically motivated and not personal. Observing non-verbal micro-behaviour is key to gaining advanced human interpretation skills. Prolonged eye contact and maintaining physical proximity, both strongly indicate mutual attraction. If you have been out for dinner with a new date, and afterwards linger to talk, a mutual relationship is building. If you have asked for help from a supposed friend, and they avoid you, they are sending you a message – they are disinterested, not supportive. If you love somebody, don't fear letting them go. If they love you, they will return sometime (if they can). Those who leave, may not have unconditional love on offer. Why try too hard for anything else? There are reasons of course, but often, they are second rate. Now you must ask, 'can I do better?'

When asking a third party for advice about an intended partner, get them to describe actions. Words are of lesser value. How they behave towards others, especially their friends and parents, will reveal much more than asking for an opinion. Secretive, arrogant, selfish and aggressive behaviours are unacceptable. Excessive vanity, constantly using others, laziness and overvaluing physical possessions are sinister prognostic features. Hardworking, loyal and supportive behaviours need to be recognised as attractive.

Those who are selfish, greedy users of others, should carry a health warning – tattooed on their foreheads. They are energy parasites, lying in wait to drain others of their resources. Learn to identify them and avoid them unless desperate for short-term companionship.

It is, of course, easily possible to misinterpret behaviour, especially when strong biases are in play. Remaining silent can avoid aggravation, but it can induce dislike or be seen as a gentle way to reduce friction. Amputating someone's leg can either be seen as an act of cruelty, part of planned torture or a life-saving measure. Assumption and interpretation without sufficient meta-information is dangerous. When judging others, come to know their motives and biases. Be extra careful about the motives of third parties whose opinion you ask. Many will tell you to 'follow the money'. This is not an unhelpful suggestion. How much money is spent – on what, and on whom, can be insightful when character and motivation are in question.

Complex behaviour will have many possible interpretations. Because the truth is easily obscured, never assume to know why someone has acted as they have, without unequivocal evidence of their motives. The tragic story of Othello and Desdemona is warning enough.

Assumption is a major cause of decision error. A marriage could be lost, or a business partnership dissolved, because of one wrong assumption. Many assume they know how someone is thinking or feeling, without enough confirmatory evidence. When it comes to calculating the odds or weighing the evidence, human minds are too easily biased. We all upgrade or downgrade the significance of the evidence presented to us, depending on our biases. In this way, even a pure act of kindness can be interpreted as manipulative; any approach from a stranger, can be interpreted as suspicious. Since many now accept the modern world as a dangerous place, these have become safe biases.

Life Change

Because we all perceive stress differently, researchers have looked at human reactions to life change. Moving to a new house, losing one's job, and divorce, can precede heart attacks, depression, suicide and strokes. Using statistics, one can calculate the probability of each life change having an effect. Statistics use large groups only, compare mean differences, and accept an initial assumption – that both groups being compared are the same – until proven otherwise (this is called the null hypothesis). If there truly is a significant difference between the groups studied, one can calculate the probability of an outside effect being real. Unfortunately, an overwhelming belief in the value of statistical analysis now exists. There is now very little faith in everyday experience and observation, even when made by an expert, experienced individual; even though there would be no science without everyday observation, and even though there can never be any guaranteed individual relevance to any statistical result.

Observers can be trained for reliability, but even so, some will imagine or amplify what they have seen, perhaps to draw attention to themselves. Most new ideas, however, start with an observation or anecdote. Deductions taken from such personal observations need to be put to the test – to see if they apply universally – something we can all believe in, rather than be dismissed.

Life Situations

As their interests and values diverge, the old and young deserve mutual tolerance.

It has been said that the only people who benefit from the law, are lawyers. It might also be said that those who write, 'How to...' and 'How to change your life' books, are also the only beneficiaries.

I doubt very much that there are any new scams; most are regenerated. Clever, tricky and smart people have always existed, alongside the gullible, straightforward and casually indifferent. With travel and cultural mixing, many are now exposed to different sets of values. When we all lived in villages, most knew one another, and what was what. In this new age of travel and ever-improving communication, many can choose to live apart, favouring anonymity. At the same time, we are becoming vulnerable, and more easily tricked.

Constant Competition

Except for hermits, modern life is competitive, and a major source of our energy expenditure. Gender equality has brought more competition to every arena – at home, and at work. Children compete for top places at school; pilots compete for Top Gun prizes; businessmen compete to become the richest; the richest compete to become the top philanthropist.

There has always been competition for one thing – for the one who is right most of the time. Others compete to have the most useful ideas or to be the one who achieves a place of honour or top status. This drives many to spend their energy. Such ego can drive us to displace good will, and to swap the benefits of co-operation for personal success. Although we call it a rat race, only humans engage in it. Rats have more important things to do!

The same driven attributes are found in most top athletes – they refer to it as the killer instinct. Their coaches will tell them that winners possess more of it than losers. Not only must athletes enjoy winning, they must enjoy some *schadenfreude* – seeing their friends and opponents fail – hence all the hand pumping, chest thumping and grimacing when they win.

Evolutionary competition is part of the biological landscape. Because the cat eats the mouse, not vice versa, a predefined predatory pecking order exists, created by the drive to survive and procreate – a fact of life (and death) all non-domesticated animals live with. Many humans like to think we have left this aspect of biology behind us. We haven't. Instead, we have adapted it, and made it acceptable – the process we refer to as civilisation. We have now evolved enough to encourage and help some of our competitors. Better to put them to use, than sacrifice them or eat them!

Defending Thoughts and Feelings

It is immature, ill-educated, and self-deceiving, not to examine our feelings, attitudes, and beliefs. So said Plato in the Republic, and many others have said so since.

> *"A fully functioning person will know fully, and without undue bias or prejudice, why he believes what he does. Because he is a non-reactionary he will allow others their opinion without malice or anger. His aim will simply be the truth, not the boost of his ego or the gain of recognition."*

Carl Rogers.

Like everyone else, a 'fully functioning person', must live with uncertainty, but possibly with less than others. In arguments or discourse, the non-fully functioning person is liable to react angrily when he finds his opinions are difficult to justify, and his ideas lack consistency. His reasons for thinking as he does, may be as much a mystery to him as they are to others. The anger evoked spills energy into a void.

Our emotions need to be examined. Questions need to be asked about the appropriateness of disapproval, and whether anger, guilt or dislike are ever justified. Why waste energy on unnecessary emotions? Wasting time and energy is costly to health and often depressing. To be able to completely justify one's feelings as 'reasonable' (acceptable to others who are not emotionally involved), allows one to relax and feel secure. Certainty about our beliefs and feelings, encourages composure and relaxation, and is a frame of mind that can engender happiness and a state of grace – a good basis for personal energy spending economy.

It is sad that few understand why they are reactionary. They may feel lost, simply because they lack insight; they feel unhappy because they don't understand themselves, and how their thoughts and feelings have become structured.

Education should foster self-examination. Coming face to face with one's misplaced attitudes and biases, may be unpleasant, but an experience necessary to achieve open-mindedness and wisdom. To achieve self-realisation, many need to be exposed to ruthless, well-meaning criticism. This may involve the un-learning of some beliefs long held and cherished. Success can be achieved once challenges to our beliefs or knowledge no longer offend us. In that state, there will be no need for conceit or egotism, only humility.

From the security of knowing everything about oneself, one can happily be sure of nothing, while keeping an open mind. The top prize is being able to enjoy all the challenges of life, without the need to win a prize.

Attention-Seeking

Few are born imbued with a selfless duty to care for others. That requires the near absence of an active personal ego, except for that needed for personal survival. This narrows the field of candidates to very few – Jesus of Nazareth and Buddha among them. I have no doubt, however, that throughout history, there have been millions of such people left unrecognised. There is an obvious reason for this. Selflessness naturally shuns attention, rejects self-promotion, and is not newsworthy.

Businesses must get noticed, if they are to sell their products and services. For businessmen, the process requires obtaining possessions, controlling employees, and making a profit in order to gain free choice. Once successful, some turn to public service, allowing them to get noticed and admired by colleagues, friends and family. The attention could bring them fame, yet more money and power.

A very famous showbiz man, who subsequently became an infamous criminal, offered this advice:

- Always be on top.

- Never give anyone a fair advantage;

- Take advantage when others least expect it.

He followed these words by saying: "How anyone can be a nice fellow and do that, I don't know". (Jimmy Saville, Radio One, 24.1.82.). After his death in 2011, it was found he had sexually abused hundreds of young boys and girls over many decades. While in the limelight, he raised millions for charity, having achieved fame, fortune and power.

In times of economic difficulty, the small businessman may have to think like Saville; ruthlessness might be the strategy he needs to survive the jungle conditions imposed on small businesses. Unlike them, corporate businessmen can easily remain faceless, leaving a lot of the day-to-day stress to their PR, sales and accounting departments. In large successful corporations, the directors can remain anonymous, far removed from the shop-floor and the immediacy of business survival.

Criminals are often cynical about society and the way business functions for most people. Few knew better about surviving criminality than the Kray brothers. One said once:

"What is straight business, anyhow? Be honest. It's just a bloody racket, same as our way of life. All of that keeping in with the right people, going to the proper school, and knowing how much you can fiddle 'an get away with. All those lawyers and accountants to squeeze you round the law. What's all of it except one great big bloody racket."

John Pearson (1973). *The Profession of Violence. The Rise and Fall of the Kray Twins*. Granada Publishing Ltd.

Limelight and Fame

"Are you rich?"

"I don't know ... but I am valuable!"

Bret Whitely, Australian Artist.

The release of energy can seem to come from the buzz of fame. When the limelight dims, adjusting to a loss of status could arise. When Winston Churchill lost his seat after the 2nd World War, he became depressed and had a stroke. Margaret Thatcher was never the same woman after being deposed as Prime Minister.

There are others, however, for whom the loss of fame will be liberating:

"I have found money, success, and fame - and they are all empty things."

Jack Higgins.*Sunday Times, London. May 1988.*

Fame is sought by many, but is not for everyone. It will be enjoyed most by self-promoting, egotistical narcissists, and rejected by the shy and modest – but with many exceptions. It can be thrust on those with a talent impossible to hide. When Irvine Berlin reached his hundredth birthday, Jerome Kern, an equally famous America composer said of him: 'Mr Berlin has NO place in American music; he IS American music'. That's fame!

Theodore Roosevelt (1856 - 1919) was born rich and led a privileged lifestyle. The lifestyle he recommended, however, was that of a 'strenuous life'. When he was young, he was skinny and weak, but determined to make himself strong. He boxed, wrestled, did dogged exercise, and won national fame as a 'Rough Rider' in the Cuban, Spanish-American War. When he left Harvard, he spent two years on a cattle ranch in North Dakota, toughening up. In a speech in Chicago in 1899, he said:

"I wish to preach not the doctrine of ignoble ease but the doctrine of the strenuous life; the life of toil and effort;

of labour and strife; to preach the highest form of success which comes not to the man who desires mere easy peace

but to the man who does not shrink from danger, from hardship or from bitter toil, and who out of these wins the splendid ultimate triumph . . .

A mere life of ease is not in the end a satisfactory life, and above all it is a life which unfits those who follow it for serious work in the world."

'A Mere Life of Ease'

Ignoble ease is the aim of many street-wise people who live life using their nous. Many of them want it for their families, regardless of the spoiling effect it might have on their children and partners. Some are self-oriented, acquisitive people. Some live to shop – principally for designer clothes, expensive cars, holidays, and trophy partners, that will make others envious. In contrast to Eric Fromm's directive on how to live life – 'to be' rather than 'to have' – they will first try 'to have', and only later try 'to be' . . . once they can afford it. Ignoble ease can be very tiring, due to under-stimulation – boring and depressing for some, but magical, exciting and a source of pride for others.

Many of the self-made men I have encountered in medical practice, have tried to 'find themselves'. Once they are rich enough to stop working, and have accommodated to the emptiness of wealth, many find themselves sad, without a *raison d'être*.

Some would say that it is impossible to 'be', without having first experienced some success or failure in life – the gift of true love and friendship; a moving spiritual experience or views from mountain tops. Those who have done little other than pursue wealth all their life, can be left bereft of anything in life that satisfies them. Having left any work and struggle behind, many return after a year or so, to start a new business. It can take time for them to realise that what they lived for most, was the challenge of engaging with others in business, and not just to gain the benefits of property and other possessions they were able to accumulate. There is much joy and fulfilment to be had, spending energy on the passions that fulfil our basic drives and needs (needs for affection, control and inclusion (see FIRO and William Schultz, earlier in this chapter).

Culture & Relationships

Western capitalism promises us future security, if only we work hard and long enough. Many insecurities can drive us to work. Unless we work, we might experience a loss of status, the loss of income, a loss of health, even a loss of life; all representing our potential for losing control. As a result, most of us spend a lot of our energy, trying to retain control. By default, we will avoid activities devoid of useful gain, even if it means giving up some self-esteem.

Care, kindliness, and love from others, can all save us personal energy. The family fold was the traditional setting for energy recoupment. The partial dissolution of supporting family ties in some western countries, must therefore, put their societies at risk from increasing strain effects. Without family and nurturing support, we risk depleting the energy we have available, and less chance of recovering it. If dissolution of family support progresses further, the result might be a more slothful, fatigued society, tired of the constant energy spending required of us. Diseases can be expected to increase again as our perception of being 'in control' diminishes. We might again have to expect reduced resistance to infection (defective immune responses), and an increase in several damaging cardiovascular problems, exacerbated by widespread chronic fatigue and exhaustion. Apart from family issues, these risks will only be reduced if politicians improve our way of life.

The animal kingdom provides many examples of family group activity, sustaining healthy existence through the minimising of energy expenditure. Acting together in packs, animals are able to hunt successfully and provide for both their young and old. Altruistic behaviour is not exclusively human. In the Serengeti, old, toothless wild dogs can be seen guarded and protected by younger fitter animals.

The strength created by some human families pulling together is clear among some ethnic groups. Jewish, Moslem and Sikh families are to be seen running self-supporting family businesses in the UK, each profiting from their family co-operation. No government social support system will ever match the support that can be provided by a close family group. It is a central tenet of Islam, Judaism, and other faiths with strict laws of observance, to care for vulnerable family members.

At home, Jewish women are the most important member of the family. Moslem children have a religious duty, as prescribed in the Qur'an – to care for their parents. The important task of maintaining the home and providing succour for all family members is a duty that will cultivate a willingness to return to the family fold.

Relationship problems and family politics can consume a lot of our energy. For 'healthily' functioning families, there is usually a net gain. Where there is rancour, there is energy depletion; where there is energy saving there is contentment. For doctors, the psychodynamics of a family unit can determine patient stress. Happy families, within which children are respected, loved, and sympathetically mothered and fathered, provide a more certain pathway to physical and emotional health; dysfunctional families will more easily create an unhealthy environment.

The Family

Island of peace and place of nurture or a sinister scene of conflict and demise? Families can provide both.

From Penelope and Odysseus to the Bennet's of Pride and Prejudice; Bob Cratchit and family, to Del Boy and Rodney – both love and nurturing are on show. There is one problem waiting in the wings. Those lucky children who have known nothing, but family love and nurture can be ill-prepared for the dog-eat-dog, every-man-for-himself nature, of modern society.

'The choice is simple', a fellow traveller once told me: 'get a wife or have a life!'

Some express the view that:

'If only we had old family values back, all the ills of the world could be resolved.'

Politically charged, Machiavellian families exist. They are not just the stuff of literature and film. Whether we suffer a dominating father or mother, or put up with sibling rivalry and jealousy, surviving a family with its own particular culture and politics, is a worthy introduction to the wider world of stress and energy spending.

Baby Bonding

After a baby is born, most mothers bond with their child as love develops. This enables the mother to look kindly on this little person whose only objective is to be fed, with no regard to the time of day or night. New mothers easily get exhausted since most will have disturbed sleep. Concern for the welfare of their helpless infant, sustains their need to make many sacrifices. The loss of calories in breast milk, adds a further physiological challenge to their energy loss. Long ago, mothers used to feed their children for a long time – sometimes to an age where they had teeth and were walking. This exhausting practice seriously debilitated them and reduced their resistance to infection, sometimes with fatal consequences.

With their first child, a new mother's lack of experience can engender anxiety. Better education and the presence of an attentive family, especially a knowledgeable mother or grandmother, will help to allay concern. The delegation of the child to a grandmother, aunt, nanny or friend, will help to retain the mother's health. Organising such support before any birth, will increase a mother's confidence and allay their anxiety. As a result, they will get more rest, and retain their health.

Surviving Parenthood

Young children cry and must be placated. Babies sleep at times 'out of synch' with normal adult routines. It helps for breast-feeding western mothers, to enjoy unstructured time – once called *otium* by the Romans; still called ησυχια (eesichia) by the Greeks. All we have to offer in western culture today is 'to take it easy', as a temporary sojourn from something some see as more more valuable – work.

Adherence to adult expectations can create frustration, conflict and poor sleep; no mother with a young baby can afford sleep deprivation. Either the child has to be delegated while the mother sleeps, or the mother sleeps while the child sleeps. Sleeping with babies is now an outlawed western practice, but still common in the third world. It can be dangerous.

> *Sleeping with babies is a known cause of cot death or sudden infant death syndrome (SIDS). Parents can roll over in sleep and crush their child.*

Whether day or night, the distancing of a child from its mother, could have later behavioural implications. A totally helpless, dependent child, has the power to disturb any adult lifestyle. Self-indulgent, previously childless couples, are in for a shock if they have a baby. When parenthood arrives, their well-ordered environment could soon be in disarray. In the west, single parents without the extended family support found in third world countries, will be exposed to many tiring stresses.

The parental situation is made challenging by a combination of experiences: caring for a new baby, loss of usual activities, feeling out of control and sleep deprivation. Seeking effective coping strategies is essential for maintaining mental health, it will test the competence of all new parents. Some mothers will cry having lost control of their lives (especially if they expected to retain it). Not all new parents are prepared enough for their new role and lifestyle.

The relationship of new parents may have to adapt. Partners can be helpful or completely hopeless as supporters. A mother's female friends can be covetous, and either supportive or disinterested. Men can meet their lack of knowledge with anxiety, aggression, dismissiveness, and distancing, especially if repeated crying (mother and baby) becomes difficult to tolerate. Some will sense that they are no longer of use. Suddenly the au pair or the flirty single girl at the office, could seem more attractive!

Having babies is a trying and testing experience for relationships. Only a strong biological drive to procreate, and the tendency to deny reality, keep parenthood popular. Child rearing spends energy by the bucket-full, with only a few westerners able to afford nannies. Not all will have supportive families, with aunties and grandmothers fighting for possession of a new baby.

Some parents are forever invested in their children, with irony often going to waste.

As an example, here are two Jewish mothers talking to one another:

"So, how's your son?"

"Oh, he's OK, but the girl he married! She is lazy and useless. She lies in bed all day, never does any housework, and avoids shopping. She's a useless wife. But enough of her, how's your daughter?"

"She's such a lucky girl. What a wonderful man she married. She can lie in bed all day if she wants. She has so much help, she never needs to do housework or shopping – it's all done for her.

She's so wonderfully happy. So lucky!"

How ludicrously ill-prepared most of us are for parenthood – one of the most challenging of jobs in life.

There is no turning back. A woman's life is changed forever by having a child; a man's life is changed for at least twenty-five minutes!

CHAPTER ELEVEN

Subliminal Stresses. The Pools In Which We Swim

Subliminal stresses abound, providing a backdrop to our everyday living conditions. One essential element they share is the lack of control we have over them. Although many go unnoticed, like the reliability of our utility and travel services, we must live with disruption as a possibility. The immediate and background stresses we face, must be dealt with, but subliminal stresses can be ignored if we so choose. Some people are unduly sensitive to environmental factors. This has led to a new personality trait being accepted – environmental sensitivity. For such people, subliminal stresses can become foreground stresses.

Subliminal stresses need not concern us, although, the political-ly-minded might embrace them, and try to change them. Many pose soft threats, as opposed to real ones. In some cities, personal and racial abuse, street crime, burglary and shop-lifting are all there, but may never involve us directly. Knowing they are there is subliminally stressful for many.

The tone of how we live can be influenced long after a major incident has occurred. The massacre of innocent Israelis in their homes on the 7th of October 2023, and the destruction of the

Twin Towers in New York, on 9/11, 2001, were both examples of heinous crimes, perpetrated by the terrorists who now live among us. These have created a sense of fear for some, posing questions such as – will similar catastrophes happen again, and might I be involved next time? On a daily basis in most cities, there will be many examples of malicious crimes against ordinary people; most of which are ignored by the news media. All help to paint the scenery – as the backdrop to our lives.

Social Factors

The rich and poor lead different lives and are subject to different stresses. The rich have more control over their living environment than the poor. There are also large differences in medical outcomes between socio-economic groups. For instance, the less well-off have three to five times more heart attacks and strokes than the wealthy. To some extent, this must result from differences in lifestyle. Few are actively aware of any difference. That is because both those who live in palaces and those who live in hovels, have become used to it. Cramped rented accommodation, with no easy transport available, only superficially compares to living in a four-bedroom detached house, with three cars on the driveway. Although those who live in different scenarios, may give little thought to either their subliminal stresses or the benefits of their existence, they are none-the-less real.

Flies occupying homes and offices, could get to see everything that happens. As a doctor, I have long believed that only flies have any chance to assess patients' living circumstances, lifestyle and true behaviour. Doctors all tend to accept what we are told by patients, but is the picture they paint accurate and true? Knowing what people actually get up to, rather than what they say they get up to, could be divergent. Without accurate information (sometimes extracted by interrogating the patient, their family and work mates), doctors might too readily accept that energy spending is irrelevant. This is understandable, but often misguided.

Although our social lives can be complicated, there are to two basic interactions:

1.   Between the **internal forces** that drive us – our desires, attitude, belief, personality, and dictates of our ego, and

2.   The **external influences,** always acting upon us – some obvious, some subliminal, many constantly changing and involving us in various ways.

Urban or Rural? Environmental Energy Spending

One can get used to background road traffic noise and other forms of noise pollution, but therein, lies a problem. The aggravation and tolerance needed to cope, spends unnecessary energy. The change from a rural location to an inner city one, can be upsetting. We can adapt our sensitivity to noise, but if the distant 'hoo' of an owl was once our greatest annoyance, the noise created by rowdy groups of drinkers and traffic, will definitely disturb our composure. And that isn't all. The most disturbing noises can come from neighbours, many of whom lack any concern for others. They will bang doors, sing and shout, whatever the hour. Those unfortunate enough to live in flats with a neighbour above, know they all wear heavy, studded army boots. Because most work during the day, their tendency is to clear out their kitchen cupboards, every night at 3AM!

Architects and builders are now required to reduce noise pollution to specified levels when building party walls. This regulation recognises the widespread economic implications of defective sleep. Moving to the countryside from the inner city also has its problems. Some city dwellers moving into the countryside, will have to adapt to complete silence at night. Profound silence takes time to get used to, and what we are used to, modifies our reactions.

There are many considerations necessary when comparing rural and urban living. One is vigilance, the other is inter-personal transactions. Because of the density of population in towns, simply walking down a street involves navigation, just to avoid others. Drivers have the same problem. In towns, they need greater awareness of other vehicles and bicycles; more navigational decisions are needed. This usually makes the town driver sharper, but potentially more tired. She needs to maintain vigilance and anticipate well, both necessitate spending energy if she is to avoid accidents.

Town dwellers have to negotiate crowds. They must sometimes battle through waves of people, especially if they travel by metro (underground or subway). Multiple, small transactions consume energy subliminally. Walking through syrup rather than water, provides an analogy – more energy is required to walk through syrup. Add to this, the frustrating vagaries of an overburdened transport system and delays. With fatigue comes a lowered flash point. The frustrated, tired motorist, is much more likely to get angry and feel road rage. If town traffic worsens further, the energy required to negotiate it will rise. Venturing out to buy a loaf of bread could come to risk life.

Because of increasing urban population density, the threat of burglary and attacks on others, is greater in urban locations. Living in a city requires vigilance. This contrasts with rural living, where front doors and cars are often left unlocked, with more dogs and geese, acting as early warning guardians. Dogs and cats can recognise the difference between known and unknown footsteps and will react early to any stranger. Less planning, vigilance, and fewer navigational changes are needed for walking down a country lane than negotiating Oxford Street in London, 42nd Street in New York or Les Champs-Elysées in Paris.

If these differences in energy spending are medically relevant, might there be a difference in the rates of heart attacks between those living in the countryside, and those living in towns? This is not an easy question to answer from the data published on the subject. In the UK, more heart attacks occur in towns (Stewart, J. 2022); in the USA, more occur in the countryside (Changanty, S.S. 2023). I suspect there are more deprived people living in the countryside in the USA, than in the UK. That could make the difference. Social deprivation is a much bigger mortality factor than subliminal stresses like crime, noise, a lack of privacy and crowding. These are all likely to be more important to health than to disease.

Town planning in the new towns of the UK has put space between people. This has created both a sense of freedom and a feeling of separation and loneliness. New towns and suburbia share one quality – they are planned to be predictable. They can provide utilitarian, but boring environments. Creating new homes that are all the same, makes them cheaper to construct – there is profit in uniformity. The result will be some loss of identity and character, as seen in the historic villages, towns and cities of the UK. Retaining character must be balanced against traffic flow, the provision of amenities and other practical considerations.

The countryside can be boring – the endless similarity of fields, hedges, and forests, for instance. At least low human density, fresh air, and the individuality of older dwellings will compensate for it. I have heard many an urban dweller remark, 'I don't know how you stand it out here. There is nothing to do. Nothing is going on!' A false, but reasonable impression.

Socrates, speaking to Phaedrus, said:

"I'm a lover of learning and trees and open country won't teach me anything, whereas men in the town do."

The thatched house I once lived in, near Saffron Walden in the UK, was built in 1666. I can say with absolute confidence – no copy of this house exists anywhere in the world. Building such an individual creation now, would be too costly (even if the craftsmen were available).

Every country I have visited, has different town planning rules. The places I would most like to live are not uniform, but then I am used to towns like Oxford, Cambridge, Saffron Walden and Chester, in the UK. I prefer uniformity to be broken up by bridges and piazze, as in St. Petersburg and Rome, rather than live with innumerable, uniform tower blocks. Every culture embraces its own style of preferred living. In so doing, architecture and town planning, can influence mental health. The more acceptable it is to us, the less energy we will spend, subliminally interacting with it.

We all value our individuality, and living somewhere unique is one form of personalisation, in a rapidly depersonalising world. Our individuality can be a source of self-esteem. The uniformity of apartments and houses in towns, makes individual expression more challenging. Given time, we can all make a house a home, but only by installing enough of our personal possessions to challenge de-personalising architecture.

All in Our Genes?

The biggest subliminal factor of all is genetic makeup. There will come a time when we will all know our health-related genetic profile, but at the moment, the details are mostly unknown, except for the clues provided by our family history.

Most people partner those from the same social stratum. As a consequence, their offspring (as a group) will retain some of the same inherited risks and benefits – perhaps preserving the gene pool and maintaining the health divide. My 50+ years of clinical medical experience, strongly suggests that those with no relevant family history (with no obvious genetic predisposition) will have fewer heart attacks or strokes than those with a family history – whatever their lifestyle – whatever their social background. They are unlikely to possess the necessary in-built, adverse pathophysiological and biochemical response mechanisms.

Damocles' Many Swords – Subliminal Threat

Every influence upon us from our surroundings, is a stress (if we define stress as any disturbance or applied force). The subliminal stresses upon us mostly go unnoticed, but are present nevertheless. Some subliminal stressors will produce an automatic response within us (like a blood pressure or pulse rate change); others will induce no obvious response at all. The stresses we notice, are most likely to be relevant biologically. It is on these, we will consciously spend our energy, whether we want to or not. Most subliminal stresses affect us subconsciously; being subject to automatic, reflex responses, with no conscious involvement needed. There are many continual background stresses that are subliminal. Even though we might ignore them, they can still elicit a physiological response. Changing air quality and temperature, vehicle movements when travelling, as well as ambient light and sound changes are all in this category.

Our mode of travel through life will determine some of the stresses we will experience. Travelling 'first-class' is designed specifically to make journeys more pleasant, with greater passenger separation – a little more privacy – and better personal service. Few can afford it or will choose to afford it. Some prefer to be chauffeured, rather than having to drive and concentrate on traffic. Apart from claustrophobia, few like being crammed into crowded spaces – their physical boundaries, dignity, and privacy could be contested.

The less energy we have available, the more taxing every stress becomes, and the more energy we will spend reacting to it. Although some stresses are constant and predictable – the same journey to work each day; the recurrent need to pay our mortgage, rent and utilities – our responses to them (the strain effects) will vary with our mood and outlook.

During the days of the cold war with the U.S.S.R., we were told that a real threat of nuclear war existed. With what is now happening in Ukraine, some feel that the threat has been reactivated. The possibilities are again being whipped up by media channels, challenged to provide enough news content. They may simply be posing questions, but the possibilities they raise can be disturbing to some. A BBC newscaster recently asked (July 16th, 2025): 'What if Russia invades a NATO country?' As something that had not previously aroused our conscious awareness, the question is enough to create subliminal stress for many.

Referring to the Vietnam War, (fourteen years before he became President of the USA) Ronald Reagan remarked:

> "I don't think anyone would cheerfully want to use atomic weapons – but the enemy should go to bed every night being afraid that we might." (July 1967. See Kaiser, R.G. 1980).

In Finland, the threat of invasion from Russia has always been heightened by proximity. At one time, 79% of Finnish 12-year olds and 48% of 18-year olds, named a Russian invasion as their foremost fear. Their foremost hope was to get a job; hope for continuing peace, they put in second place. These subliminal stresses were common to many (Solantaus, T. et al. 1984).

Advertising

I doubt many of us realise the full extent to which advertising influences us subliminally (some would say indoctrinates us), until we travel somewhere too backward to have any. Few such places are left!

In a capitalist world ruled by supply and demand, adverts are essential, and their influence inescapable. Adverts not only inform us about products, they can create new desires or offer solutions to all our problems. By motivating us to work hard, we might someday be able to afford these products. Advertisers know we all have unsolved problems, and enough of us want to improve our status and want our dreams fulfilled.

The motivation to buy, can be driven easily – suggesting necessity or scarcity. 'Hurry up. Buy now or miss out'. An awareness of unfulfilled desires serves as a subliminal stress for many. All serve to quietly drain our energy, little by little.

Some sample adverts I once collected together, were enticing and amusing in various ways:

Perhaps you're not sure of what you are entitled to?

> *"After a lifetime's slog*
>
> *one's entitled to relax*
>
> *and play a little golf."*   (Insurance Ad.)

And what about your fate?

"Death by missing adventure?" (Insurance Ad.)

If travel is the thing, why not choose a car whose:

"16 valves

pump pure adrenalin."   (Car Ad.)

Or for the high-flying, why not snatch:

"A few hours grace

before the madness starts all over again."'   (Airline Ad.)

One insurance advert I found showed some unusual insight into the work predicament, listing some fictitious companies, clearly set to damage health:

Stress Inducers Ltd.

International Coronary Manufacturing Co.

Nervous Exhaustion Associates

Constant Aggravation Ltd.

Working Weekends Ltd.

Breakdown Hasteners Ltd.

Stab in the Back Enterprises.

Midnight Oil Burning Co.

The advert went further by suggesting that one could avoid 'stress disease' by investing wisely and accumulating sufficient capital to make an early escape from a dangerous occupation. Albany Life, the American Insurance Company responsible (now Canada Life), should have been congratulated. In one advert, they highlighted a major source of stress, linked it to major disease, and prescribed an effective preventative strategy. Adverts can sometimes inform and educate, and perhaps even reduce our stress by making life easier. Unfortunately, their greatest appeal usually lies elsewhere.

At least this advert conceded that high blood pressure and heart trouble were 'stress-related' diseases, even though many doctors still remain unconvinced. Fashion in medicine, as with hemlines, requires general acceptance. Only those doctors who have had their jobs threatened; have had experience of significant tax demands or have suffered bereavement or divorce, will readily accept the connection of disease severity to stress.

Information

Throughout my life, the available sources of information have greatly increased. It now seems as if we must resist intrusion, with so many media outlets now available, even on our mobile telephones. If we allow it, we can be bombarded by information – stories, reels, and numerical data, most of which will be irrelevant to our personal life and work. Some are addicted to it, hoping not to be left out or be thought out-of-date. Many hope to find one golden needle in the many haystacks full of information chaff, presented to us each hour. Even those who try to ignore it completely will be aware of its possible significance. Sometimes the feeling of possibly missing out, provides a minor subliminal stress.

Information can range from the boring and irrelevant, to the stimulating, exciting, and sometimes life-changing. Pertinent information is crucial to decision-making, so the need to access it can be motivating, although, often a waste of time and energy. That's life, but there is a problem. Once we get interesting information, we then need to appraise it intelligently, using experienced judgement to assess its relevance. AI can help with our search for information, but who is going to supply the wisdom needed to interpret it; put it in perspective, and help with our decision making?

The Pleasure Principle

Our subconscious minds must react and deal with many subliminal stresses – those that need not interrupt our conscious thought. Sigmund Freud thought our subconscious was made up of desires, impulses, and wishes that need to be fulfilled. This primary wish-fulfilment drive, he called 'The Pleasure Principle'.

"I want what I want, and I want it now!" If young babies had words, these would be their most useful. Freud's interpretation would have been, 'I never want pain or discomfort.'

Hunger is a discomfort which neither babies nor some adults want to suffer. Babies cry - young children have tantrums – adults go to the larder or wine rack; others go to their doctor. Not all adults need immediate satisfaction: some have learned patience, and quiet sufferance. To suffer purposefully, as with righteous self-denial, can be a source of self-esteem and another form of self-gratification.

A suckling baby gets quiet gratification; relaxed and without pain or discomfort. During equivalent periods of adult life, we probably unblock overused neuronal channels in our brain and spend less energy on problem solving. The biological survival imperative, however, is ever-present – to save energy and seek gratification, rather than pain or conflict.

To avoid pain we can use many pathways. One path is to avoid anything that might induce fear – often motivated by a fear of fear itself. To avoid fear, we must avoid danger. By avoiding physical pain, we avoid any feeling of our vulnerability. The desire to avoid pain is an inherent human characteristic.

Petrarch (Francesco Petrarca), the Florentine lyric poet of the 14th century, wrote:

> "My brother chose the steepest course straight up the ridge, while I weakly took an easier one which turned along the slopes. And when he called me back showing me the shorter way, I replied that I hoped to find an easier way up on the other side, and that I did not mind taking a longer course if it were not too steep. But this was merely an excuse for my laziness; and when others had already reached a considerable height I was still wandering in the hollows."

> Petrarch (AD 1304 -74). *The Ascent of Mount Ventoux.*

Subliminally, much of human endeavour is directed to achieving self-gratification. We all spend a lot of energy on it. Some seek wealth in order to stay in comfortable five-star hotels, with helpful staff, always on call. Some buy expensive cars, and travel in first-class comfort – to minimise their physical discomfort and gain privacy. Many wealthy people born poor, dedicate their lives to accumulating money, just to get as much gratification as they can without discomfort.

I have a psychoanalytic question. Can money ever replace the experience of clutching our mother's breast and suckling; can it compare to the succour it once gave? My guess is that some want to accumulate money, friends and servants, to help them regain this feeling of succour, while avoiding any painful or tiresome hard work.

Capitalism comes with many benefits for some – helping to protect the financially successful from unpleasantness. Partly to preserve profits, we are kept from seeing the death of animals, lest we lose our interest in buying meat. We are kept from the truth about death, lest we get depressed, give up work, and stop buying profitable products. Any energy we spend on accumulating assets, we can recoup while savouring the comfort and pleasure we have bought. The poor, contented man, can find himself in the same position, but with fewer resources (money and energy).

The Wealth Paradox

A rich tourist approached a poor farm worker sitting on a turnstile.

"You ought to get yourself a proper job mister," said the rich man.

"Why?", said the poor man.

"Because you could travel the world, enjoy yourself, and take it easy, like me!"

> *"But I have always taken it easy", said the poor man. "I usually enjoy myself, and I'm content to remain in this beautiful place. So why would I waste my time and energy on a job, when I am already content? "*

With limited choices, the poor might find it more challenging to achieve contentment. The many more choices available to the rich, however, cannot guarantee their happiness or contentment.

There is no doubt that the rich and poor often lead different lives. There is also no doubt that the rich are healthier than the poor – the health divide.

One amazing fact needs an explanation. Why do the poor have three to five times more cancer and heart attacks, than the rich? Instead of poverty and wealth being the key factors, perhaps being content or discontent; happy or miserable, might be more important.

There are contented people among both the rich and poor. That's because the gift of contentment cannot be bought.

Past Experience as a Stressor

Some people live beneath thick black clouds of anger, guilt, doubt and resentment.

> *Mary was a middle-aged woman with two children. For years, she had been fearful and angry with many people. She often felt anxious and depressed.*

> *She was asked to imagine the time when she first felt anger. Describing the scene, she said she saw herself in*

a hospital corridor with her parents walking in front of her, stony-faced and silent. She was 15-years old and had become pregnant as a result of her first sexual encounter. Her parents found out too late, made her have her son, but then offered him for adoption.

The moment of her greatest grief was in that hospital corridor, walking away from her baby – something that would stay with her for the rest of her life. She had been manipulated by her parents to hand him over for adoption, and still resented them for their lack of support. She wanted to keep her baby, but they would not agree. She hated herself for not being strong enough to stand up to them – to stand up for her child and have the courage of her convictions.

At 47-years of age, she was hoping for a re-union. She wanted the chance to ask her son for forgiveness. She wanted to lay her resentment to rest with her parents, but her father had died many years before. She now realised, that in the more formal days of her youth, her father must have felt ashamed. The social mores of the time were very different. She reasoned, however, that had they truly loved her, they would have acceded to her wish to keep her son.

For 32-years, Mary spent a lot of her energy on rumination. As a result, she had never known life without constant tiredness.

PART THREE

MEDICAL ENERGETICS

CHAPTER TWELVE

Medical Causes of Fatigue

A statue at Saranac Lake, honouring the physician E.L.Trude au, states some ancient goals of medical practice:

"To cure, sometimes. To help, often. To console, always."

"The great mystery of medicine is the presence, in a machine of exquisite design, of what seem to be flaws, frailties, and makeshift mechanisms that give rise to most disease."

Nesse, R.M., Williams, G.C. 1995.

Many diseases feature fatigue as a symptom. As they advance, most diseases require increased energy expenditure, and could affect ATP energy production (not addressed here). During an active disease, like those causing a temperature (representing energy loss), more energy than usual is required to maintain bodily functions. The diseases that pose the highest risks – atherosclerosis, hypertension, and cancer, do not often present with fatigue until advanced.

Even though fatigue is not an early feature, they are all, nonetheless, potentially fatal.

Tiredness not only results from the toxic, poisoning effects of alcohol and various drugs, but also from heart, kidney and lung disease. The process of cell re-cycling (apoptosis), itself employs some very toxic substances, made by the body and used against it. Some made by our white cells (leukotreins), are especially dangerous when in excess. When produced inappropriately, tissue necrosing factor (TNF-alpha), promotes inflammation. Similar chemicals (cytokines) released in the brain can cause neuro-inflammation – a likely cause of fatigue with viral infections, Alzheimer's and Parkinson's diseases. Their involvement in everyday stress-related, fatigue and depression, is unknown and much less likely.

With brain inflammatory conditions (like AIDS, etc.), interferon-alpha is produced in the brain. It is neurotoxic and could be responsible for fatigue and depression, partly by decreasing the amount of serotonin present. Since serotonin acts as an anti-depressant, its reduction is likely to cause fatigue; an excess relieving depression. Some anti-depressants are selective serotonin re-uptake inhibitors (SSRI's), allowing the build-up of brain serotonin.

Anaemia, whatever its cause, is an infrequent cause of tiredness. Anaemia is more often associated with shortness of breath, although untreated severe anaemia (where the amount of haemoglobin in the blood is less than 50% of the normal range) can cause fatigue at rest. Active gastrointestinal bleeding, as a cause of anaemia, can itself cause fatigue.

Physicians faced with a chronically fatigued patient will face an age-old diagnostic challenge. Is it psychological or physical? If physical, has every diagnosis been excluded? How much investigation is appropriate? Many patients will face a diagnostic grand-tour, being tested for every conceivable medical condition, often without a positive finding. At the point where such searches seem never ending, it will be pertinent to review the patient's relationships, circumstances, their psychological and behavioural characteristics. Although most experienced doctors are aware of the need, they may not have the time or inclination for social enquiry.

Among the physical causes of disease I found as a doctor, were leukaemia, myxoedema (underactive thyroid), Addison's disease (low or absent cortisol), EB (Ebstein-Barr) virus infection (glandular fever), chronic renal abscess, Weil's disease and Lyme disease. In all other cases, ongoing stress and disturbed sleep, most often explained tiredness, fatigue or exhaustion.

> *Addison's disease affected one renowned US President. While in London in 1947, the President to be thirteen years later, John F. Kennedy (then aged 30-years), was diagnosed with the condition. He had to take treatment for the rest of his life.*

The Causes of Fatigue

Very few people complaining of tiredness, fatigue or exhaustion, will have a medical cause for their symptoms (apart from being a side-effect of the drugs they were taking). Only 1.5% of 1000 patients who came to my clinic for medical screening, were found to have an organic cause for their fatigue.

Not every defect or disease causes fatigue or death. Those involving inflammation, like bacterial infection (kidney infection and pneumonia) or viruses (COVID-19 and glandular fever), consume energy fighting them off. The core body temperature rises, and energy is lost as heat. This indicates the presence of an infectious agent with the upper hand.

Heart disease and cancer involve little inflammation, and because they consume little energy in the early stages, create little tiredness. As a result, cancers often remain undetected for ages. In the end, with cancer widespread and the body fighting it, tiredness and fatigue become common. The same happens in progressive heart disease. As the heart fails, tiredness can sometimes become profound.

To remain conscious, the brain must have enough blood oxygen and glucose. A lack of either, will cause tiredness – and even unconsciousness, if either gets too low. A high blood glucose (hyperglycaemia), as occurs in uncontrolled diabetes, also causes tiredness, although some patients will get used to it and not complain. Diabetics who accidentally inject themselves with too much insulin, will also get drowsy if the blood glucose drops too low.

An excess of carbon dioxide (CO_2) in the blood, as happens with some respiratory problems, also causes drowsiness. This can be associated with obesity, if extreme enough to reduce breathing (sleep apnoea). Tiredness and even sleepiness occur, as CO_2 builds up in the blood.

In Victorian times, when nutrition was poor, tired people were often diagnosed as anaemic. Many were prescribed beer as stout – black, because of its iron content. Many patients still regard anaemia as a possible cause for their tiredness, although this is now only rare. Minor degrees of anaemia do not cause tiredness, but the presence of anaemia might point to another medical cause for fatigue.

The heart and circulation are responsible for the delivery of oxygen and glucose to the brain, so any failure of heart pumping action (heart failure) is liable to cause tiredness and fatigue. The commonest symptom, however, is shortness of breath. When not enough oxygen reaches the heart muscle, chest pain can occur while walking (angina of effort). When not enough oxygen reaches the leg muscles, calf pain (claudication) can occur. When insufficient blood reaches certain parts of the brain it can cause fatigue and dementia (vascular dementia).

In other forms of dementia, brain cells are either reduced in number or there is too little neurotransmitter (acetylcholine) for normal brain activity. Brain function can be disturbed by abnormal protein accumulation (Alzheimer's and amyloid dementia). Whatever the pathological features, fatigue is common.

Mental activity (cognition, emotion and executive functioning) requires the presence of glucose and oxygen, and high-energy chemicals in neurones to be released. Fortunately, the supply of these high-energy chemicals never runs short (unless disease takes over). Daytime mental activity will progressively block some neural pathways – the most likely cause of tiredness in healthy people. Restful (slow-wave) sleep unblocks them, but dreaming (REM) sleep, may not (REM sleep is more likely under stressful conditions).

Power is spent constantly on maintaining brain activity but is modified by psychological factors: whether the activity brings joy and satisfaction or is tedious and unfulfilling. In the latter case, our resistance to the activity spends more energy, and is the more likely cause of tiredness and fatigue.

Any medical condition that disturbs replenishing sleep (sleep deprivation), will cause noticeable next day tiredness. Not only stress and worry do this. Difficulty in breathing and joint pains are among the many medical causes. If the resulting sleep deprivation is prolonged, fatigue will develop into exhaustion. Although unlikely in those without a predisposing problem, exhaustion can risk a medical catastrophe, like a mental breakdown (the sudden onset of failure to cope mentally), schizophrenia, depression or panic attacks. As a result, other medical conditions can suddenly get worse – like migraine, gout, psoriasis or eczema. Angina can start to occur with less effort, peptic ulceration can become recurrent, repeated infection can begin, and the treatment of hypertension can become more challenging.

I have seen all of these in my long career, but many patients develop them without any preceding tiredness or fatigue. For a medical catastrophe to occur, I strongly suspect that a predisposing medical condition is necessary before it will happen. Many patients who experience tiredness, fatigue and exhaustion will remain well, albeit with many experiencing a worsening of their established medical problems. Most experience a lowered resistance to infection – if only recurrent herpes simplex or other minor viral illnesses. As Florence Nightingale observed, this is a common outcome among those who are stressed.

Because chronic fatigue can forewarn of a heart attack or stroke in those predisposed, I always advocated heart screening for those who were stressed and had a family history of heart attacks, angina, high blood pressure or strokes. Screening is even more important for those with established heart disease and high blood pressure. Many inherit their high blood pressure (with muscle thickening of their arteries – arteriosclerosis) or a tendency to 'fur' their arteries (with cholesterol and calcium compounds – called atherosclerosis). The earlier these pathological processes are detected, the better.

Significant problems face physicians interested in prevention. They need clinical expertise to make early diagnoses, but also need an interest in psycho-social matters (to discover and evaluate patient stress). Unfortunately, many do not regard this as part of their job description. Also, few have enough time to spend on the lengthy, in-depth patient consultations, required to fully evaluate every patient's personal circumstances. Although patient continuity is invaluable, few doctors in the UK, now know their patients or their families well enough.

I frequently found that in-depth enquiries, helped to solve cases of fatigue, when every routine test was negative. Investigating patients with tiredness, chronic fatigue and exhaustion, needs to explain why certain individuals become ill; why some remain ill, and why some deteriorate unexpectedly. Although this might have been obvious to family physicians sixty-years ago, the UK medical profession today, has taken to developing anonymity. Many blame 'the system' they work for – for not providing the time they need with patients. There is a simple solution to that, but very few in the UK are inclined to consider it. I had to remain a private physician and cardiologist to solve the problem. I was then able to provide the consultation time needed.

The Sleep Paradox

Many live with a sleep paradox – unable to sleep well, when they need it most – when tired by the stress of unresolved problems. From an evolutionary perspective, the incitement of more REM dreaming sleep during stressful periods (perhaps for problem review), will reduce daytime energy and performance. This reduces the likelihood of successful problem solving. In some instances, as in wartime or times of civil unrest, it can compromise survival.

Exhaustion causes diminished performance. Perceiving this, increases arousal, fear, anxiety, and restlessness; problem rumination then makes getting to sleep (sleep induction) more difficult. The paradoxical sleep that occurs in response, could be broken by periods of anxious wakefulness, nightmares and panic, accompanied by sweating and palpitation (tachycardia). Even though some dreams are disturbing, they may need to be repeated if they are to generate a new idea or helpful strategy. They can be counterproductive, causing unrefreshing sleep, daytime tiredness, and a reduced inclination to act or solve problems.

Myalgic Encephalitis (ME)

ME is one form of 'Chronic Fatigue Syndrome' (CFS). It is characterised by constant physical and mental tiredness (for more than six months), not improved by rest and sleep. No consistent reasons have been found for it, despite many viral and brain MRI studies. The official US government website (cdc.gove/me-cfs/hcp/clinic al) recently reported 3.3 million sufferers in the USA (2024).

One question arises regularly about ME. Is it psychosomatic or caused by true brain disease? Various explanations have been given: traumatic life events; exhaustion of nervous system energy or neurasthenia (Beard, G. 1898); a neuro-immune disease, a psychosomatic disorder; a viral illness; mass hysteria; 'Yuppie Flu' or a biosocial syndrome maintained by illness beliefs. The World Health Organization (WHO) has classified ME as a neurological disorder (International Classification of Diseases. ICD-10: G 93 .3; WHO, 1992)(ME Society. Nursing in Practice: June 2016).

Although tests rarely reveal a specific viral cause, 80% of cases are thought to be post-viral. The viruses detected include: Ebstein Barr virus (glandular fever), and other herpes infections; parvovirus B19, Coxsackie B, enterovirus and Borna disease virus (BDV), together with SARS-CoV-2 (the cause of COVID-19).

Hwuang, J-H. (2023), found evidence for more viral infections in cases of ME/CFS (antibody and antigen detection), than in control subjects (two to three times more for BDV when 5000 ME/CFS subjects were compared with 9000 controls). The viruses most frequently found were BDV, parvovirus B19, and Coxsackie B. These findings suggest, but do not confirm, a viral cause.

Some patients with ME were found to have raised blood inflammatory markers, autonomic imbalance (blood pressure changes on standing and fainting episodes), and occasional brain changes on MRI scanning. Similar brain changes are also found associated with anxiety and obsessional-compulsive disorder (OCD), and post-traumatic stress disorder (PTSD), so they are not specific to ME.

Many have suggested that ME is a psychosomatic condition needing psychotherapy. Except for an increased risk of suicide, a review of the all-cause mortality of ME, showed no difference from normal people. In common with all others complaining of fatigue, there is no single physical diagnosis that accounts for most cases. In many studies, cognitive behavioural therapy (CBT) was found effective for reducing fatigue symptoms in ME. How fatigue, virus infections, living circumstances, sleep, and stress might interact in ME cases, needs to be studied. These are not issues which doctors offering only 10-minute consultations can address (like many GPs in the UK).

Not every ME patient will have experienced inescapable stress or suffered depression, although established fatigue can be depressing. It occurs more in twins than expected, although no genetic predisposition has yet been found. It is not officially considered a psychological illness, although the thoroughness of each psychosocial enquiry needs questioning.

Not all patients experience a full recovery, although for younger patients, the chances are better.

Chronic Ebstein-Barr Infection

(Glandular Fever or Infectious Mononucleosis)

Many healthy subjects have had glandular fever – an Ebstein-Barr virus (EBV) infection – without knowing it. I found raised EBV antibodies present in most of the CFS/ME cases referred to me. I was never sure whether the antibody changes they had, represented recovery or active infection. This is because I was unable to measure their viral antigen (evidence of virus presence). I gave many with raised antibodies, a two to three-week course of doxycycline or oxytetracycline. Eighty percent of them reported improvement. Without a double-blinded trial, I remain unsure of any placebo effect. I was encouraged, however, by the fact that only 20% of subjects treated with placebos, usually report improvement. I was also encouraged by the fact that most patients had previously tried several other medications, without success.

Tetracyclines have multiple uses, one of which is to treat Dengue fever, COVID-19 and SARS-CoV-2. They have an antiviral effect related to the inhibition of RNA function.

Other Infections

In everyday GP practice, a common explanation given to patients with fatigue, is that they have a virus infection. Fatigue is common, days before and during a virus infection, whether it be a common upper respiratory tract infection, influenza, herpes simplex, herpes zoster or an unidentified virus. Using only nous and guesswork, a viral diagnosis will prove correct within a day or two. The problem is to differentiate trivial infections, from the more serious ones causing pneumonia, myocarditis, meningitis, and septicaemia.

Chronic, but active infections, like brucellosis, TB, Weil's disease, Lyme disease, and those with abscess formation, have long been known to cause fatigue. Now we can add chronic EB virus and COVID-19 infections to the list. All are easily missed.

Florence Nightingale suffered years of debilitating illness after returning from the Crimea. Many others who went there developed a similar condition, so it was named Crimean Fever. It is now thought she might have caught brucellosis from drinking unpasteurised milk. She was also a driven person – working day and night on her research, writing, and always engaged in projects to help others. It is reported that:

"She was full of self-doubt, manifesting low self-esteem, self-depreciation, and a sense of guilt. She also displayed narcissistic and obsessive-compulsive tendencies, and suffered from tormenting depression, religious hallucinations, and suicidal despair. Nightingale was an artful manipulator of people, and many of her achievements were only won through threats and subduing people to her will."

Rajabally, M. H. (1994)

In the same era, TB was rife. This caused prolonged fever and progressive weight loss. The young were most susceptible. Before the introduction of TB vaccination, those older people who were exposed to it when young, became immune.

Chronic hepatitis sometimes causes fatigue. Weil's disease is contracted by swimming in rivers polluted with the infected urine of rats. I saw only one case. Other forms of viral hepatitis, including hepatitis C, can all cause similar debility.

Lyme disease is caused by infected tick bites. Walking through fields where tick-infested deer or mice have roamed, presents a risk. It was first found in Lyme, Connecticut, USA. I once saw a woman who caught it on a walking holiday in France. Like syphilis and Weil's disease, it is also caused by a spirochete bacterium. Although the only case I found had positive Lyme disease test results, she was also suffering from being trapped in an unhappy marriage. The positive diagnosis allowed her an alternative, more acceptable, explanation for her demise.

Infectious agents are the cause of many chronic illnesses; some are known well only to specialist doctors. Tropical disease and fever medicine are specialist subjects. Some fatigued patients will need to be referred to such a specialist.

Post-Traumatic Stress Disorder (PTSD)

> The DSM-5 (Exhibit: 1.3-4). Diagnostic Criteria for PTSD (2014), defines the diagnosis.

PTSD occurs in some adults after a traumatic event, especially if exposed to the possibility of death, injury or violence. Repeated exposure is likely to occur in those employed in policing, the fire brigade or the armed forces.

The symptoms can include fatigue and disturbed sleep, with distressing dreams and daytime flashbacks. Other features are a defective memory, and feelings of negative self-worth, sometimes with persistent anger, fear, and guilt. Some reduced social involvement is a feature, as is the inability to feel closeness, happiness or satisfaction. Irritability, reckless behaviour, and startled responses are common. De-personalisation and de-realisation can occur to those who fail to engage with others.

Fatigue and exhaustion are associated with disturbed sleep. Fatigue is made worse by persistent negative thoughts, with fears and concerns related to adequacy and future security.

Menopause

The hormone changes associated with the female menopause commonly induce fatigue, even before the cessation of periods or hot flushes begin. Fatigue can be profound, and not always adequately reversed by hormone replacement therapy (HRT)(oestrogen and progesterone preparations). Some women will gain daytime energy if also given androgen supplementation. Many younger women suffer short-term fatigue and irritability when pre-menstrual.

Many menopausal women get tired and depressed. Some experience irritability, anxiety and panic attacks. Some will also have high blood pressure for the first time. Although these can be related to hormone changes, they might also relate to contemplating the end of their reproductive life. Many women will gain improved energy and well-being from HRT, with others helped by the addition of testosterone to their treatment regime.

Do men have a menopause? Could this account for a change of mood or reduced vitality experienced by some middle-aged men? Between the ages of 40 and 50 years-of-age, circumstances can change substantially for men. These changes are unrelated to their blood testosterone levels. Many come to view themselves as 'passed it' or 'on the way out'; less able to attract young women in the absence of fame or fortune. Their diminishing physical prowess and greying hair will depress some, but a source of pride for others. Depression (and stress) can be associated with reduced blood testosterone levels, and some men are revivified by testosterone implants.

Since a hormone alone cannot reverse social and ageing factors, boosting blood testosterone levels is unlikely to provide a magic bullet. Some men continue to have work stress, are unfit, have a changing role with age, and have less sexual stimulation. Both patients and doctors prefer quick and easy 'fixes', rather than attempt an understanding of the feelings and attitudes involved. Changing the causative situations is not a quick fix, but only by reversing evoking situations can real benefit ensue. After that is done, there is nothing wrong in trying a hormone for additional help.

Other Hormonal Conditions

The thyroid gland is partly responsible for our rate of metabolism (our mental state is also involved). If damaged (usually due to auto-immunity), the thyroid gland produces less hormone, and the whole body slows down. Lethargy, weight gain, feeling cold in warm weather, impotence, hair loss, and dry skin are the features of an underactive thyroid (hypo-thyroidism or myxoedema). The pulse usually slows as energy levels fail. This relatively common condition must be tested for in every patient with tiredness and fatigue. There are two thyroid hormones – T4 and T3 (the number indicates the number of inclusive iodine atoms in each molecule), and one pituitary driving hormone – TSH – thyroid stimulating hormone. All three need to be tested, although T4 deficiency will be more commonly found in Europe and the USA. The symptoms are quickly reversed by taking thyroxine (T4), sometimes with additional tri-iodothyronine (T3) medication if necessary.

Diabetes (ineffective or deficient insulin) can present with tiredness (diabetes fatigue syndrome), associated with hyper- or hypo-glycaemia (high and low glucose levels). Some with uncontrolled chronic diabetes, accommodate to hyperglycaemia without much tiredness.

Addison's disease is a rare cause of profound tiredness, restored completely by cortisone. A lack of adrenal cortisol hormone occurs in Addison's Disease. Once caused by tuberculosis, it's most frequent cause now is an auto-immune reaction (the body producing self-damaging antibodies). Fatigue is associated with weight loss, skin and mouth pigmentation, and low blood pressure. Symptoms may be corrected, but the condition is not cured by taking cortisone. The only patient I saw with it was able to control his energy by adjusting his cortisone dose. If he wanted to go to an all-night party, he would simply take an extra tablet. Since he only rarely did this, it had no long-term adverse effects.

To what extent cortisol variations contribute to normal levels of tiredness, I am not sure, but I would guess they are significant, since together with the hormone adrenaline, cortisol features in every bodily response to stress. These hormones have been referred to as the stress hormones.

Heart Failure

Heart failure is more prevalent and riskier than cancer.

> *"Heart failure is a debilitating and deadly syndrome that commonly occurs in those who have suffered high blood pressure over a long period of time and/or suffered a heart attack. As the term suggests, heart failure means that the heart is permanently damaged leading those who are affected to experience debilitating symptoms and remain at high risk of being hospitalised and/or suffer a premature death."*

European Society of Cardiology Congress (ESC). 2009.

One important symptom of heart failure is tiredness. A more relevant, important symptom is shortness of breath. Ankle swelling can occur, but is non-specific, being much more common in those who consistently sit for too long. Feeling breathless while lying down is a symptom of serious left heart failure. It must never be ignored and should be urgently investigated.

Since the heart and circulation exist to deliver oxygen and nutrients to each of our cells, it is hardly surprising that tiredness occurs when the heart fails to pump efficiently. It occurs as heart muscle ages or becomes weaker after many decades of high blood pressure. Heart muscle weakness can be inherited, but it's more usual cause is narrowed coronary arteries (for more information see my book: *'Heart-Smart'*).

Brain Biochemistry and Fatigue

> *Exhausted bees are quickly revived by giving them honey or glucose solution. Putting them onto a flower is better. They can then feed on nectar (Quinlan, G. et al. 2023). In humans, tiredness and fatigue are not so easily reversed.*

Brain glycogen (derived from glucose as a source of chemical energy) decreases in amount during memory tasks and with sleep deprivation. Exhausting exercise depletes both muscle and brain (astrocyte cell) glycogen. It is possible that both severe mental fatigue and physical fatigue, are associated with reduced brain cell glycogen.

Those debilitated by illness find physical activity challenging during their recovery. They become easily exhausted and breathless and can have fast heart rates after minimal effort. They will spend much more energy than normal, accomplishing simple tasks. This will hold back their rate of recovery. Following physical exercise, they can also feel mentally fatigued. Gaining physical fitness increases the ease of exercise, increases stamina and promotes vitality.

Age

Fatigue in those over 70-years of age, will depend on their daily physical routines and on their medical condition. In one study, 77% of those over 70-years old, reported fatigue. Other studies have supported a connection between physical activity and perceived energy. The relationship between physical activity and fatigue is bi-directional – that is, fatigue levels impact physical performance and *vice versa*. At all ages, there are mental health benefits to be had from exercise. Fatigue in older subjects is usually exercise dependent, so it will get worse with frailty and infirmity.

Premature ageing: a haggard, unkempt tired look, is quickly noticed by others, but rarely mentioned by the sufferer. Tiredness and exhaustion can arise from the demands of everyday life, and as such, attract little public sympathy. A notable exception arose when it appeared in the face of an exhausted, prematurely aged, American President.

> *"Two years elapsed between the Watergate break-in and President Nixon's final resignation. It must have been an intolerable burden for the man who had his finger on the button, as we say, but even before that, there had been signs of psychological strain, of his appearing depressed or incoherent in public, not to mention his tendency to develop clots in his veins, possibly at times of particular crisis."*

> *Beyond Endurance: Survival at the Extremes.*

> Glin Bennet

Glin Bennet's fascinating book is filled with numerous examples of mentally and physically exhausting situations, and how human beings have coped with them. What is much less appreciated is how personal, social, and medical disasters, occur every day to ordinary people – those simply trying to make ends meet; running a business or bringing up a family. Such daily disasters are not newsworthy. Editors are at liberty to ignore them. Their jobs demand they know how many care.

Causative Circumstances

In a society bereft of good Samaritans, who will take responsibility for those driven to exhaustion, many of whom have been rejected by their acquaintances, family, colleagues, bank managers, social services, the police – and I am ashamed to say – the medical profession.

> *I well remember a grandmother who developed pneumonia, after her son's marriage failed. She worried that she would never see her grandchildren again! Her depleted immunity – the result of ineffective sleep – combined with her inherited COPD, predisposed her to pneumonia. I admitted her to hospital and had to enlighten her son about what caused her demise. That it was partly his fault, came as a shock to him. Why had he not seen this for himself? Unfortunately, many are blinded by personal issues.*

When busy, we all have a natural tendency to see only the foreground – for physicians, the illness in question. Many will assume that the background is not their concern. Physicians are mostly caring people but can suffer from social factor blindness. Blind or otherwise, many will argue that a patient's background is neither their concern nor their field of expertise. In a clinical team, the practice nurse or ward sister may be the only one to take an interest.

Can any patient fully recover without a satisfactory resolution of pertinent social matters? The grandmother mentioned before was not depressed, just miserable and 'worried sick'. Following her pneumonia, she recovered fully, but only after being assured of seeing her grandchildren regularly. The description of chronic (meaning long-term) misery – rather than depression – would better fit cases like hers. Many who suffer fatigue, have no history of depression. Many depressed patients will, however, suffer fatigue. The features of fatigue and depression overlap, but can be differentiated (Balog, P. et al. 2017)(Kop, W. 2012).

Labels matter. Do the labels – depression, misery, 'flat battery', 'burn out', energy depletion syndrome or fatigue – matter? They do, for one simple reason. The wrong label can lead to inappropriate treatment. It is the excessive spending of mental energy, and its effects on sleep that determine fatigue, not the flattening of any battery or the burn-out of any biological system. These terms have led us up an intellectual *cul de sac,* all wrong in their conception.

Psychiatrists can use the diagnostic label – 'exogenous depression': depression arising from environmental circumstances. Potential danger lurks here. By labelling any complaint as a 'medical condition', it could be a disservice to the sufferer. He might come to think that all he needs is medical treatment, needing to take no responsibility for his circumstances. The chance of his recovery then remains remote. Inappropriate anti-depressive therapies could be offered. Although they can help sleep, they can also diminish coping ability and lead to hangovers. What is more often required for 'exogenous depression', is relief from the inducing circumstances, together with lots of refreshing sleep and relaxation.

Dietary Influence

Some mineral and vitamin supplement manufacturers inform us that calcium, magnesium, manganese, and selenium depletion in the diet, cause fatigue. If so, such depletion must be rare in the western world. The placebo effect of taking vitamins and minerals, means that at least 20% of those taking them, will report improved well-being.

Real relief from fatigue is more likely to occur with stress relief and exercise, with dietary adjustment a minor issue. Obesity is a major cause of tiredness and fatigue, simply because it consumes extra energy, and restricts exercise ability – a major factor in achieving the improved energy status many seek.

Vitamin B6 (from poultry, pork, some fish, oats, and wheat germ) is a known co-factor in the production of one neurotransmitter – GABA (gamma aminobutyric acid). Taken in excess, it can relieve anxiety and reduce responses to stress (Duranni, D., Idress, R., et al. 2022). B6 deficiency, however, is rare in western countries where protein deficiency is uncommon. Its deficiency is most unlikely to be relevant to any tired adult in the western world, although in some deprived parts of the world, it can cause tiredness and confusion in adults and seizures in infants.

Therapeutic Causes

The job of some drugs, like tranquillizers and anti-depressants, is to reduce the aroused state. Some tiredness as a side-effect is almost unavoidable. The same happens with some older types of anti-histamine, and pain-killing opiate-like drugs (fentanyl, tramadol). Patients report tiredness as a side effect of many other therapeutic drugs. Some, like the beta-blocker propranolol, can cause fatigue by disturbing sleep – inducing vivid dreaming during REM sleep.

A lot of individual variation is in play. Patients should always check the drug information that accompanies their medication, especially if they operate machinery or wish to drive. Most patients are aware of the many adverse effects of drugs. Some will stop them, contrary to medical advice; others will request a change. Many patients quickly come to know the side-effects of their drugs; often better than doctors appreciate. The individual variance in patient responsiveness to drugs is so great, no doctor can say with certainty – 'this drug doesn't do that', (meaning, 'not supposed to').

Recognising Fatigue in Others

All doctors, nurses, paramedics and care workers, should be able to recognise tiredness of all degrees. They need to be alert to the fact that it may be associated with dangerous levels of high blood pressure, cardiac ischaemia (not enough blood getting to heart muscle), cerebral ischaemia (not enough blood getting to the brain), hormonal disturbance, depression and infection.

Tiredness is always associated with mental inefficiency: a defective memory, poor concentration, dithering while making decisions, reduced patience and irritability and a failing sense of humour. These signs worsen as tiredness progresses through fatigue to exhaustion.

Many fatigued subjects will robustly deny such changes. Many suffering unavoidable relationships will choose to suffer them and not mention them. The symptoms need not be urgent, unless important decisions need to be taken. They might then portray knight's move thinking – jumping to whatever conclusion takes their fancy at the time – just to reduce further energy spending. Holding incorrect assumptions is common, as is being unduly biased and not using common-sense. Tiredness can divert our attention from important issues, making our decision making unreliable. Unfortunately, only close friends and relatives, may be party to such behavioural changes.

Rest, relaxation and sleep, may need to be enforced by using sedative drugs. Occasionally they can be life-saving. Doctors who are traditionally interested only in physically related signs and symptoms, might only suggest pills to lower the blood pressure, (which may not work well if the patient is exhausted); pills to relieve angina (which can make the patient feel worse) or headache pills for migraine (which do nothing to alleviate the antecedent causes), rather than aim to treat the patient's fatigue or exhaustion.

Rehabilitation

The chronic fatigue that occurs with unrelenting stress or post-viral fatigue syndrome, can continue for months or years. Depression and apathy can be reasons, but the continuing need for the close attention of a partner, mother or child, can also prolong the condition.

Once recovering, difficulty will lie in overcoming any apathy and unfitness. Only by being pushed out of their rut, will some decide to leave ill-health behind. Those who are unfit and ill, easily get stuck. It can become a Catch-22 situation. Because they are unwell, they may not be able to exercise; being unable to exercise, they will be less able to overturn their medical condition.

The job of convalescence and rehabilitation is an expert one. Rest is an invaluable element of recovery after every illness but must not be too protracted. When the time is right for training, the patient can slowly gain strength from it, although, often relapsing at times. If undertaken too early, training can cause regression into a weakened state. The 'trainer' has to be strong enough to counter any resistance to improvement and encouraging enough to inspire progress. Patients without much personal discipline will take longer to return to normal. Those intolerant of an unhealthy body image, will make faster progress.

The potential for recovery will be linked to the cause of demise. If the patient has been worn down by an unhappy marital situation, only by addressing reconciliation or resolution, will the patient want to push for fitness. If his prospect is to return to the unaltered situation, his motivation and commitment could dissolve. Only once all the socioeconomic and relationship problems have been resolved, will full recovery be possible.

It's a pity that some must get ill, before they are prompted to understand the unhealthy nature of their lifestyle. Wisdom is usually gained only by marinating knowledge in the flavours of meaningful experience.

When the author and playwright, Rex Edwards, had a heart attack, he became determined to find out why. What mistakes had led to his demise? He found it incredulous that the eggs and butter he had eaten (the prevailing theory in the 1970s), could be the cause. He found that nobody would guarantee his escape from another heart attack, unless he stopped eating them. In the end, he concluded that his heart attack had much more to do with his long-term frustration and overwork, than the food he had eaten.

He recognised the exhaustion he had before catastrophe struck. He took the heart attack as an opportunity to learn, eventually deciding never to overwork again. Only after that realisation, did he feel it worthwhile to rehabilitate himself back to health. In his book, *'A Coronary Case'*, he details his quest for answers and the methods he used for rehabilitation.

Apart for the lost or fugitive, illness always involves several people – either as leading characters or those playing an anonymous role. Quite often, the players involved will not understand their contribution. They can be involved positively, neutrally or negatively; they might have created situations that caused the illness or promoted its progression. Others might promote a cure, fostering successful rehabilitation. Every patient's condition needs to be viewed as part of their personal circumstances. Only from this perspective can appropriate management be planned.

CHAPTER THIRTEEN

Ill-health, Disease and Medical Catastrophe

It is in the nature of all things to remain unaltered for ages, and then to change suddenly – sometimes catastrophically. The suddenness of change is real, but the idea that all catastrophic events 'come out-of-the-blue' is an illusion. This comes from our failure to notice the small changes that will bring us step by step closer to a cliff-edge – a place where falls can happen.

Technological advance can seem to happen overnight, but it always takes time to develop a new idea or invention. By contrast, the benefits and disadvantages of progress are always gradual. The introduction of the internet and email took time, as did the removal of physical libraries, telegrams, and fax machines. The introduction of robots and AI have already caused job losses, with many more to come. The adaptive processes in the film industry took decades to develop, but the showing of one film, changed film entertainment overnight. 'The Jazz Singer' (1927), introduced film with sound for the first time, and at once, the expectation of audiences changed forever. Will the return supersonic travel and the use of quantum computers benefit us quite so quickly?

Medical Catastrophe

Many doctors enjoy emergencies. Could that be why some are not keen to prevent them? That seems unfairly cynical, but is it?

Doctor A: *"What's your problem Mr. Kenny?"*

Mr. Kenny: *"I was just sitting quietly at home, when I had this sudden, terrible pain in my chest. I don't understand where it came from. It just happened 'out of the blue'."*

Doctor A: *"I am afraid you've had a heart attack, Mr Kenny.*

Mr. Kenny: *"But how is that possible? I have always been so well!*

Doctor A: *"If an obstructive clot forms in a heart artery (coronary thrombosis), blood might not get through. A small piece of your heart muscle can get damaged as a result. That's a heart attack. We'll give you treatment, and you'll be OK. Just relax and take it easy!"*

That's usually as far as any explanation will go. But is this explanation satisfactory? It might sound so, until one starts to think about how this could come about. Not every patient is disposed to ask further questions. I wonder if the desire to ask them, is commoner amongst potential survivors. Survivors need to know why they failed, in order to prevent repeated failure.

Doctors motivated to prevent disease must know about the many progenitors of medical catastrophe. They might ask, when was the patient last well? What circumstances might have contributed to their demise, and are they still pertinent to their recovery and rehabilitation? Might another attack (perhaps to be the last) be prevented? To get reliable information, he might choose to interview the patient's spouse, children, and even work mates. The doctor should be a detective – in relentless pursuit of the truth and understanding.

Not every physician has an interest in preventative medicine, especially if overburdened by a workload of established disease. Not every physician needs an interest in the social and psychological factors affecting disease onset and progress. Unfortunately, many in the past, have had little inclination. Their role demands they focus on physical disease, even if they might want to engage with patients as whole sentient beings. Most doctors are fascinated by physical disease, a fact pre-empted by choosing medical students whose grasp of biology and the physical sciences has been proven.

Patients are the ones who most need to be concerned about survival. They alone have the ultimate responsibility for their fate. Each should ask some vital questions like, 'Why did I have a heart attack? What can I do to prevent another? The answer they get must first be centred on interventions of statistically proven benefit, like taking anticoagulants, statin drugs, stent deployment and coronary bypass. Only rarely, will personal issues get considered alongside statistical acceptable considerations. The medical profession has defined its role and has successfully left personal enquiry behind.

Anyone wishing to look further, should read Rex Edward's' book, *A Coronary Case*. He claimed to have discovered the truth about why he had a heart attack. When I met him fourteen years after his heart attack in the 1970s, he had had no further attacks – anecdotal evidence at least, for his having found some useful truths. Although not the same as universal truth, it might provide a useful clue. Since he wrote his book in 1964, there has been very little shift in what doctors believe about heart attacks. Many continue to believe that diet (high intake of cholesterol and saturated fat), is more important than fear, worry, bereavement or divorce. That is convenient, because few doctors want to consider such personal matters.

Let's return to Mr. Kenny, with another doctor who has a broader interest in him as a person. He interviews Mrs. Kenny, for some further insight.

Doctor B: "How long has Bill not been quite himself, Mrs Kenny?"

Mrs Kenny: *"Since you ask doctor, it's been a long time really. At home, we have had a difficult time with him. Our teenage girls mustn't say anything about going out in the evening. That just makes him angry. He says they don't understand the dangers. He has been incredibly irritable for some time.*

Doctor B: "Has he been tired at all?"

Mrs Kenny: *"Exhausted, more like. Tired all the time. Falling asleep watching the TV in the evenings.*

Doctor B: "For how long has he been tired and irritable?"

Mrs Kenny: *"About a year really."*

Doctor B: "Have you noticed anything else?"

Mrs Kenny: *"Yes. About six months ago, he started to look much older and started to forget many things. It's worse when he's had a bad day at the office. That's the trouble really. About 18-months ago, he thought his partner was double-crossing him. It all blew up the week before his heart attack. He finally faced his partner with the facts, and the police were brought in. He hadn't actually slept well for a year. I'm glad he's had a heart attack. It might make him rest. You will tell him to rest, won't you doctor. He won't listen to me!"*

Doctor B: "Are his business problems over now?"

Mrs Kenny: *"Not quite. His partner has yet to appear in court. At least he has admitted his guilt. Without him, there's extra work to do at the office, although our manager and I can do all that. Our customers have been wonderful. Very supportive. Many were worried about him – noticing the changes in him. We can sort it out. It will be difficult, but everything will be all right in the end. If only he had faced up to his partner a year ago, when he discovered some evidence of fraud, none of this would have happened. Instead he got more and more stressed but took no action."*

Doctor B: "You must protect him in future. If you see him changing again – not sleeping, and becoming irritable, let me know. Don't wait for chest pain to come. I would sooner waste my time checking a normal person, than treating a heart attack."

Mrs Kenny: *"I'd sooner that too."*

Timidity and meekness often underlie human catastrophe. After the event, many become ashamed of their indecisiveness or their tardiness in making a decision. This can make interviewing third parties useful.

Some doctors will regard this approach as interfering, perhaps unethical; 'none of their business!' I understand their point of view, and respect it, because not everyone can be expected to have an interest in the psychosocial, humane components of disease. If preventing disease is not their mission, their disinterest is understandable. Individual patients and doctors are not always best suited to one another.

Those patients who have sustained a medical catastrophe, such as a heart attack or stroke, should recognise which doctors have an interest in prevention. They should not allow meekness and timidity to stand in their way – their life could depend on it.

Experts of all sorts are now being scrutinised and handled with suspicion by the public. Until a patient has cross-questioned the expert advising them, and understands where their expertise lies, they should not assume they know enough to help them.

Is Stress Always the Cause of Heart Attacks?

It would be easy to give the wrong impression about the cause of heart attacks. It is true they are caused by coronary artery blockage, but not true that tiredness always precedes them or that adverse life situations are always a dominant factor. Many people are unlucky enough to have inherited the progressive 'furring' of their arteries (atherosclerosis). In time, many of them are likely to sustain an artery blockage somewhere – the result of inner arterial changes, as well as changes in blood biochemistry (like increased blood coagulability). It can be difficult to exclude personal circumstances and psychological factors, but they should always be scrutinised and put into perspective. By doing so, surprising facts will often emerge that could help with clinical management and future prevention.

Order and Catastrophe

Many try to confer order on life, whether it's tidying-up after their children or tying their shoe laces. Nature isn't tidy. Left untended, everything becomes disorderly. Unfortunately, few have enough personal energy to maintain their environment in perfect working order. The obsessive neurotics among us will try the hardest. There is some sense to it, since unattended systems tend to change suddenly. Suddenly, a pile of books will topple over; plates and cups will unexpectedly fall out of an overstuffed cupboard. Although all these events are catastrophic (if only in a mathematical sense), few will be life-threatening.

Many choose to keep their car in running order but will ignore their body. Is this why more people call on doctors than on emergency motoring organisations? Those who care too little for their car, can end up stranded with no water in their radiator, no petrol in their fuel tank or a flat battery. Those who take too little for their body, might first attend hospital with a heart attack, stroke or advanced cancer. Doctors as patients themselves, are common among them.

The Seeds of Catastrophe

One of the objects of science is to make the future predictable (through an understanding of how natural systems work). Predicting the next big Californian earthquake, and knowing when a heart attack is imminent, would advantage many. At the domestic level, all we need is vigilance to prevent our bath overflowing or stop our bank account going into unarranged overdraft. Predicting heart attacks and earthquakes takes a little more science.

Catastrophe can occur when a system is bi-stable. That is, two states of existence are possible – unchanged and stable or altered and possibly broken. All it takes is one small stimulus to change a precarious state into a catastrophic one. One minute you could be standing on a cliff edge. After taking one small step forward, you could be at the bottom of the cliff in pieces (but only if the cliff is high enough). One archaic idiom of Biblical origin is apt – it takes only one straw to break a camel's back. Some situations are one-way only.

There are electrical circuits that flip back and forth, from one state to another. This is a two-way catastrophic phenomenon. The pacemaker function of the heart serves as an example.

No catastrophic event occurs 'out-of-the-blue', although it may seem like it. The Wall Street crash of October 1929 in the USA; the overflowing of a bath and the fall from a cliff, might all have been predicted if enough relevant information had been known beforehand. Unfortunately, few will bother to enquire beforehand. Not everyone looks before they leap.

In the case of any cliff, it is always unwise to approach the edge without support. Those who sail boats need to be aware of the prevailing wind speeds and their direction; they could otherwise be at risk of keeling over. Those holding shares in any stock, need to be as well informed financially as they can be, aware of any adverse economic warning signs.

In the 1920s, Joe Kennedy was once given stock tips by his shoe-shine boy. He returned to his office and placed orders to sell all of his shares. That was just prior to the Wall St. stock market crash. His thinking was simple. If buying shares is so popular, it must be a good time to sell.

In the case of heart attacks, some patients will experience a period of increasing tiredness, fatigue and exhaustion, before their eventual sudden demise. I have tried, in writing my book *Heart-Sense*, to make more people aware of this.

When our temper runs out, after having been tortured, teased or pushed around, the situation can quickly change – we can become bi-stable. Calm can quickly change to rage. The result – road rage, baby-battering, wife-beating, murder or suicide. Like elastic, our temper will take only so much stretch before it snaps. These catastrophic phenomena can all be prevented, although not necessarily with ease. One problem is – many see prevention before an event, as boring or uninteresting. It is perhaps seen as 'worrying too much' or 'being too pessimistic'.

Life is not possible without taking risks. Unfortunately, assessing the risk of situations is something only a few consider. Everyone can appreciate the need after an adverse event. Life has always been a minefield, littered with unseen IEDs. Without being able to predict the future, all we can do is use intelligent planning, undertake surveillance, and try to calculate the risks and benefits. Lucky people have an advantage.

Who would walk through a minefield without a map, knowing that a map was available? Those who wish to appear macho, brave, and irreverent of risk are likely candidates. Many get away with it and get away with it often. They are the ones who regard caution as neurotic.

The most important counterparts of assessing risk are luck and statistics. With luck, you can beat the odds; without it, the statistics will beat you. To tell someone that their chance of surviving a minefield is 100 to one, is to tell them that it is unlikely. Some ignore this, and will go ahead anyway, regarding the risk as 50:50 – in other words, they *may* or *may* not survive.

A few British and Commonwealth battle survivors have been awarded the Victoria Cross when their feats of bravery went beyond the call of duty; often in complete deference to the odds of success. In so doing, they raised the honour and aspirations of other fighting men. At the opposite end of the spectrum are those who catastrophise unnecessarily, always thinking the worst. They will visualise that their end is nigh, and when they do arrive safely, it will only be by God's grace. This degree of anxious neuroticism or fear of death in quite ordinary circumstances, can make life unbearable. The problem we have with 24/7 newscasts, is inducing fear fuelled by many anecdotal examples of catastrophe.

In 1985, an Air India flight disintegrated in mid-air, 120 miles south-west of Shannon. This fuelled the anxiety of every fearful flyer the world over; their worst fears became tangible. Three hundred and seven passengers, and 22 crew, fell 31,000 feet into the Atlantic Ocean. At that altitude, most would have died once they hit the cold thin air. Within hours of the disaster, the Sikh Students Federation, the Dashmesh Regiment, and the Kashmir Liberation

Army claimed responsibility. A suitcase bomb was thought responsible.

In July 2025, another Air India flight crashed soon after take-off from Ahmedabad. Two-hundred and sixty died in all. Somehow, both fuel switches became turned off. For many, this will have further magnified their fear of flying.

In 1984, Jim Fixx, aged 52-years – the man accredited with 'inventing' jogging, died during his daily jog. This was two years after a divorce. He had run 80-miles each week for 15-years prior to his death. In 1978, he wrote a book, 'The Complete Book of Running', which earned him more than one million US dollars.

He was found dead on the roadside, outside the Vermont mountain town of Hardwick, dressed only in running shorts. His second wife said his doctors had found him to have serious heart disease. She had urged him to have regular medical check-ups, but he was negligent and rarely went to his doctor.

One can speculate about what happened to Jim Fixx. He most likely had gradually developing, narrowed coronary arteries, well before his heart attack. Then, in an instant, a cholesterol plaque within the artery might have ruptured. This would have attracted clot, causing all blood flow to stop. That would have damaged his heart tissue and perhaps incited a sudden, fatal rhythm disorder – ventricular fibrillation. This would have brought his effective heart pumping action to a halt.

Having been diagnosed with coronary heart disease, I doubt he was warned about the dangers of extreme exercise. So, did he run in the face of danger? After all, it was exercise that helped him change from an unfit overweight man (95+ kilograms), smoking 40 cigarettes daily, into an athlete. One could, of course, argue that his running had kept him alive, and that he knew best. A life of inactivity and without exercise discipline, might have been too great a price for him to pay. It is one thing to have catastrophe thrust upon us, without prior knowledge, and another to chance a catastrophic event once it has been predicted.

The Benefits of Catastrophe

Many of us have experienced one minor, transient, but impressive cardiovascular catastrophe – a faint (vasomotor syncope) – a blackout due to low blood pressure, with not enough blood reaching the brain. The sight of blood, witnessing an accident, being in pain, standing for a long period packed into a hot train, can all induce a faint. But what purpose does it serve?

Fainting results from reflex changes in the body that lower blood pressure and slow the pulse at the same time. Reducing blood flow to the brain causes failing consciousness. All of our physical activity stops during a faint. We save energy while unaware of our situation. Without the intervention of ill-informed bystanders, whose first inclination is often to sit the victim upright and pour brandy or warm sweet tea down their throat (risking asphyxiation), many will find themselves in a prone position. Left to their own devices, many subjects will collapse to the floor, with their head at the same height as their heart. Blood will then more easily flow to the head and brain, and consciousness should return. Escape from an unpleasant situation has been achieved – at least temporarily.

Mrs. Cohen was a Yiddish speaking, older patient, with a poor command of English. She had experienced multiple faints. Two professors of medicine failed to find any cause. Both admitted some communication difficulty. One of them decided to refer her to me for heart reflex testing. I too, found nothing wrong with her physically.

Those working in medical centres of scientific excellence, are not always inclined to ask patients what they think has caused their problems. On this occasion, my use of this question, solved the mystery.

"It's shame that's making me collapse" she said. "My son left his wife and my four grandchildren. He has run-off with a girl in his office. I shall continue to collapse until he does his duty and returns to his family. It's shame that's making me collapse!"

This begged some questions. Can stress lower our threshold for fainting? Technically, can it affect our cardiac reflexes enough to make low and high blood pressure more likely? It had to conclude that it must.

During wartime, soldiers injured in action seemed capable of walking to safety, despite horrendous injuries. At the first sight of help – a Red Cross tent in the distance – they would collapse, unable to take another step. Del Boy (of Fools and Horses fame), collapsed once he realised that the watch he had found was far from worthless, and was being sold for millions of pounds. The shock caused him to fall backwards. This is but a famous comedy sketch, but it can happen.

When one partner in a close relationship suffers from a prolonged illness, the other partner will usually find the strength to cope. If the health of the sick partner returns, the helper will then risk collapse – something they were unable to do while needed. In this way, ill-health and illness can alternate between partners. Only by getting both well at the same time is it possible to break the circle of alternating illness.

Each collapse can be seen as a medical catastrophe – a sudden change from being able to cope, to not coping – caused by stress. A 'collapse' can take various forms: pneumonia, acute agitation, shell-shock, psychosis, acute migraine, a fractured leg or heart attack Whichever it is, it will successfully inhibit the need for further coping.

This world has witnessed many catastrophes, but none so great as one in pre-history. It is supposed that a large meteorite strike,

65-million years ago at the end of the mesozoic era, extinguished 96% of all species. Mice, insects, some plants and our human forebears survived. What actually occurred remains the subject of debate. One explanation is that the earth was struck by a massive meteor, causing the skies to darken under the subsequent dust cloud. Reduced sunlight from masses of volcanic ash and dust, could have caused the large-scale extinction of plants and plant-dependent life. The herbivore dinosaurs died first; the extinction of large carnivorous dinosaurs then followed.

Thinking of what might happen next can remain a subliminal stress or be an active one, slowly draining the energy of some people.

CHAPTER FOURTEEN

Unlocking Energy: Rest, Sleep. and Traffic Analysis

"And sleep that sometime shuts up sorrow's eye, Steal me awhile from mine own company." Helena. *A Midsummer Night's Dream: Act 111. Scene 11.* William Shakespeare.

Sleep and Rest

Our brain is always switched on, even during peaceful, untroubled sleep. In the background, the brain controls breathing, and affects heart activity, hormone production, sweating and bowel activity. While asleep, we can build energy reserve chemicals like glycogen as well as neuro-transmitters, with the generation of high-energy chemicals like ATP, continuously produced and in infinite supply. Some believe that the fluid bathing the brain clears away waste products during sleep – some like Tau protein are thought to cause dementia. Poor sleep might cause a build up of these waste products and contribute to daytime tiredness.

During the day, brain activity will progressively cause many of our neuronal channels to block, causing tiredness. It is the opening of these neuronal channels during restful (slow-wave) sleep that restores our energy, ready for the next day. City traffic forms an accurate analogy. During the day, voluminous traffic will block the roads. During the night, traffic flow diminishes, and roads unblock, ready for use next day.

If these concepts about waking and sleep function are new to you, you might want more detailed clarification. For this, read my more technical book—*Tiredness, Chronic Fatigue and Exhaustion: Neurophysiology and Cardiovascular Risk.*

During peaceful periods of relaxation, meditation and non-REM sleep, our brains 'tick over', spending minimal amounts of energy. During REM or dreaming sleep, we spend lots of energy – almost as much as when awake. This active phase of sleep is often associated with a rapid pulse, and a raised blood pressure – the same as being stressed. Dreaming sleep perhaps affords us time to 'think-through' current and future scenarios, perhaps to find solutions to vexing problems. Through dreaming, we might achieve some psychological adjustment. Through the more relaxed, non-REM sleep (slow-wave sleep), which alternates with dreaming sleep, the unblocking of neuronal channels should allow us to awaken refreshed, ready for the next day's cognitive action.

Contrary to popular belief, reinforced by advertising, morning energy does not come immediately from consuming breakfast cereals, vitamins or medicinal tonics. The now old-fashioned Wincarnis tonic wine, claimed to cure 'brain-fag' and to act as a 'nerve restorative'. It also claimed to be effective for depression, sleeplessness, and 'mental prostration'. At one time, 10,000 doctors recommended it (loiselsden.com/2015/03/10/tonic-wine/). Boosting vital energy with vitamins, minerals, omega-3 oils and fresh air, will perhaps work a little for those who believe in them. Many are desperate to enliven their spirits. Here is a secret that can help make it happen – take some active physical exertion, followed by undisturbed, peaceful sleep.

One vitamin – vitamin B6 – is involved in the synthesis of the neurotransmitter glutamate. It has long been prescribed by doctors for neuropathy and other nervous system problems. Might it help with neuronal unblocking and energy release? It is harmless, but is that good enough reason to try it?

Similar replenishing activity often goes on in factories at night. The night staff have time to re-stock items needed on the shop floor, ready for the following day. At night, the batteries of fork-lift trucks are plugged in for recharging. This occurs while the day staff are sleeping and readying themselves another day's work. This analogy is not applicable to the brain, since we have no need to recharge or replenish. More than enough brain energy is always available in neurones (brain cells). If we were to run short of cellular energy at any time, we would be reduced to a fragile state, constantly at risk of death.

Because evolution favours the fittest, those species still in existence, must have overcome their need to create, store, and discharge energy as required. Animals and humans have thus developed a system that will create chemical energy instantly and in abundance, available to each cell, all of the time. Depleted chemical energy storage cannot, therefore, explain normal tiredness. The blocking of brain cell channels (neuronal pathways) by daily cerebral activity, is a much more likely. These channels are re-opened only during minimal energy spending states – non-REM sleep, meditation, relaxation, and to some extent, sporting activity.

Perceived Energy Gain

Exhilarating situations boost our perceived energy. For most of us, such moments are infrequent. A roller-coaster ride; finding someone we feel attracted to or holding your newborn baby for

the first time are all invigorating. But where does this boosted
energy come from? Could the feeling of energy release come from
brain transmitter chemicals like serotonin and dopamine, from
endorphins or from hormones like adrenaline and cortisol? It is
likely they all are involved together.

Proud moments with raised self-esteem; winning and achieving
success, will all do it, especially if the unexpected has been accomplished. These moments are often attended by excited vitality; our
cup of joy seeming to spill over. At these times, anxiety, conflicts,
frustrations, and unhappiness, will all be replaced by the feelgood
factor. Many chase such moments, hoping they might continue
for ever. Those who fail in this quest, might turn to drugs like
amphetamine and cocaine.

Gymnasium training; finishing the final paper of college examinations; sharing a laugh and a joke with close friends, can all carry
us on a train of energy flow that makes us feel complete, healthy,
energetic, vital, and simply glad to be alive.

Exhilaration can be viewed in many ways. Some prefer the poetic
and romantic; others, the scientific. Although the feelings and
essence of poetry and literature, come from brain chemistry and
neurophysiological activity, few will have any desire to understand
the underlying science. After all, we humans have survived for
millennia on romance and poetry alone, without scientific insight.

'All Shook Up'

Elvis Presley appeared to age prematurely. He seemed to deteriorate physically, on a downward spiral of drug use – combining
'uppers' with 'downers'. The illusion of super energy he once portrayed, had to come to an end. He possibly died from the effects
of drugs and exhaustion. Although it feels good, exhilaration (expressed in one of Elvis' songs – 'All Shook Up') spends energy
by the bucketful. Unfortunately, it cannot arise without having

periods of calm detachment, effective sleep and exercise. I have not included diet in this list; food being more often soporific than exhilarating. Although our diet provides the substrates we need for cellular, high-energy, chemical production, our diet is many steps away from influencing our perceived energy levels.

After exhilarating activity, most of us will sleep well, with beneficial effects that may last for days. As we grow older, moments of glory can be relived; even whole families can benefit from reflected glory.

Experiencing exhilaration is worthy energy expenditure: 'what life is all about', some might say. When you spend energy like this, you are living to the full. Those who have never experienced exhilaration or fascination, passion and drive, have not experienced life to the full. Many must content themselves by replacing any peaks of exhilaration and success, with promoting their status or earning more money, readying themselves for the day when they too can have some fun and enjoy themselves! Few will achieve it, many working harder and longer to pay for their mounting living expenses and taxes. Unfortunately, world insecurity is growing. We now live with many growing threats, one of which is the threat of jobs lost to technology.

Energy Saving

The only way we can save our energy is to reduce our mental and physical energy expenditure.

Achieving dominance over others, can save us spending our own personal energy. Those who create demands in shops, more often get what they want. They usually get it quicker than others, and with fewer complications. Most shop staff will recognise the no-nonsense, assertive customer. They are likely to react quickly to save themselves humiliation and embarrassment. They will either quickly satisfy the customer or delegate the task to someone more competent. The uncompromising customer knows exactly what she wants, and often gets it. My co-worker Noreen Connolly had the perfect question for any agitator found in my practice: 'What must I do to make you happy?' she asked. Strangely, few had an answer. Do agitators simply enjoy agitating others? It could be that their only source of self-esteem comes from their successful domination of those around them.

The softer, compromising 'nice guys', can get overlooked. They risk being ignored while more dominant customers get all the attention. The nice guy could feel unexpressed anger or frustration but must learn to deal with it. He might be told to come back later, go for a walk, ring back or even be dismissed until a manager (or someone who really knows what they are doing), returns from lunch. At this stage, the nice guy could start to regret his character, especially in the face of objectionable, frequently successful, dominant people. He may regret not being like them. Any resentment could lead to his anger and aggression (usually with somebody he doesn't fear) – his wife, children or subordinates at work.

There are, however, truly nice guys who genuinely have lots of patience and time. They are rare but do exist. I have met three in 50-years! Most despise dominant behaviour so much, they would never want to emulate it. From their standpoint, dominant characters burn energy unnecessarily. Who, therefore, is the more efficient? Is it the nice guy or the dominant character? Given the amount of energy spent, the dominant character may be the more efficient – if he achieves what he wants quickly and without wasting time. In addition, he may get a degree of elation from his success. The nice guy is often uncomplicated and can enjoy life – happy to be an amused observer; untroubled and taking it easy. While achievement may be the dominant person's only objective, the enjoyment of 'being' can elude them. 'Being', rather than achieving, will content the nice guy more.

Travel is a superb, but expensive form of education. It allows us the opportunity to meet those with different lifestyles, practiced at spending and conserving their energy. While visiting different cultures, we have the opportunity to observe the whole spectrum of human behaviour and activity.

Many object to cultural generalisations; they will lead to false opinions about some individuals. I regard them as useful presumptions, held before getting modified by experience. Take one naive generalisation – that all tigers are dangerous. This does no justice to edentulous tigers without claws. Assuming this, will usually be lifesaving when approaching tigers in the wild. The generalisation that all Scots are frugal, will have many exceptions. If you loosely assume it to be true until proven otherwise, you will find the presumption useful on a daily basis.

Strongly held, bigoted generalisations, can have social consequences. They can be unduly biased for the wrong reasons, and usually lack much supporting evidence. Some people are not given to relinquish their views, even when faced with reliable evidence to the contrary. Charlie Kirk was shot and killed for no good reason in 2025. He was adept at exposing people with false assumptions. He chose to debate those who disagreed with him, easily exposing the frail basis for their strongly held beliefs. When human rights are affected, the bigoted holder of a generalisation can be dangerous. Although the stuff of racism, this should not displace the fact that generalisation can hold useful validity.

The ability to generalise in an evidence-based way, is a gift that can aid survival. It enables one to identify dangerous elephants – even if they are invisible but filling the room - and even if pink or white. Our minds can use generalisation to identify possible dangers. Using the generalisation process, enables us to see the wood for the trees. If what we are told does not fit our idea of generalised truth, suspect inaccuracy and misleading or false information. In the absence of confirmatory, objectively obtained evidence, a generalisation may be all we have to rely on to make decisions.

The Holiday Effect

The point of some holidays is to spend less energy and become revitalised. Any need for assertive behaviour usually arises at the start of a holiday. The booking and travel tickets may be incorrect. There may be no alternative flights; the airport may have become non-functioning; the wrong hotel may have been booked or the booked hotel may be over-booked and have no rooms. Couples who have not known one another for long, will be exposed to more than they anticipate. Bad weather can throw them together, with previously unnoticed behaviour, causing unexpected conflict. With so many opportunities for frustration and high-energy spending, holidays can become a major source of stress.

> *Warren Buffett has for decades been one of the world's richest men. He owns a private jet company. He once declared one luxury he enjoys – not having to queue at airports.*

Obvious to most travellers is that different nations have distinctly different cultures. They will hold distinct values and behave differently. They may differ in friendliness, approachability, acceptance of others, and helpfulness. They will vary in their sense of humour and affability. They will vary in how they value time, money and family. All cultures naturally include pleasant and unpleasant characters, but there is often a general demeanour that becomes apparent soon after arrival. Despite our culture, we all share more similarities than differences.

To what extent we are pure Homo sapiens or a mixture of other human species, is not usually known or discussed. We do know that many of us harbour some Neanderthal genes within our genome. That could partly account for different physical appearances, and our values, beliefs and outlook that differ. Evolution cannot be transgressed for long, but it does require us to survive for at least eighteen years (in western societies) – before we can legally procreate and go on to produce further generations – to assure the survival of our species.

The other factors influencing survival, relate to our need to adapt. First to climate. Cold climates need strategies for survival not needed in hot climates. Climate will have affected cultural development. Those in hot climates could roam free, but those living in cold climates must once have needed to huddle together. This suggests that affability and togetherness might have been favoured by cold climate survivors. In addition, they would have needed the skill to light fires and make warm clothes.

In hot climates there are different dangers. Scorpions, deadly snakes, lions and tigers. These roam more in hot climates than in cold ones. Being able to out-smart them, with an ability to stalk and kill them, would have been a great advantage. Separate cultural attitudes must thus have evolved.

The circumstances experienced by immigrants to a new country will challenge them. Having signed up to work as a cardiologist in Holland, I made an assumption – that there would be no significant cultural differences between me and Dutch people. The differences were small, but some I needed to adapt to.

The Dutch I came to know, had a more Teutonic attitude to work and money than me. I regarded rules as guidelines for discussion;

they took rules to be immutable. Some thought that honour was old-fashioned and negotiable. They regarded us reclaiming   the Falkland Islands as pointless. 'What's the point?', they asked. 'It's a matter of duty and honour', I replied.

> *I once ask one of my colleagues to image a scenario where a decision had to be made. Imagine standing in front of a very long, wide patch of grass. A boy is struggling in the sea beyond, but on the grass in front of you is a sign: 'DO NOT WALK ON THE GRASS'. The question is, what will you do. My Dutch colleagues were torn between obeying the written rule and saving the boy's life. I was not.*

I asked my Dutch accountant to declare my share of some private earnings, made in our cardiac department. Having no mortgage in Holland and no other legitimate business expenses, I assumed I could not claim tax relief. 'Do you have a mortgage in the UK?', he asked. I asked if that was of relevant. He told me that Dutch law states: 'If you have a mortgage, you can get tax relief.' 'Yes, but, how can that apply here?' I asked. 'Let me repeat myself', he said. 'Our law states – if you have a mortgage, you can get tax relief. There is no mention of where it originates!' Another cultural lesson learned.

What you will find in the tropical Caribbean, is often a 'take it easy attitude'. Having travelled extensively through the Caribbean islands, from St. Thomas to Trinidad, I found this attitude as endearing as the weather and scenery – both relaxing and infectious. Many active, 'ready to get up and go' westerners, some demanding instant self-gratification, could find Caribbean attitudes challenging.

Don't expect western, speedy service in the Caribbean. Taking time is an advantage they like to preserve. Shop assistants won't be rushed; in any case, they are not easily perturbed by time-urgent holidaymakers. They have a way of handling fretful, impatience visitors – they smile and giggle openly. I have seen some newly arrived tourists get furious. For the Caribbean-adjusted, western tourist, taking time should add to the pleasure of being there.

Demanding western behaviour, usually takes five to ten days to dissipate. Westerners might have to learn or re-learn to enjoy every moment. Why rush through precious moments, diligently photographing them but not enjoying them to the full?

I once encountered a good example of unnecessarily aggressive behaviour. I was on my way to Antigua. Mr. Nasty stood out from the crowd. I noticed him first in front of the check-in desks. He was pacing about, looking tense. Because it was a large 747 flight departure, check-in was slow. A long delay had arisen by the time I arrived; something to do with a faulty aircraft. Clearly it was in everyone's interest to wait quietly while the safety of the aircraft was checked. A twenty-minute delay ensued. Directly the delay was announced, Mr. Nasty was on his feet, asking for a manager at the check-in desk.

"I've never come across anything like it," he said loudly enough for everyone to hear, "Every time I travel with your airline, something like this happens. Delays, delays, delays. This time I'm writing to the CEO to complain. Bring me a pen and the appropriate form immediately!"

Sensing this poor chap must have had a bad week, the check-in operator dealt sympathetically and calmly with his unreasonable behaviour. He was handed a complaint form and a pen. Form in hand, he strode back to his wife and three children, who seemed embarrassed. Muttering loudly, he announced he would never again be travelling with this airline. Once he had completed his complaint form, he paced back to the reception desk, ready to unleash another tirade. This was met with equanimity and reasonableness – a style that seemed to ruffle him. He was looking for a fight. Several times he strode back and forth, giving every bystander the benefit of his vast travel experience.

Why so angry? He was off on holiday, to a place with nothing more to do than sit on a beach and sip piña coladas. Perhaps he was fatigued from overwork; irritable, and badly in need of a holiday. Perhaps he was just a nasty person. Perhaps he could have done with a few more parental admonishments as a child. Why did his wife seem unperturbed? My guess was, she was used to his behaviour. She was allowing his 'spoilt-little-boy' drama, to have full reign. Perhaps she had helped to induce it; sending him like a ferret down a rabbit hole, to achieve her objectives.

Having spent all his days at work, he was clearly not used to being with his children. His drive to the airport with them, might have been aggravating. His de-

*manding, dominant behaviour will have saved him
from further argument and discussion.*

*On the long, eight-hour flight, I don't think he sat
down for more than a few minutes. He paced around
the whole time. Luckily for him, it was a large airplane.*

*While on holiday, I didn't see much of him. I oc-
casionally saw him playing with his children, swimming, and playing tennis. When next I saw him up
close, we were at the airport ready to return home. His
behaviour had changed completely. He was smiling.
He looked relaxed, happy, and healthy. His previously
tight, expressionless, mask-like face – one that so often
accompanies aggression and fear – had disappeared.
He could be seen happily passing time with his children. He looked as if he had left any tiredness and
tension behind. The last of his worries was when the
airplane was to take-off and return him back to work.*

One could name the conversion of Mr. Nasty to Mr. Nice Guy,
the 'holiday effect', although, I have seen the same phenomenon
with the patients who were subjected to a period of bed rest and
sedation in hospital. The conversion involves a change – from
high-energy spending, to one of energy economy.

The Sleep Paradox

Few people can cope with unresolved, on-going background problems, and yet have untroubled sleep. Perhaps those who can, lack

anxiety and obsessiveness. Perhaps they have an ego that allows a clear conscience. Whatever the reason, few escape the paradox suffered by the most stressed and distressed – the inability to sleep well, despite any fatigue caused by excessive personal energy expenditure.

Healthy survival can depend on combatting a vicious downward spiral – increasing tiredness caused by defective sleep; then fatigue resulting from agitated sleep, sometimes leading to exhaustion and insomnia.

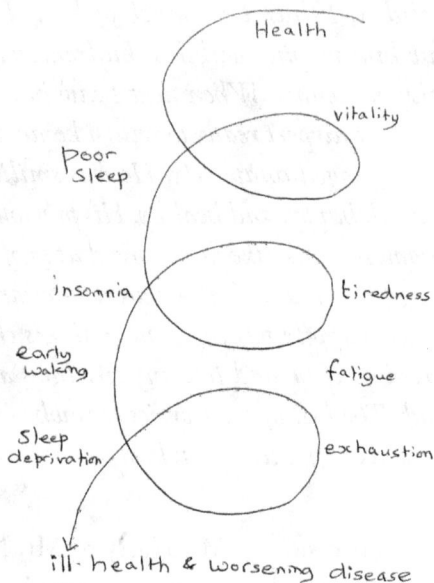

Fig. 4: Sleep Paradox

The Sabbath: A Divine Biological Function?

The fast erosion of a weekly Sabbath for non-practising Christians and Jews, has occurred simultaneously with seven-day working, and 24-hour shopping and entertainment. This has meant the loss of time for revitalisation. Even secondary education has succumbed.

The headmaster of a comprehensive school in Great Horton once wrote:

> *"The youngsters have a tremendous thirst for work and when I offered them the Sunday morning classes they nearly bit my hand off . . . We are trying to tap into their motivation; and for them to come in on Sundays affirms the strength within themselves to do well."*

The Times
16.12.96.

You don't need religious conviction to appreciate the health significance of observing a Sabbath as a day of rest; a day for swapping our usual activities for a day of relaxation and contemplation. In fact, any change of routine can be refreshing for those leading an unrelenting, repetitive existence. Since those with a religious faith will spend their Sabbath in prayer and spiritual refreshment, they can gain both energy and self-esteem as rewards for being dutiful and observant. Solace and comfort are also to be found in some non-religious rituals.

Days off work are important for mental and physical health. This allows time for reuniting with family and friends, for sporting activities, reading and other hobbies. Some recognise no need for this: they are fully and happily engaged with their work, with no desire for diversions. A friend of mine has five children. When I asked him what he was going to do after the weekend, he said, 'I'm going back to work for a rest!'

For the lonely, time can drag when unstructured. Solitude can be stressful – a time those unhappy with themselves can find unbearable. For the untroubled and self-contented, solitude can represent valuable time for thinking and creating.

More work can be achieved by the productive, with planned work and rest periods. Marathons are won by those who pace themselves, not by the pacemakers employed to rush away as fast as they can. The tortoise can sometimes beat the hare (according to Aesop).

The Uncomplicated Life

Is discipline essential for survival or is it OK to be lax and pampered? Perhaps both are essential, at different times. The longevity of monks and nuns suggests that rigid discipline, relative solitude, security and contemplation, are survival factors. From the longer survival of the rich and pampered, one might conclude that a life free of any control by others, with financial freedom and security, most fosters health and longevity.

The Russian cosmonauts on the Mir space station initially regarded their American visitors as too soft. Instead of creating problems, they admitted to getting on with the difficult or messy jobs, without consulting them. It made their life together easier. Russians, brought up during the Cold War, were more likely to know deprivation than those from the USA or Europe.

Never having to lift a finger for anything, safe in the knowledge that someone else will be responsible, minimises energy expenditure. The result (in keeping with the health divide) is the likelihood of a longer life, albeit unfulfilled.

An article in the scientific journal Nature, suggested that total pampering was the reason why queen bees lived longer than worker bees. Laurent Keller and Michel Genoud compared 43 species of colony-forming insects and found a strong link between the longevity of queen bees and the social structure of the colony. Life for the queen is simple and risk free, once the colony is established; her life can then be extended.

While a typical ant can expect to live no more than a month or two, their queen will typically live for ten years – for some species, it can be 28-years. Some termite queens live for eleven years; for honey-bee queens, five to six years is usual.

The longevity of the rich, in comparison to the deprived, needs explanation. The extent to which humans might parallel insect longevity, is interesting to consider. Could it be that many royal families, billionaires, and Lottery winners, have a more care-free pampered life, than those who need to work for a living? Regardless of social status, few feel free; free of worry, with no need to make decisions. Although poor, some will have extensive family support. The rich can get the same from servants and those they employ. None, however, can claim to be pampered like a queen insect. The perception of security and knowingly being in control are major factors (The Whitehall II study (Marmot, M.G. 1991).

Humour

"From quiet homes and first beginning,

Out to the undiscovered ends,

There's nothing worth the wear of winning,

But laughter and the love of friends."

Hilaire Belloc. *Dedicatory
Ode.*

I suspect that a sense of humour is health promoting. Unfortunately, it cannot be relied on to predict longevity.

Comedians, apart from Bob Hope who lived to 100-years of age, have not fared better than average. I reviewed ten famous comedians, famous in my lifetime (Tommy Cooper, Arthur Askey, Bob Monkhouse. Peter Sellers, Max Miller, Max Wall, Groucho Marx, Benny Hill, Jack Benny and Dick Emery). I calculated their average length of life to be 72.5-years.

At least a good sense of humour suggests a healthy attitude to life. A person who can laugh freely, is often less burdened by the troubles of life. Some light-hearted people, however, have a remarkable ability to ignore their troubles.

Laughter can arise freely but is not always unburdened. Some laugh to hide their feelings; others laugh when embarrassed. I suspect that living in circumstances that provoke laughter, could promote health. Disease prevention is another matter. I much doubt that a sense of humour has much to do with the occurrence of disease, although it might lessen its impact. Because diseases are mostly caused by genetic predisposition, viruses and bacteria, any connection with a sense of humour is tenuous. That there is a connection between laughter, humour and feeling healthy, we can take for granted

*Ridiculum acri fortius ac melius magnas perumque
secat res.*

(Humour achieves more than force.)

Horace

*In 1997, Jeanne Calment celebrated her 122nd birth-
day. She said she enjoyed everything and had spent her
life with a smile on her face. She expected to 'die laugh-
ing'. She died seven months later in August 1997.*

The Times
26.1.97.

What we cannot easily assess, is how many happy-smiley-people
have died young, from adverse inheritance or catastrophic circumstances. A good sense of humour undoubtedly promotes well-being and improves quality of life – it would be laughable if it didn't!
But does a good sense of humour prolong life and prevent disease?
Nobody knows.

Does a miserable, depressed life, reduce longevity? Apart from
suicide, I have not noticed this to be the case among my patients,
but the statistics suggest I am wrong. At 18-years of age, depressed
people can look forward to only a further 28-years of life (on
average); the non-depressed can look forward to double that – to
a further 56.8-years of life. The causes of death were not suicide
(0.4%), but stroke, heart disease, diabetes, hypertension, asthma,
smoking and inactivity (Jia, H., Zack, M.M. et al. 2015).

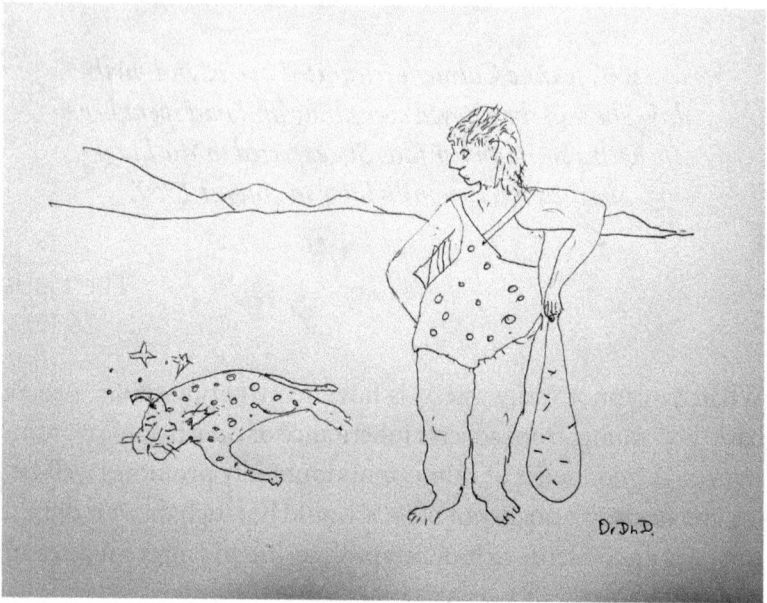

Fig. 5 The 'Simple' Life?

Through the experience of living with the Yequana tribe, living deep within the 'impenetrable' jungle near Venezuela's Caroni river, a tributary of the Orinoco, Jean Liedloff came to learn the origins of her western hang-ups and neuroticism.

Within the tribe, there was no obvious unhappiness. She came to wonder just how that could be, given the absence of any modern conveniences. She observed them deriving joy from accepting the world as it is. She learned that right and wrong, good and bad, efficient and inefficient, were artificial in Yequana culture. She found that unnecessarily critical judgements, as they are applied throughout western life, are first initiated by parents and later by peers. Not so for the Yequana. By comparing the two, she concluded that it is mostly negative issues that drive westerners to perform.

She once suggested constructing a pipeline for water carriage up to the village. This, she thought, would help their progress. The women, who so enjoyed three trips a day with their children, washing clothes and fetching water, saw no point to it. During these leisurely, free of time-pressure trips, they could enjoy one another's company, commune with their children, and enjoy the environment. Having a pump installed would not have represented 'progress' for them. The Yaquana had no wish to change their established routines. They had no need for speed, efficiency or novelty, all of which drive western life.

Having compared lifestyles, she wrote:

> "But soon my sense of emancipation gave way to the tyranny of habit, to the great weight of conditioning that only sustained conscious effort can countermand."

Jean Leidloff. *The Continuum Concept*

The Siesta

Taking a nap is an important strategy. It can help avoid sleep deprivation and unlock energy for what follows – especially in hot countries, where they work early in the day and during the late evening. An afternoon sleep can unlock as much energy as night-time sleep.

There are two common misconceptions about siestas. First, many people think if they sleep in the afternoon, they will not sleep at night. This is incorrect, because the relaxation effect of an early sleep, allows for improved night-time sleep induction. Second, many think it 'a waste of time'. They might say, "I've paid a lot of money for this holiday and I'm not going to waste it in bed!" If being healthy means having more available energy, the advantage of a siesta should not be missed. Some people, more concerned to get their money's worth than preserving what money cannot buy – their health – may not agree.

Those who are tired and fatigued may need a siesta for at least five consecutive days, before feeling refreshed. The 'holiday effect', of gradually reducing arousal, makes taking a siesta easier. Uptight mothers and fathers, fresh from the fatigue of work, will take at least five days to reach the point where nothing bothers them. Taking a siesta then comes more easily.

The benefits of a comfortable bed and a quiet place to sleep, can be taken for granted. Individual taste will prescribe variants between a hammock and a water bed; a king-sized bed of duck-down, and a sandy beach with a rolled-up towel for a pillow. The ambient temperatures preferred can range from icy: windows fully open – in Scotland – in February, to the tropical heat and humidity of Singapore. When trying to survive, being adaptable helps. Unfortunately, it is adaptability that is quickly lost with fatigue and exhaustion – with too little energy left for adaptation. Overly fussy, energy-starved people are easily aggravated, and can't always sleep anywhere. Like Goldilocks, everything has to be 'just right' for them, before they will consider sleep. An irritable state can defy relaxation and sleep induction. Unfortunately, irritable people quite often find it difficult to admit to an over-aroused state.

CHAPTER FIFTEEN

Exercise, Nutrition and Vitality

Physical and Mental Training

High on the list of our original survival priorities was that we developed the capacity for physical exercise – to escape predators. Muscles are capable of great feats of endurance, especially after being trained to increase aerobic exercise (enabling the efficient use of oxygen). The change achievable is incredible – from being able only to run only one hundred yards (91.4 metres) with considerable effort, to running twenty-six miles (41.86 Kms) in a marathon race without stopping. Obviously, special changes must happen to make this improvement possible.

Weight training will lead to increased strength, but proportionately, not to the same extent seen with aerobic training. One might eventually be able to lift three to four times more weight than before, but this is a small proportionate increase, compared to the 45-times increase in running distance achievable with aerobic training. Training enables the same work to be done, with less oxygen used as fuel. In other words, exercise training increases the physical efficiency of the body as a machine. Change in muscle metabolism is only part of the explanation; improved heart and circulation efficiency, will also have to occur.

Training our memory, intelligence and mental endurance, only works to a limited extent. Those who have trodden the path of studying for school examinations, through to a university degree, will know how much more mental capacity develops through study. Those used to solving problems can become faster thinkers and retain more knowledge. The improvement is small however, when compared to the improvement in physical prowess achieved by sports training. There is some interplay between the two – those who get fit, seem to gain improved mental capacity and endurance, perhaps because of their positive attitude.

Since the 1960s, there have been many attempts to demonstrate improved intelligence using different forms of mental training. General intelligence, it seems, can only be slightly improved. Memory training can improve in the short term, but not by much (approximately 11% improvement. See: Jaušovec, N. 2012). The long-term training represented by schooling (during which time, our brains are maturing), might be the most effective, although, age may not be the limiting factor we once thought. It is possible to learn a new language at any age, but first one has to be motivated and then to believe it is possible. Perhaps older people should stop thinking – 'I'm too old for this!'

Take the case of UK black-cab, taxi drivers. They need to store large amounts of spatial information over several years. Some parts of their brain have been shown to increase in size (the hippocampus. See: Maguire, 2000). Some older performing musicians will develop an enlarged auditory area in their brain (Pantev, 2003). It was once thought the brain didn't change after a certain age (said to have limited plasticity), but this has been shown to be false.

Physical training can improve several mental functions, including confidence. It can result in aggressiveness but is more likely to create quiet confidence. It is associated with better sleep, improved libido and vitality. Training can also enable us to maintain interest and concentration for longer periods. These advantages are obvious to anyone who has experienced fitness and unfitness at different times. Fitness can produce a positive mental state, not dissimilar to the euphoric effects of some drugs; an experience that can create the desire for even greater fitness. Unfitness for some can be associated with physical and mental lethargy.

Whereas the physically unfit person is inclined to 'take it easy', the typical trained athlete will be active. One reason is that those who choose to train physically are more active in the first place. Untrained, physically inactive people, like Winston Churchill when older, are not necessarily lazy. Are both laziness and natural vitality inherited? Both seem potentiated by natural tendency – taking it easy for the naturally lazy; exercise for the physically vital.

The conception of fitness we each have, can be different. First, there are biological, gender-driven differences. Fit men more often boast about their athletic prowess than women. Women more often see fitness as a resource. With it they gain vitality rather than strength and endurance. Men often exaggerate their fitness, seeing themselves as they once were at school or in the army, rather than as they are.

In medical practice, women seem to have less need to boast and are more realistic. Most women, for instance, accurately know their height; men more often over-estimate theirs. After many decades of measuring patient height, I found this to hold true 90% of the time. I sometimes met patients at our local gymnasium. I nearly always found the performance of my male patients, to be far less impressive than their claims.

One very overweight patient of mine, once told me he couldn't understand why he was unable to lose weight, given his frequent attendance at the gymnasium. I once observed him on a treadmill. He walked so gently, he was able to read a book at the same time. He boasted he never became breathless while exercising, but at the rate he usually walked, there was little chance of him losing either his breath or his weight. When I challenged him about this, he said he didn't know one needed to get out of breath to advance fitness. I explained, that to get aerobically fit (reducing the oxygen needed for active exercise), he had to get breathless. The more often we push our limits, the more we will advance our exercise efficiency. He was so obese, I advised him to lose weight before increasing his exercise.

False impressions abound when trying to assess patient fitness. There are those who don't regard themselves as fit, but they are when tested. Just occasionally, when doing treadmill exercise testing for cardiac risk assessment, I encountered untrained people with a remarkably high exercise tolerance. The usual explanation was that their daily work involved lots of exercise. Some did manual labour; others were required to run up and down many office stairs each day.

On one occasion I was completely misled by a patient. He told me he could play two rounds of golf in a day – without tiring or getting breathless. On the treadmill, he became breathless after two minutes of low-level exercise. He also had ECG changes, strongly suggestive of a narrowed coronary artery. One aspect of his history was true. He could play two rounds of golf, but only if he used a motorised buggy – he only got off to hit his ball!

Exercise training can increase exercise capacity, even for those with a physical defect like angina or arthritis.

In the early 1970's, ex-Olympic coach Alistair Murray, started exercising those who had suffered heart attacks. The medical establishment thought him reckless and would not support him. The prediction was – the majority of his clients would drop dead. He showed, using gradually graded exercises, that fitness training presents no problem to heart patients. There were no casualties among his first 100 cases, and most achieved improved exercise tolerance. Although they progressed at a much slower pace than expected for healthy people, the patients he trained increased their performance in parallel to their healthy contemporaries. The training benefit to those with coronary disease and heart failure, became obvious to those working with them. After many years, it was finally proven to be safe.

Exercise induces both increased adrenaline flow in the blood and increased sympathetic nervous system activity. The latter is mediated by noradrenaline at nerve endings. These hormones, together with cortisone from the adrenal gland (and many other chemicals such as endorphins and kinins), are chemical responses to exercise. They cause increased blood flow to every organ, an increase in blood pressure, and improved oxygen delivery.

Mental stress stimulates the body in much the same way, although, the mixture of chemicals produced is a little different. Perhaps it is not surprising – physically trained people have bodies that seem to better withstand mental stress – perhaps after constantly exposing themselves to increased hormonal loads. In addition, physically fit people gain in confidence and composure, helping to quieten their mental responses, and to reduce palpitations, panic attacks and hyperventilation, simply because they have become used to the stimulation. Unfitness can make some more susceptible to stress. Because unfit people are less used to the effects of adrenaline and other hormones, they are prone to have adverse symptoms when stressed.

Poor self-image, anxiety, and a lack of confidence can all exaggerate stress responses. Anxious people will respond to the same amount of adrenaline-like substances, with a faster heart rate than those who are relaxed. This is why a tranquilliser like diazepam, reduces palpitations in the anxious and unfit.

There is great variance in how each person responds to mental or physical stress; a fact which makes 'stress' an interesting concept, but not specifically useful for clinicians.

Nutrition

The subject of nutrition, and its connection to health and disease, is a minefield of misdirection, misinterpretation, conjecture, exaggerated claims, and advertising, all of which has successfully created a billion-dollar worldwide industry. The gullible who are unable to grade and interpret scientific research, are easy prey for those promising better health and a longer life. There are, however, hidden within a fog of baseless contentions, some – not to be missed – conclusions of value. Even if one is gullible, and not persuaded by science, at least most supplements are harmless (except perhaps, when they include excessive amounts of vitamins A, D and E).

Throughout my career, the value of nutrition in fostering health and preventing disease in western societies, has become steadily exaggerated. Few in the western world suffer from malnutrition, so the focus has changed from having sufficient food, to valuing various food components. Others point to the detriment of excess (in particular, of saturated fats). Public interest has gone beyond the basic need for fat, carbohydrate, protein, vitamins and roughage, needed for health. It is now thought that food can help prevent and treat certain diseases, the latest rationale for which is that food interacts with our bowel bacteria – with our gut microbiome.

In my medical experience, working solely in the western world, I have seen nutrition greatly improve health, but with only marginal effects on the progress of disease. The appropriate diet can reduce obesity and help control diabetes, kidney failure and blood pressure (with sodium salt restriction) – it helps, but will not cure. Adequate nutrition (with all the necessary nutrients) undoubtedly fosters health, but its effect on disease is a different matter.

In terms of allowing us more vitality through promoting better sleep, individual preferences and responses to food, need consideration. For instance, caffeine in drinks will disturb sleep for some, but not for all. Big meals can be soporific, but not for all. Sugar does seem to worsen dental caries and acne, but first you must have the predisposition.

The time we eat is said to affect us. Some even invent eating schedules. The subject abounds in hearsay, so sensible conclusions about the value of eating habits and health, are hard to come by. For instance, we are told that roughage and green teas can prevent bowel cancer, but a major problem of interpretation exists. When an individual adopts a regime that has been proven statistically (shown to apply 'on average', calculated from analysing a large group of random subjects), it may not apply to any specified individual. With food prescriptions unnecessary, what we eat remains the choice of every individual.

I have not learned much more from studying the chemistry of diets and heart disease, than my grandmother once told me (see the two books I wrote on food and the heart in the bibliography – email me, if you want a copy). When I asked her if there was a secret to living a nine-decade, healthy life, she replied, 'hard work and good food!' By good food, she meant fish and meat protein, together with a range of fresh vegetables. She had never taken a supplement in her life, but lived into her 90s.

Can food improve our energy, vitality, physical fitness and mental capacity? Many who take supplements believe so. This billion dollar worldwide industry, supplies minerals, vitamins, and additional substances (like Q10, ginseng, phytosterols, and ginkgo) which no diet readily supplies. Many of the supposed benefits are backed by no more than hearsay and pseudoscience; some are culturally specific, like rhino horn and sharks' fins.

Vitamins are essential to healthy life. There is no argument about that. Problems arise when nutrition pundits try to make a case for excessive doses, claiming they can prevent cancer, give us extra energy, better eyesight, and younger skin, while staving off dementia and preventing heart disease. The only way we can verify such claims is to do animal experiments, and some interesting findings have arisen, yet to be validated in humans.

So far, a 'balanced diet' would seem to offer most of the advantages, although there are some exceptions. Animal experiments have shown a significant reduction in heart disease in those given selenium supplements. Selenium is found in nuts, and in some populations where its intake is minimal, there are increased cardiovascular outcomes. Similar evidence has been found for magnesium, manganese, omega-3 and 6 oils, flavonoids (dark red and purple fruit), and fibre.

One study that once intrigued me, concerned natural vitamin E. Was it possible that vitamin E, acting as an anti-clotting agent, might prevent heart attacks? The argument made, was that only 'natural', not the synthetic vitamin, would work. Too much might cause bleeding and strokes, more likely in those with high blood pressure. I was unable to resolve the truth of this issue.

The B vitamins, because they can reduce a blood risk factor called homocysteine, are thought to reduce cardiovascular risks. B6 is involved in the production of glutamate, a neurotransmitter. Its absence in the diet might cause tiredness and fatigue, but in countries where this occurs, there are many other causes of fatigue. In excess, it can cause problems like neuropathy – with tingling fingers and toes – often the reason given for taking it in the first place.

Linus Pauling, a double Noble Prize winner, became convinced that vitamin C could prevent both cancer and heart disease. He founded the Linus Pauling Institute in Oregon, to help prove his theories. As yet, not much evidence supports his theories. The Institute does, however, provide valuable information on nutrition and disease, all available on the internet.

The search for a universal elixir of life – to be drunk from vessels other than the Holy Grail – continues. The direction medical research is taking, suggests it might be better to get the opinion of a geneticist than a shop assistant selling supplements!

PART FOUR

ENERGY EXPENDITURE, ENERGY BALANCE, AND THE LIFE
EQUATION

CHAPTER SIXTEEN

Energy and Quality of Life

"We are pre-occupied with the past, that has already happened, and we are pre-occupied about the future, which doesn't yet exist. We worry about what will happen and we think about various things that make us feel anxious, frustrated, passionate, angry, resentful or afraid. While we are so pre-occupied, our awareness of the here-and-now slips by and we hardly notice it passing. We eat without tasting, look without seeing, and live without perceiving what is real.'"

No-Nonsense Buddha for Beginners.

Noah Rasheta (2018)

Although I have dealt with the disease, morbidity and mortality of patients, all of my working life, what has always counted most to my patients has always been their quality of life. Many factors must combine to improve or diminish it, and I will consider some more of them in this chapter.

The negative factors which affect quality of life most, are fear, anxiety, obsession, frustration and resentment, which spend our energy most, and positive factors like relaxation, meditation and enjoyment which spend it least. One object of this book is to point out the relative energy-spending function of each, especially when the origin of personal fatigue remains a mystery. For each of us, there will be separate antagonists and protagonists.

Healthy individuals will often have enough energy to experience a full, high-quality life: through work, travel, and interacting with others. By doing so, they will create their own book of memories. Creating that book is what many young people hope to do; older people may have more time to review their book and reminisce.

One experience with the potential to ruin our quality of life, few will enjoy, is the development of a disease. An exception exists – active attention seekers may gain from it. But how are we to know if we have a disease? Diseases often grow unseen and unsuspected until they cause pain, inactivity or disability. None come 'out of the blue', although some may appear to. Eventually, most will cause tiredness and fatigue.

We all approach life differently. Many spend their energy fruitlessly, with no prospect of getting it back. Others do very little and receive nothing but benefits and rewards. Rather than luck alone, our talents, vitality, ambition and drive, have a lot to do with it.

Something other than luck is needed for success and an improved quality of life (success being always self-defined). Some achieve it with little more than a pleasant speaking voice, a beautiful face or an ability to kick, bat or throw a ball. Some achieve success with a talent for maths, science, languages, art and music. An affable personality, networking skills, and executive functioning will raise our perceived profile. Elon Musk, as a man of ideas, became a success in business by taking chances, and selling his dreams to others. First, the idea that cars could be made fully electric. Second, that life on Mars is possible – a bolthole for humans, supposedly facing extinction. To succeed in striving towards such goals, one needs energy, talent, and strong motivation.

There are many ways for us to spend our energy. As discussed in Part 2, they range from reacting to immediate foreground issues, solving long-term problems, and facing many subliminal factors in our environment that can affect us subtly. In the foreground are transient needs for fast-thinking – whether to turn left or right and what to buy for lunch. In the background are issues that need slow thinking, like what career to pursue or whether to marry Jack or Jill. The subliminal issues we live with may not affect us consciously but are ever-present. Where we live, and our exposure to the local social and political environment, may require us to respond.

The human body is always working, even during sleep. Alone and inactive, we talk to ourselves, devising ways to cope with life challenges. The current, background challenges we face, differ a lot between western and other societies. How we perceive them, will vary with our personality, intelligence and several other factors. The environment in which we choose to live or cannot escape, presents us with challenges both obvious and subtle. In the west, we may have been born free, but are forever in the grip of social and official regulatory demands; our energy, like the money we earn, is not all our own. Every citizen, signed up to a society, is required by law to spend some of what we have on compliance and duty to others. This is not freedom, it is accepted control, with very few able to find an alternative.

The circumstances of our life, which greatly influence the quality of our existence, will depend on the social and political state of our country. The quality of life of those experiencing war, is far removed from those living in a stable, peaceful country. Whatever country we live in, we all (the undersigned citizens of western societies) tacitly agree to spend our energy and money, contributing to 'the system' and helping anonymous people, even though it diminishes our vitality and quality of life. We have legalised those in power, to extract what they need from us – for 'the greater good'. For many such reasons, the wealthy live longer than the poor (the health divide).

Because western societies are actually managed by the anonymous, no one person can be made fully responsible for the pond in which we swim; as citizens we have resigned our control (unless you believe that voting helps). This suits those in power, whose control partly depends on harnessing our energy, and restricting our choices. Is all this worth it? Should we citizens continue to pay this much for the right to swim? If the situation continues, and the control over us expands, might dis-ease, tiredness, fatigue and exhaustion become even more common? Maybe not, since over time (measured over several decades), we in all western societies, are progressively living longer.

The quality of our lives depends a lot on exactly where we are born, where we choose to live or where we have to live. Two of the most important factors shaping quality of life, are our circumstances and the relationships we have, some of which are helpful; some of which are unhelpful and even pathological.

Remember 'The Life Equation'

Without balancing the energy we spend, against the energy we have available (through unblocked neuronal channels) – the result of effective sleep and relaxation – we will all suffer tiredness. If any imbalance continues, we will experience fatigue and then exhaustion; possibly going on to suffer an accident or a medical catastrophe.

We spend our mental energy in short bursts or consistently over the long-term. We all sleep either deeply and refreshingly or fitfully, with marked dreaming and nightmares. The result is always daytime tiredness, likely caused by persistently blocked neuronal channels in the brain.

The problems we pay attention to are either in the foreground of our consciousness or in the background. They are simply 'part of life'. Spending energy on solving longer-term problems can get complicated and vary from person to person. The problems that drain a lot of our energy are background issues with no quick fix. Unfortunately, the energy we spend may not be matched by what we need most – refreshing sleep. This paradox, I have named the Sleep Paradox (see Fig. 4).

Some background issues will risk our security. We might lose our job, not be able to afford our rent or mortgage, and have to move home. At the other extreme, a person who has just won the lottery may need time to consider their options, most of them pleasant rather than worrying. The many and various background situations we find ourselves dealing with, will not only spend our energy on thinking, analysis, consideration and decision making, but also on feelings and emotions. Fear, frustration, anger, guilt and resentment are among them.

Some worries and concerns are ever-present, hanging over us like a slow-moving, dark cloud; some are like a never-ending storm. With disturbed sleep, we will not regain our energy. In a low-energy state we will be less able to think straight, especially if experiencing irritability and a short-temper. A lack of concentration and defective executive functioning, sufficient to make effective solutions difficult to formulate, will make our life even more difficult.

Handling Stress. Constitutional Characteristics

Fuel consumption is a characteristic we all share with our vehicles. Drive hard in some vehicles, and one can watch the fuel tank(s) indicator empty. Thirsty cars and lorries often have two fuel tanks! It's not surprising that many fuel-thirsty individuals, prefer fuel-thirsty cars, dashing around with no time to spare. They can be seen accelerating from one traffic light to the next, burning gas and tyre rubber, getting only a little further ahead. They are rushing through life.

Other fuel wasters are to be found worrying about every detail in their life; meticulously adjusting their clothes, their children, their bank balance, and everything they encounter. Beware of overly obsessive characters – they can exhaust everyone around them.

Worry, worry, worry. Some people worry about everything and nothing of consequence. With nothing to worry about, some will invent concerns. Neurotics burn so much energy, they can have energy crises. Neuroticism is only beneficial when it focusses on detecting danger and its avoidance.

> *Mavis came from a long line of over-anxious people, all of whom were terrified of hospitals (in Great Britain, this is not entirely unjustified). So fearful was her father, he suffered a duodenal ulcer for twenty years, without ever consulting a doctor. Too scared to call for help, he died from one massive internal bleed.*

Aggression throws energy to the wind. Some people, like piranha fish, are naturally aggressive; others are aggressive only when let down, led astray, disrespected, used or abused. For some, it is only a transient feature when they are tired, fatigued or exhausted.

Can the important components of our responses – our constitution – be altered? If by constitution we mean genetic pre-disposition, the answer must be 'no'. If we mean, the ability to adapt to circumstances, then the answer is 'yes', but only to some extent. Take Michael's response to stress:

> *Michael ran a big business, a big car, and a big appetite for life. He drove a Rolls Royce, was in his early forties, and had incompatible business partners. He smoked and drank enough to acquire bronchitis and cirrhosis. Both his blood pressure and blood cholesterol were raised. After a medical screening examination, we discussed his unhealthy state. He resolved to stop drinking, stop smoking, start exercising, and to follow a low-fat diet. His motivation was such that he built his own gymnasium and became an 'exercise freak' (his words, not mine). Most importantly (in his opinion), he decided to leave his partners and started again in a new business. By making all these changes, he regained control over his life, having formerly lost it due to his lack of discipline, and delegating decisions to less than competent partners.*

Nine months after his medical check-up, his physical build looked athletic. His pulse had slowed, and his blood pressure and cholesterol had normalised.

In his opinion, giving up the aggravation associated with his former stressful business relationships, explained his improvement. He had regained control of his destiny and was able to stop his undisciplined use of food, cigarettes, and alcohol for self-gratification. He came to recognise that these had not been helpful replacements for his lack of resolve. The changes he made, empowered him further, and through self-discipline, he earned self-esteem. He also changed his body image, from fat to fit.

Exercise, it seems, can toughen our elastic – our constitution – and modify our responses to stress for the better. Social re-adjustment can lighten the load, but one needs to be enlightened enough, and courageous enough, to attempt it.

The most essential elements of a good constitution are psychological – ego, self-worth, discipline, adherence to hard work and persistence, to name a few. Judgement and intelligence can help us decide what to cope with first. Those with good judgement and foresight, will usually take a planned, easier path through life; at least, a path they know they can handle with ease.

Self-Induced Stress

"My problem lies in trying to be at least four different people."

Professor Heinz Wolff (1928 – 2017).

Wolff's point was to suggest that with a computer, it is possible to perform the work of four. Although appealing, it often fails in practice. Give me diligence, persistence and intelligence anytime! I have yet to see computers reduce work. They are simply better and faster than humans at boring and repetitive tasks. Furthermore, however much work one person does on a computer, it is always the work of one. The desire to do more and more, in less and less time (Type-A personality), can double the risk of heart attacks (in those prone to them).

"Working is the modern super-tribesman's equivalent of hunting for food and, like the animal zoo inmates, he frequently performs the

pattern much more elaborately than is strictly necessary. He creates problems for himself."

The Human Zoo. Desmond Morris.

The zoologist Desmond Morris, called this human specific trait of self-stress, the Stimulus Struggle. The object of the struggle is to obtain 'the optimum amount of stimulation from the environment'. With insufficient problems, we tend to create some, just to keep occupied.

Involvement in this struggle is not obligatory, but few now opt out. A few opt out because those who control profits have promoted their insecurity (at least in western capitalist societies). Even the most scrupulous organisations can require their employees to move house, take on a large mortgage, and make themselves dependent. This assures job commitment and corporate mastery over employees. Employees are thus required to accept Morris' Stimulus Struggle.

Different nationalities agree to the Stimulus Struggle with different fervour. Westerners, imbued with the 'Protestant work ethic', will eagerly embrace it. The Japanese are similarly driven. From my own limited travel experiences, I would say that natives of the Caribbean and Fiji, love it least. Once they found oil, the need to struggle left some Arabs and Eskimos. Since striving, and rushing around to achieve acquisition, can relate to the incidence of heart attacks and strokes, the western way of life has also been called 'the western way of death'.

Self-stress can be motivated by ego, desire for status, avarice, and many vain aspirations. These human characteristics are common enough to be regarded as 'normal' traits. The fact that they might lead to illness in those susceptible, is not something many ponder.

Unfortunately, both success and failure are traps:

"Sir, there are two tragedies in life.

One is to lose your heart's desire. The other is to gain it."

Man and Superman. Bernard Shaw. *1903.*

"What do the UK honours OBE and MBE stand for?'"asked Tessa's granddaughter.

"Other **B**uggers **E**fforts, and **M**y **B**loody **E**fforts!", she replied.

Tessa Ransford. Scottish Poetry Society.

Fear

Apart from anxiety and obsessionality, fear also spends lots of human energy. It is hardly good for our health. Since the Second World War, many have lived with the threat of nuclear conflict. Many remain at war over disputed land; some are considering war to define which culture should predominate. Living in fear, diminishes quality of life; achieving happiness and contentment, improves it.

Fear can be inhibiting or motivating. Among our fears are those of death from disease and aeroplane crashes. We might also fear being abused, being burgled or attacked on the street. Most fear being out of control. Others fear loneliness and poverty, with parents fearing for the safety and health of their children. Many fear failure, getting into trouble with the law, and the demands of taxmen. Others fear marriage and pregnancy. Many fear the loss of status and a diminished standard of living. Then there are the many neurotic fears – of heights, small spaces, large spaces, spiders, thunder, being dirty, public speaking, drowning, suffocation, and starvation. What many fear most is being judged by others. If they knew themselves better, perhaps they would have no need to fear it.

Shyness creates fear, based on the prospect of being made a fool of or unacceptably becoming the centre of attention. For others, not being the centre of attention is what they fear most.

As Oscar Wilde famously said,

> *"There is only one thing in life worse than being talked about, and that is not being talked about."*

The Picture of Dorian Grey. A Novella by Oscar Wilde (1891).

We have all felt one or two of these fears from time to time. Why is it that fear, as one potential cause of medical conditions and mental ill-health, is mostly absent from medical textbooks?

The Fate of a Good Samaritan

> *Jim came to Cheryl's help when she was divorcing her husband. It was a friendly act to start with and should have remained so. She needed his help and she took it freely. Through his cloud of romantic fantasy, he didn't see how good she was at taking, and how poor she was at giving. As the months rolled by, she expressed her friendship and love for him, despite not being 'in love' with him. Unfortunately, he had fallen in-love with her – a dangerous mistake.*

Cheryl found a man she really liked and told Jim how supportive he had become. Despite this, she continued to come back to Jim, every time she needed money, advice or solace. Jim should have said 'no' to her sooner but blinded by love he tried hard to underrate her shameless duplicity.

Beware of romantic liaisons that begin with helping an emotionally needy person.

Thereafter, Jim found it difficult to engage in other relationships. He didn't want to risk being used and hurt again. Perhaps Jim needed lessons in how to judge people and their motives. That might have saved him lots of heartache, money and energy. Unfortunately, love can be to blame. It can blind us to the obvious and give others free access to our emotions and bank balance.

Delegation, Cooperation and Help

Delegation reduces personal energy expenditure. Achieving success requires energy, but much less if we delegate and behave in a relaxed way.

Everyone develops their own style of cooperation. It is shaped by personality, social background, learned behaviour, and several other factors. With appropriate training, we can use ourselves in different ways. Initially, rôle play can help. Thereafter, we might learn to incorporate new, helpful or empowering behaviours. The teachings of Dr. Robert Sharpe and David Lewis (authors of *'How to Thrive on Stress'*) will help those seeking this ability.

By using ourselves efficiently and appropriately, we can gain personal and collective esteem. The latter will boost *esprit de corps*, improve collaboration, and reduce personal effort.

Suffering quietly, without intervening or cooperating, will often make things worse. Few changes happen in organisations without someone complaining. If nobody reports poor service in a restaurant, improvement is unlikely. The business could close – a 'no win' situation, when restaurant facilities are in need. The facility may deserve to close, of course, but sometimes a helpful, constructive word in the manager's ear, could save it from collapse. Many could benefit from one simple piece of feedback.

Self-Worth

Some become excessively clean and tidy, trying to maintain their image of worthiness. The core belief is, 'I am a good person, because I am clean at all times.' Working continuously might maintain our image of diligence – an important form of worthiness: 'I have achieved a lot to-day, therefore, I am a worthwhile person'. These attitudes, driven hard by western culture, do little to improve our sense of inner worth. That is because the promise of western life can be false – that we can all find happiness and contentment – as long as we work hard and obey the rules set by others (thereby, maintaining their power or luxurious existence, if not ours).

Courage is required to give up a successful career, even if you feel it is killing you. It is just as difficult to divorce a partner who gives you no love and tries to deny you the right to be yourself. To grow up, and no longer comply with your parents' every wish, requires courage and confidence. To change faith or fall in love, requires commitment and some courage derived from self-worth.

> "... not only does love for oneself provide the motive for
> such major changes; it also is the basis of the courage
> to risk them. It is only because my parents had clearly
> loved me and valued me as a young child that I felt

sufficiently secure in myself to defy their expectations and radically depart from the pattern they had laid out for me.

Without that security of my parents' love reflected in my own self-love, I would have chosen the known instead of the unknown and continued to follow my parents' preferred pattern at the extreme cost of my own uniqueness. Finally, it is only when one has taken the leap into the unknown of total selfhood, psychological independence and unique individuality that one is free to proceed along still higher paths of spiritual growth and free to manifest love in its greatest dimensions.

The highest forms of love are inevitably totally free choices and not acts of conformity."

M. Scott Peck (1990).

'The Road Less Travelled'

Those who cannot or will not follow this path, are often racked by guilt, parental discord or resentment – all of which are expensive in terms of life energy expenditure.

Feel-Good Factor

Feeling good about life for whatever reason – your successful mission or the success of those you love – can give one a feeling of

self-esteem, happiness with contentment; fulfilment with satisfaction. Its effect is to allow relaxation, effective sleep, and easily
refreshed energy. No major event need be involved. A remark made
in passing, a look, a touch, a word of understanding, are all able
to induce a feeling of well-being; in fact, anything that induces
contentment. For me, the pleasure of helping others to get better,
has been a lifelong source of contentment. At the end of my career,
UK medical regulators did their best to diminish it, but failed.

Religion

There can be unmatched value in the security of purpose and
self-esteem achieved by following the edicts of a religion; doing
one's duty to God. Many humans need piety and ritual, devotion
and service. They need the composure they gain beneath the wings
of omniscience. Jews, Catholics, Muslims, and Protestants, and
many others, have this as their purpose; at the same time providing
the support, recognition, admiration and reward deserved by their
fellow supplicants.

The same level of self-esteem arises for soldiers who have fought for
their country. Camaraderie comes from having joined in a collective purpose; one that gives an identity to all fellow contributors.

A Primitive or Advanced Lifestyle?

The Venezuelan Yequana tribe, described before, have no word
for work. Western views of leisure and work are not distinctions
they make. The western assumption that progress is essential; that
children belong to their parents; that life must be governed by
sets of rules, and that it is better to be young than old, have no
significance for them. The Yekuana do not regard happiness as
a right, and unhappiness as unfortunate. Neither do they regard
it as a right, for everyone to experience every possible form of
happiness, during their lifetime.

Jean Leidoff, who visited the tribe, found no pressure to perform physical feats in order to prove herself equal to their men. She wrote:

> *"Anchu gave not the slightest sign that I ought to walk faster, that my prestige would suffer if I kept a comfortable pace, that I was being judged for my performance or that time on the path was in any way less desirable than time after arrival . . .*

> *Gone was any sense of competition, and the physical strain turned from an imposition upon my body to a satisfying proof of its strength, while my teeth-gritting will-power in the face of martyrdom no longer applied.*

> *Perhaps I was catching a glimpse of the Indians' secret of outdoing our well-nourished strongmen (Europeans) despite their generally inferior muscle power. They were economising their forces by using them only to do the job, wasting none on associated tensions."*

> *The Continuum Concept*. Jean Leidloff

The Yequana value wakefulness and sleep equally. Quite often they will wake in the night, share a joke or the observation of a nearby wild-boar pack. They will then return to sleep instantly, with no sign of annoyance or discontent.

The minimised energy spending requirements of the Yequana, contrast significantly with what westerners feel they need to spend, if they are to progress and succeed. For reasons related to security and a need to comply, we are forced to help maintain the structure and stability of the societies we inherit. From the Yequana point of view, westerners have lost the plot.

Different Lifestyles

Simple Living. High Thinking.

The 'simple living, high thinking lifestyle' is preferred by many educated altruists. My guess is that most people, trying to emulate the rich and famous, would like the opposite: an easy life characterised by high living and low thinking.

The 'simple living, high thinking lifestyle' was portrayed by John Wayne in several western movies.

> *"Every man should live by a code 'a law: I won't be wronged. I won't be insulted, and I won't be set upon!"*

John Wayne.
Film: *The Shootist.*

Such a person would be attracted to Erich Fromm's idea – choosing to 'be' – rather than 'have'. The sage, guru, priest and academic, occupied by the intellectual, moral or spiritual, will often have little interest in anything other than basic living. Plain food and accommodation; rooms full of books, and the pursuit of knowledge gratify their existence. Self-esteem and status are implicit. In parts of England, a priest still has more prestige than a billionaire. This has been a stable British outlook. It still exists but could disappear with the cultural dilution of immigration. What other cultures would claim the wealthy and powerful to be less prestigious than a country vicar?

This style of life benefits from low energy consumption; little or no energy being spent on the vanities of life that engage the majority. Instead, energy is spent on ardent pursuit and the possibility of worthwhile achievement. Energy is more easily used efficiently when one has the respect and appreciation of others.

High Living. Low Thinking

Imagine a life, portrayed in some Hollywood movies. A long drive up to your house. A splendid entrance. A butler to open the door and greet you. Inside, a sweeping staircase with murals on the walls. Several separate rooms for receiving visitors, a dining room for 20 guests; a separate library, bar, TV room / cinema, art gallery and snooker room. Both front and back, having tended, immaculate gardens. Two tennis courts and garaging for six cars. A swimming pool, with its own bar and lounge area. I know this house well. It was built in Majorca by my friend and patient Gerry Couch, who died tragically some years ago.

Such a lifestyle costs a fortune to run, with very few able to afford it. It can be engaging, once it becomes a way of life – a lifestyle in itself.

More than a few of my patients lived this lifestyle, so I am well acquainted with it. They all owned successful businesses; none of them were employees. The main thinking and focus supporting this lifestyle is making a profit; the money required to live like this needs a plentiful cash flow.

One could downscale to arrive at the front door of a modest detached house or a well-designed semi-detached home or apartment. Whatever the architecture, the aim is to have a comfortable life at an affordable cost. Ideally, there will not be too much to think about – something some will want to delegate to a lawyer, accountant, interior designer, a gardener or doctor.

We must all decide where on the spectrum between simplicity and opulence, we would choose to live. Obtaining it could then become a life-consuming, energy-spending quest.

Energy and Timetables

Our bank and credit card accounts detail every penny we spend and earn. They also detail where, when, and how we spend our money, and sometimes why we spent it. Unlike the money we spend, the details of all our personal energy transactions are neither recorded nor available.

As a crude measure of personal energy expenditure, we might choose to access personal diaries, and look at time-schedules and the activities involved. We would need to assess the number and type of decisions made; the degree of satisfaction or dissatisfaction experienced, and the interpersonal friction and gratification involved at each point in time. Even if this were possible, it is unlikely we could make a reliable quantitative measurement of the energy turnover. If we could, we might go on to compare various occupations and lifestyles. In turn we could relate this to the occurrence of heart attacks, strokes, and the risk of other diseases.

Without a scientifically acceptable device to measure human mental energy in real time, in a fully mobile, unhindered way, we are left only with thousands of years of anecdotal observations. Although collected by millions of people, none help us to decide about energy in a scientific, unbiased way. So, let's look at the two extremes possible – at the difference between two people; one who spend lots of energy, and another who spends very little.

Mr. Slowburn is a retired man, living in the countryside. He paid off his mortgage many years ago. His children, who left home long ago, are happily married with healthy children of their own.

Mr. Slowburn gets up in the morning, whenever he feels like it (no time pressures); makes tea for his wife (as a creature of routine, no thinking is needed). Every day he reads the same newspaper and watches the same TV breakfast show (he remains in low-gear, in switched-off mode). Later on, he and his wife will decide on the day's activity (amicably shared decision-making reduces energy expenditure).

Later that morning, his telephone will ring with bad news. His broken lawn-mower will cost much more than expected to repair. Should he pay, think about it, get a second opinion or simply get a new one? (At this decision point, his energy meter will whizz around). Trusting in the competence of experts (a suspicious nature burns more energy), and knowing he has plenty of money for payment (security minimises energy expenditure), he agrees to the repair, even before asking the price (reflecting his financial security). Both he and his wife, thereafter spend a pleasant morning shopping for groceries.

Mrs. Slowburn has always been a relaxed, peace-loving, well-organised sort, who well knows her husband's habits, needs, and thinking pattern (his original choice of partner, permanently reduced his energy expenditure). Before boredom sets in (avoiding energy spent on frustration), they go to lunch (planned relaxation) to a quiet country pub (with no annoyance from loud music or unruly children). With no rush to meet their next appointment (Type-B energy sparing behaviour), they can both enjoy unstructured time (albeit, a major stress for some).

Every night, both sleep peacefully, feeling secure and totally in control of the life they lead together. Both will awake refreshed, ready to enjoy another day.

And now, a somewhat faster lifestyle:

Mrs. Fastburn is the mother of two young children: ages four and six-years of age. Her husband works 'all hours', so she is constantly on duty, coping with three other people. The children are at different schools. This requires a strict timetable for dropping them off and picking them up after school (unavoidable duty creates tension, maintains energy expenditure). Mrs. Fastburn has no relatives living nearby who might help at times. This was caused by them moving closer to her husband's place of work (a big life change spends lots of energy on adaptation and anticipation processes). She knows nobody, with whom she can share her duties. There are neighbours, but she has chosen not to get too friendly. Pride makes it difficult for her to ask for help. She is a poor delegator. (Both sustain high-energy expenditure).

Every morning is rushed (exhibiting Type-A behaviour). After dropping off the children at school, she rushes round the supermarket, often without a list (being rushed, she often forgets things, and shopping can take her twice as long). Because she is often tired and irritable, she finds it hard to remember all she needs (being inefficient burns more energy). She finds it difficult to decide what food to provide for her family each day. She wants to avoid being accused of monotonous food choices; always taking the easy way out – always preparing the same, pre-prepared dishes (decision making is impaired by tiredness). When most tired, she admits to buying only easy-to-prepare options. This causes arguments at home and raises family tension (more energy spending).

She has a part-time job, in a demanding estate agency. She likes her desk to be in order, (obsessive characters can do high quality work at high energy prices). Her clients are very demanding (high energy output required), and the paperwork must be done on time (two jobs at once, multiplies energy expenditure). Her boss, worried about his turnover, imparts anxiety to all his staff (possible insecurity leading to energy drain). Buyers have to be chased, documents have to be signed, mortgages have to be arranged, vendors have to be placated, and a happy working relationship maintained (many areas of coping, together cause increased overall energy expenditure). She rarely has time for lunch. Work takes priority (more Type-A behaviour).

At the end of each day, she still has lots to do. She usu-ally goes to bed late, despite her tiredness. She often has vivid dreams that leave her tired on waking. And so, her life seems like a constant drudge, full of repetition, with no respite in sight (seemingly, no way out).

There can be no doubt about who is spending the most energy. No need for measurement; it's obvious. In these simplistic examples of lifestyle and behaviour, I have compared two unlike age groups on purpose. The parents of young children lead very different lives to those grandparents who have stayed the course – surviving parenthood and middle-age life – a time of life, when the calls on our coping ability are maximal. That is not to imply there are no grandparents who will start a new business and be as busy as any 30-year old – at least those who do more than play computer games or watch TV all day.

Which style is more representative of those who get heart attacks and strokes at an early age? Might they be the ones who spend the most energy? Could socio-economic status, and the lifestyle it allows, make a difference? The answers are not highly predictable, although statistically we are certain about which groups have most medical problems – those less in control of their lives. That comes down to the security they feel and directly relates to their financial position, job status, and how happy and contented they are.

The predisposition to heart disease and cancer is a big issue. No-body has suggested that stress and lifestyle has much to do with causing either, once smoking and exposure to toxic chemicals are removed from consideration. There are pathological characteristics, completely independent of circumstances, that are predetermining. It is those with high blood pressure (and arteriosclerosis) who get more strokes. It is those with 'furred' coronary arteries (atherosclerosis) who get the heart attacks. By adding personality, stresses, behaviour and lifestyle style as accelerants, maybe we can better predict the risk of demise.

What have I observed while practising cardiology for over 50-years? Most doctors feel that strokes and heart attacks come 'out-of-the-blue'. Once it was pointed out to me, however, I started to see those who had experienced progressive changes beforehand – from once having energy, to slowly developing chronic fatigue and exhaustion, months before their heart attack or stroke. Not all patients will experience this (if they are to be believed) – there are undoubtedly those with inherited, severe arterial pathology, who are at high risk and who will get a heart attack or stroke, regardless of their psycho-social or behavioural issues. Usually, however, it is some circumstantial event (the straw that breaks the camel's back) that pushes them over the medical catastrophe, event horizon.

Stress & Frustration

> *"I don't buy this about stress. The only time I feel like I'm going to have a heart attack is when I can't behave in the way that I'm accustomed. The frustration is in holding yourself back."*

John Humphrys. *The Times. 26.1. 97.*

Unless intentional, failure to communicate often causes enormous frustration. Because expressing yourself accurately and meaningfully is difficult, it occurs as much between people who speak the same language as those who do not. Feelings are particularly difficult to convey with words, since no language has a sufficient vocabulary. Instead, it can be better to interpret behaviour – especially facial expressions and demeanour (micro-behaviour). In some instances, the failure to express thoughts, ideas, and feelings adequately, can get dangerous. Such a failure between a doctor and patient can have dire consequences. They can relate as much to what is omitted, as to the words chosen.

> "A good therapist doesn't listen to the content of the bullshit the patient produces, but to the sound, to the music, to the hesitations. Verbal communication easily conceals the truth. Real communication lies beyond the words."

Frederick Perls.

Gestalt Therapy Verbatim (1972)

Those who wish to address this theme further, need to study the thoughts of Ludwig Wittgenstein.

The most important failure of communication we all make, is with ourselves. So how might we do it better, in order to decide on what to do; on what to think and feel; all sufficient to stand the test of time? To do this, it will help if we critically examine our true needs, overrule our biases and be less impulsive. (See Appendix 1, for my list of biases). With deliberate slow thinking, we need to acknowledge that our biases are always in play during the process. (see: Daniel Kahneman. *Thinking Fast and Slow*). This might save us from that regret, so often experienced in the days after an ill-considered, impetuous decision.

For a further discussion of biases (for patients and doctors) see my book, *The Art & Science of Medical Practice*, 2024.

Common Driving Forces: Hope and Vanity

Both hope and vanity drive achievement. In all capitalist societies, the thrust of business and politics, is to keep it that way – providing the means to achieve goals (at a cost), should we choose to jump the many hurdles placed before us. When not satisfied, hope and vanity are among the sources of our disappointment and depression.

Vanity will help to maintain our personal standards, rather than to give into entropy – the natural process of disintegration. Hope and vanity often wane with age. The result can be an unattractive personal appearance that will not inspire confidence.

The first of the four truths taught by Buddha was, 'Life is suffering'. Put another way: 'Life is full of conflict', 'Life is difficult', 'Life is testing'. Whatever life is, it is an energy spending experience, with challenges to be met, questions to be answered, and conflicts to be resolved. A life without suffering, would spend the least energy. Calm composure might then be possible. Who, given the chance, would choose such a life – one that included little joy and excitement?

One way to minimise our energy spend, is to blame other people for our problems. Politicians, 'the rich', and our adversaries are convenient targets. The rich get richer as the poor get poorer, so they are an easy target. Few politicians stay in power long, so they are usually only transient targets. Without an opportunity to blame others (some of them, deceased adversaries and family), there will always be righteous indignation and resentment to drain our spirits.

Children are often blamed for their parents' demise, and *vice versa*. "If it wasn't for you, I could have made something of my life". "If it wasn't for you, I would have been rich by now. You have ruined my life!" Some blame society; some their age, their gender, their race, their social class; the luck they have; even the weather. Failed scapegoating strategies can re-enforce those with cynical and resentful traits. They might then spend even more energy ruminating about them.

Blaming the past is one alternative to admitting failure. Blaming age and gender, are self-defeating, cop-out strategies. Martyrs and blamers do not always healthy people make. They should consider who cares. It is healthier (and spends less energy) to take personal responsibility for our mistakes, and to free ourselves from resentment and conflict.

Everything that happens in life is a challenge, exposing our conflicting attitudes, our faults, weaknesses, biases, misconceptions, and flaws of character. It is strangely difficult for us to see ourselves as having these flaws, and even more difficult to accept any need for change. For these reasons, counsellors and psychotherapists will not be out of work any time soon.

Self-Image

Our perceived quality of life can be reflected in our self-image.

How many are content with their self-image? Are they happy with what they see in a mirror or the feedback from others? How many would like to change what they actually see and hear? If so, how much time, money, and energy are they willing to spend on maintaining or improving their self-image? For some, this is all-consuming and all they care about. For the few who are content, there is no need to spend extra energy on it.

It is easier to be oneself than to maintain a mask – in an attempt to be someone else. Taking on the beliefs, attitudes, and behavioural styles of others, will be stressful. Since we all have an in-built instinct for survival, part of which is to conserve our energy, reversion to type can be expedient. Since energy is spent overcoming any resistance to our wishes, the easiest path could be the best choice.

Human beings (like Mendel's sweet peas) tend to revert to type. Only conditioning of the most influential sort, undertaken over a prolonged period, holds any hope of changing us permanently. Some of course, change their ways and beliefs, after one cathartic moment – Damascene or otherwise.

The vision of where we belong in any hierarchy, helps to determine our future achievement. For young adults, self-image can affect their future – whether they stay put or rise in status. The illusions of status will least concern those happy within themselves: they will be happy, whatever their position. This is not the commonest state of mind of most people. Most are driven to achieve status and security through self-promotion.

There was a simple test given to naval officer cadets which, despite its simplicity, has proven highly predictive of the final rank they will achieve. They were asked how they would deal with a theoretical crisis at sea. They were asked to imagine an aircraft carrier entering a war zone. The question posed was, 'what would you do if the lift transporting the aircraft from below decks to the flight-deck, gets stuck at a time when there are incoming enemy aircraft?'

There are a number of possible solutions, all of which display self-image and the aspirations of every naval cadet.

> *If the cadet says, 'from my desk at the War Office, I would speak directly to the Captain . . .', he sees himself as an admiral. If he says, 'I will first grab my bag of tools, he sees himself as an engineer on board. If he orders engineers to the scene, he sees himself as the captain in command. How we see ourselves, influences our progress in life.*

It would be wasteful of energy and a vain fantasy, to aim for high office or stardom, when one has only modest talent. The fact that so many with modest talents have achieved fame, is no secret. It does, however, fuel the disappointment of those with talent who get overlooked. There are many who populate organisations who feel bitter about being passed over for promotion.

There are also, many highly talented people who do not see themselves in high office and will not try to achieve it. Some highly talented people despise promotion, knowing that the only real advancement worth having, is personal growth and development. In the film, *'Good Will Hunting'*, this mindset is portrayed by the young mathematical genius (played by Matt Damon), who despises money and recognition.

Others feel entitled, and feel they were born for distinction. The *Good Schools' Guide of Great Britain*, once said of the boys of Eton College: 'they are imbued with impending greatness'. We all have our destiny – but don't waste energy pursuing the wrong destiny.

Many methods exist to boost self-confidence and self-awareness. Some magnify the fantasy that everyone, given the right conditions and help, can achieve all they want. While this is possible for those with talent and energy, for many it will remain a vain hope. They risk being challenged by disappointment, once fact meets fantasy. Hopefully, they might find a genuine, truthful guru, to provide some realistic insight. Worthwhile friends, gurus and therapists, can help us face reality. Hopefully, they will also expose our true potential.

The Quest for Happiness

When undecided and unsure of what to do for the best, it helps to know what it is that makes us truly happy. An acceptable quality of life and a sense of fulfilment often engender happiness – but try asking people what makes them happy. Most will need to give a lot of thought to their answer. Surprisingly few will answer immediately. Among the answers will be relief from stress; acquiring something, travelling to somewhere or having a successful relationship. Most want money, enjoyable experiences and thus an improved quality of life. To answer the question truthfully in order to gain genuine insight, some will have to put their selfishness aside. Feelings of happiness, contentment, satisfaction, and fulfilment minimise our energy expenditure. Happiness, and a sense of humour, are as important to health as exercise and what we eat.

To sense happiness in a relationship, our natural psychological need for affection, control and inclusion must be satisfied. This involves the giving and receiving of just the right amount of affection, control and inclusion, within our relationship with another person.

If we have a giving nature, a happy relationship will come only if our partner wants what we have to give. If we love to receive, then only by getting the necessary affection, control or inclusion from our partner, will a happy relationship result. The amount and quality of what we give and receive are important, but first we must find a compatible partner – one mutually fulfilling all the giving and receiving requirements. I previously estimated the odds of finding such a person in an arena full of randomly chosen people. It was somewhere between 64 : 1 and 6400 : 1! (see Chapter 8 – family and relationships).

Human Complexity

It is fashionable and egotistical to think we humans are complex – even unfathomably complex. It is not often you hear someone refer to themselves, like Professor Higgins of Pygmalion fame, as 'simple'. Nearest to the truth, and something best hidden, is that we are all painfully simple – as far as most of our thoughts, feelings and deeds are concerned. Once the masks of delusion and illusion we have created are stripped away, what's left is mostly straightforward. Any difficulty we might have with others will usually lie in overcoming their defences – the defences they put in place to protect their projected image – of being deeply mysterious, fascinating, overwhelmingly sophisticated and desirable.

Why do we all feel the need to spend so much energy keeping up false appearances? The fear of exposure and vulnerability must have some evolutionary purpose. Perhaps it's because would-be predators would otherwise more easily discover our weaknesses and attack. Defiance and the appearance of strength must once have best suited our survival. Even Plato, 2,400 years ago, has Socrates discussing the idea that appearing good and just is more advantageous than the truth (Plato. *The Republic*).

When people appear complicated or complex, they are best re-garded with suspicion – subjects needing further revelation. It will rarely be that they are unintelligible, mystical and unknowable. There is joy, however, in finding a person who is open, modest, simple and uncomplicated; a straightforward person, totally true to themselves.

When one has known someone as a friend for a long time, and been regularly exposed to their every foible, it might then be possible to generalise about them – to describe their true essence in one or two words: 'John is greedy; a self-centred person. He always wants his own way'. To be of value, our understanding needs to be predictive – able to accurately predict their behaviour at different times. I have only met two people with the 20/20 insight required to understand others fully after meeting them once.

The best solutions to any problem are nearly always simple: with enlightened ease, the correct solution will readily explain all of the positive and negative aspects. Think of a crossword puzzle. How satisfying it is to interpret the clue and find the correct word. How obvious it all is, once the correct answer is found.

Solving Problems & Survival

In human affairs, the solution to a problem might be easy to formulate, but difficult to accomplish.

A businessman, stressed at work, with an unhappy marriage of long-standing, might wonder what he should do for the best. One answer would be to sell his business and get divorced. That's the easy way out, some might say. They could, of course, carry on trying to find an acceptable compromise. The best solution may be unacceptable – it might take too much courage, be insensitive or disrespectful. Also, the financial implications might be too serious to contemplate. The action taken will usually depend on the personal values held, the feelings of others or the money involved. They might conclude: 'I can't do it – the costs are too high'.

Conflicted people can repeatedly create the same problems. Had this businessman known he was about to have a heart attack, he might have taken a different view. Realising that his life depended on it, he might have found the necessary courage to enact a solution. Unfortunately, it can take a heart attack or stroke to make such changes justifiable. Heart attacks and strokes, however, are not yet as predictable as we would like. Cardiologists might suggest that the odds of having one are high but will not be able to predict the timing of any catastrophe. A danger for doctors is that we scare patients unnecessarily.

Survival often involves selfishness. As unattractive as this may be to altruists, the human jungle has rules that are easily ignored by the self-interested. Matters of honour, pride, and duty may come into question. They will be evaluated for their expediency. The strength of character it takes to keep honour in place, could prove lifesaving, foolhardy or fatal, when tough survival decisions have to be made.

Emotional and rational issues occurring at once, complicate decision making. Mr Spock, of Star Trek fame, could always be relied upon for an objective answer in a difficult situation. Because he always thought logically without emotional overlay, he could be relied on for clarity. Few humans are capable of this, except perhaps, the autistic. Elon Musk, who has admitted to having Asperger's, uses it to explain his dispassionate, direct nature. Every counsellor or psychotherapist is at their best when independently objective, focussed on the key questions of conflict, and able to separate the emotional from the rational.

With perfect judgement, nobody would ever make a mistake. There would be no need for conflict or heartache, and no need for corrective behaviour. If it existed, perfect judgement would always lead to correct decisions that stand the test of time. In reality, few people excel at judgement. As a result, many will have to make regular adjustments to what they think and do. All too often, human stress results from poor prior judgement. We will pay for this with energy spent on heartache, recrimination, guilt and regret. We will spend energy correcting our mistakes or suffering the consequences – in an unhappy place with little quality of life.

All too often there is insufficient information on which to base good judgement. Who, for instance, insists on a compatibility test or a relationship analysis, before going on a first romantic date? Unfortunately, our future happiness and contentment, unhappiness and energy expenditure, can depend on the judgements we make today.

Cultural Constructs

Conflict spends energy and can reduce our quality of life.

Can a culture be strengthened or weakened by progressive cultural mixing? History records a lot of cultural mixing after successful military invasions. The UK has withstood the invasion of the Romans, Vikings and the French in 1066. The UK is now struggling to cope with the substantial immigration of peoples from the Middle East and Asia whose cultural differences might be seen as challenging.

We are all brought up from childhood to adulthood, exposed to our family culture. Thereafter, we might be exposed to several other cultures. In multicultural UK, many are questioning the prevailing culture. Donald Trump has said that immigration can destroy a country from within, but can cultural mixing be advantageous? Whether it sources advantage, stress or illness has yet to be explored.

The person we become is mostly inherited (we inherit our personality, intelligence, height, eye colour, etc.). Our outlook, attitudes and beliefs, might also be decided by the values and beliefs we choose to accept from our environment and cultural background – adopted from our family, friends and those who educated us. If our culture is represented by the beliefs and values of our ethnic, faith and family group, it is not surprising that clashes between cultures will occur. The violence of these clashes will depend on how strongly our values are held and how compatible they are with others. The potential for such clashes is now a constant background drain on the energy of many UK inhabitants. Those who feel they belong, spend least; those who feel foreign – like a fish out of water – spend most.

Each culture has its own constructs. Those with their own culture are not restricted to religious or ethnic groups; they exist for family groups, professions, and whole nations with whom we are said 'to identify'.

Consider the culture of criminality and the associated values held. In the UK, criminals are expected by the police and lawyers, to have little regard for the property of their fellow citizens. Once apprehended, however, judges and citizens in the UK, expect them to show remorse. I am not sure why. What good does it do the criminal or their victim(s)? Nevertheless, for British culture, it is obligatory for convicted criminals to show remorse, guilt, and a need for forgiveness, if they want leniency.

Why commit a crime in the first place, if you are going to feel guilt and remorse afterwards? The reasons are many, all laid bare in the pages of crime fiction. Remorse is not expected universally; some cultures don't care much for it. I have chosen not to name them. It is certainly not a requirement for those employed as spies or assassins. Remorse can be respected if genuine but is too easily feigned.

Compare the criminal culture to that of Judeo-Christianity. Instead of valuing the rule of law, criminals often abide by a separate set of rules. Transgressing these rules, like police informing, can be so contrary to the accepted criminal construct, that harm or death may come to the perpetrators. Informing on criminals, and upkeeping the rule of law, however, is seen as the duty of every law-abiding citizen. These are values set apart from the values espoused by the criminal fraternity, but there are paradoxes. Criminals very strongly support their friends and are strongly loyal. Among one another, honouring compatriots is *de rigueur*.

Law abiding, fairness, mutually respectful behaviour, reasonableness and honesty, are highly valued, traditional British constructs; many require 'thank-you' to be said in response to any kindness;

we almost all insist on forming orderly queues, considering those who jump them, on the road or otherwise, as outsiders. All visitors and immigrants to the UK, need to know this. They will otherwise upset a lot of 'traditional native Brits' (my strong definition – those whose eight great-grandparents were all born in the UK, representing as it does, a lengthy exposure to British values – not just those required for nationalisation. A more sensible, weak definition would include only grandparents).

Personal Energy Assessment

You might want to undertake an assessment of your personal energy spending characteristics. If so, go to Appendix 2. There you will find a questionnaire. Simply by answering it, you should gain some insight.

Better still, get a friend to answer the questions with you in mind, then discuss the results to compare your self-image with that of someone who knows you well.

CHAPTER SEVENTEEN

Factors of Consequence for Society

SOCIAL ASPECTS OF FATIGUE AND THE HEALTH DIVIDE

All organisations have the strengths of their weaknesses.

Pugh's Principle

Running parallel to the energy spending of individuals is that of societies. The authority to spend energy on behalf of a society is vested in only a few political figures. The more developed a society and culture, the more energy needs to be spent maintaining it. We have moved from sharing energy expenditure with our families and tribes, surviving as hunter-gatherers, to functioning as a global society. Fortunately, only a small proportion of the vast mineral and oil energy reserves we have, has been spent on this quest. All societies delegate control to those who seek power, and to gain from it personally. Some will improve the lot of those they serve, but many will not. Most people have remained hunter-gatherers by nature; spending their lives solely in the pursuit of food, shelter and possessions. In many societies this is a challenge not always met by those we call the deprived.

Both the diseases we suffer (morbidity), and those that cause our death (mortality), have an overriding aspect that multiplies their occurrence three to five-fold – social deprivation. Morbidity and mortality occur most in the poor and ill-educated, wherever they live in the world.

Apathy about solving deprivation and its abandonment in favour of more engaging projects, has afflicted the bureaucrats of all nations. As a poisoned political chalice, many will think it best avoided. When, for instance, is deprivation ever featured in any daily news served to us; unless as a by-product of something more dramatic and newsworthy – like war, an earthquake, flooding or a large building collapse. No agency wants to claim responsibility for it, and most avoid discussing it. This consideration alone, makes this chapter somewhat irrelevant. It will, however, help the educated and endowed to fine tune their advantaged status.

You might ask if I am qualified to write about both deprived and the privileged. I think I am. I started life among the underprivileged of Walthamstow, in East London, where I first went to school, and where I first worked. I ended my working life among the financially privileged of Loughton (solely in private practice), and the financially privileged of Battersea and Chelsea in London.

Energy and Civilisation

Big changes occurred during the Renaissance, but they never involved the working man, except to incur his labour. Only a privileged few, gratified their artistic and scientific whims, sponsoring those with new ideas: scientists like Galileo Galilei, and artists like Michelangelo and Raphael, to adorn their palaces. One such person, who must have spent a lot of his energy achieving this, was Frederigo Montefeltro, the first Duke of Urbino. Young courtiers would come to learn at his court – how to walk, how to speak in a refined manner, and how to behave in a manner that avoided making others feel inferior. They learned that refined behaviour marked the gentleman. It still pertains in some sectors of society today.

During the Renaissance, experiences of fine art, music, science, and gastronomy, were distributed to those far removed, helping to break the chain of monotonous everyday experience.

It was Pope Julius II who spent energy convincing Michelangelo to paint the Sistine Chapel, even though he had said he disliked painting! Had it not been for Julius' gift for talent-spotting, Raphael, then 27-years old, would not have had the chance to paint murals in La Stanza della Segnatura (the Pope's private library), an art-form he had scarcely tried before.

From the standpoint of entropy – the tendency of all things to disintegrate in time – such formal, courtly manners, were unlikely to survive. It takes lots of energy to create refined structures. Sophisticated buildings, oil paintings, murals and nuclear reactors, do not come about by chance. That is why none are yet visible on Mars. Lots of energy and talent is required to create them – energy that will be released later, unless enough energy is spent maintaining them. The entropic process is one of natural recycling – energy once spent on constructions is later returned to nature. Fortunes are now spent daily on behalf of world society, maintaining our most revered treasures.

The more energy spent on creating magnificent constructions, the more a society can be said to be 'civilised'. This embodies the essence of the Renaissance and man's heroic will – the belief that apart from any Divine intervention, man can understand and conquer all.

"There must have been a time when it (the Tuscan landscape) was all forest and swamp - shapeless, form-

less; and to bring order out of chaos is a process of civilisation."

Kenneth
Clarke

Civilisation. 1969.

Social Energy Demands

Many are concerned about the social and political nature of their society. They may see many wrongs to be righted, and much injustice to be swallowed. How many are satisfied with what they see going on about them – things that can be ignored by those in power who live far, far away, from the common man. Although governments change, and just about manage to rearrange the furniture of society, they only rarely improve our social wellbeing. This impotence is something we must all live with.

Has a money dominated world, caused us to lose some social responsibility? Have we lost concern for our neighbours? After all, many don't know their neighbours, and may not want to know them.

We all know our rights, and know what society has to offer us, but do we know our social duties? The more we live in isolation, separated from one another, the more anonymous we could become. Anonymity helps to resist intrusions into our privacy but can detach us from any civil duty. What is more, society is now geared to keep it that way. In many western societies, citizens have become takers – as a right – with little sense of duty or need to contribute.

These matters vary with culture. When I was a young man in the UK, there was no need to define traditional Britishness; only a small minority of residents came from another cultural background. With native values now being rapidly diluted by extensive, even overwhelming, cultural mixing, Britishness is becoming difficult to define, and morphing further within each generation. Whether the new morphs will bring us something better or worse, only time will tell. This subject – a new social stress – is beginning to tax many older traditional British people. What magnifies the stress, is that no politician is offering a way out, although, maybe there is no need. Eventually, integration could greatly advantage us all.

Both immigrants and natives must spend time and energy adapting to change, negotiating mutual acceptance. The cultural adaption needed will add to our energy consumption, but more for the antipathetic than the welcoming. In many modern societies there is a notable loss of sensibility towards other people; especially if they are foreign or less well-off. My name might not be Jack, but I am fully aware of the 'I'm alright Jack' attitude – an attitude that denies any personal responsibility for others.

There is much to cause unrest (stress) among the citizens of the UK. It is our social duty to pay our taxes and vote for those supposedly 'trained' to manage our national funds, yet patients are still dying on NHS waiting lists, and elderly care is unsupportable. The expensive computer systems NHS bureaucrats bought, have not helped with connected thinking and social management. Many have benefitted, but few of them are patients. With evidence of wasteful UK government spending, perhaps it's time for a major re-think of what we expect from a democratic society. Instead of democracy, perhaps one of Plato's suggestions might work – a philosopher king might suit us better as a leader.

Because the problems of the world are only rarely solved by one individual, many join political movements; some gaining self-esteem from being affiliated with a philanthropic purpose. Getting used to our impotence at solving societal and political problems, like deprivation, war, abuse, criminality, homelessness and elderly care, allows for no pride or dignity to be had from any political party.

The situation in the UK is not all negative. At least, we have safe water to drink, efficient waste disposal, excellent fire services, and street lighting, all of which we take for granted.

That Selfish Social Gene

> *"The Public be damned. We like to do everything possible for the benefit of humanity in general, but we do first see that we are benefiting ourselves."*

William H. Vanderbilt. 1882.

With knowledge should come improved awareness. With awareness may come responsibility and duty. Self-esteem can come from fulfilling our duty, and guilt from rejecting it. Gaining knowledge consumes energy, whether we try to acquire it, use it, retain it or disseminate it. Because it consumes much less energy, some prefer to remain ignorant. It could be healthier mentally.

> *"To know too much is to decay."*

Chuang-Tzu. *The Inner Chapters.*

As we grow in knowledge, we might get to feel we are progressing towards knowing everything. That's an obvious illusion, of course. Characteristic of those who know most about a subject, is humility. They may know all that is known, but still feel they should know more, with so many questions yet to be answered.

Captains of society – those who choose what we are exposed to – influence our world. They can create, manipulate or hide information. Fashion buyers tell us what we will wear next year; news editors censor the pictures we are allowed see and the stories we get to read. Fashion, political biases and discrimination, are all manipulable. To some extent, our values are shaped by bureaucrats who believe their judgements are best. Commercial corporations also manipulate us, as long as we credit them with supplying our needs and desires. They exist only to make a profit or if charitable, to help the needy and pay their executives large salaries.

Only a few create the fashion; most others follow. The aim – to be found acceptable by our peer group; a fashionable insider, not an outsider; one of us, not one of them. The desire is to be BCBG (*Bon Chic, Bon Genre*) for not only the fashionable French. Is this not all wasteful energy consumption?

Many of us have a need to be fashionable and accepted, ensuring that most of us will comply. There are advantages. Many of us believe we get respect when committing to fashion. As committed followers, few will entertain alternatives. Some might say, 'Everyone is wearing it or doing it, so who am I to rock the boat?' And so, we are controlled, as if in chains. I wonder about J.J. Rousseau, the philosopher responsible for stating that 'Man is born free and everywhere he is in chains'. As one of the accepted French elite, living in Paris after 1742, my guess is that he was BCBG. *Aucune ironie perdue*?

Social Status and Disease

The first Whitehall study of British civil servants, clearly showed that the lower the pay grade of an employee, the higher the mortality rate. This might be explained partly by differences in standard risk factors like smoking, blood cholesterol, blood fibrinogen level and the tendency to clot, blood pressure, obesity, and physical activity.

The Whitehall II study found that the amount of control each employee had, correlated with their heart attack and stroke risk (Michael Marmot. 1991). The more each felt 'in control', the fewer the cardiovascular consequences. The volume and number of demands made of them at work, did not correlate – whether highly demanding or easy to cope with. This observation is consistent with other findings of occupational mortality. Those occupations that afford least control, are most often associated with an increased cardiovascular mortality.

Compared to men in the higher employment grades (administrators, but not the top jobs), men in the lowest grades (clerical and office-support staff), had the greater chance of developing a new cardiovascular condition (increased 1.5 times). The largest difference was for angina (2.27 times more). The odds for women rather than men getting such problems was 1.47 times greater.

Control at work is not the only important issue. Lower financial status individuals will have different home conditions and will often experience a different lifetime pathway, both educationally and socially. Although all of these might contribute, having little or no control over circumstances (and its associated insecurity) is the most important factor (Marmot. M.G., et al. 1997).

Perhaps contributing to the mortality predicted by the health divide, the Whitehall II study found those of lower status had higher blood clotting factor concentrations (raised blood fibrinogen, as found in those prone to heart attacks and some strokes). The differences were not accounted for by measures of childhood circumstances (height, father's social class, and participant's education).

Environmental Energy Spending

Tolerance to road traffic noise and other noise pollution, is likely to develop faster in those with no option to avoid it. It can be made more bearable by adaptation, but there remains a constant, sub-liminal stress, appreciated more when it stops. Noisy communities are a constant source of stress (increased energy spending) capable of increasing our blood adrenaline levels and blood pressure (Sei-dman, M. D., Standring, R. T. 2010).

Making a change from living in a quiet rural location, to an inner city, can be disturbing. For those living in the countryside, the 'hoo' of a distant owl might be the loudest sound they hear. In urban locations, many live engulfed by noise, much of which comes from traffic and the proximity of others: noisy neighbours practising their singing and bonhomie at 3 AM.

Urban dwellers who move to the countryside, can also find it difficult to adjust. They will need time to adjust to the silence. Although this soon passes, it may leave rural dwellers more sensitive to noise when experienced elsewhere – when travelling or staying in hotels, for instance.

One difference between country and town living, is the need for vigilance. A comparison of crime rates indicates that urban living is more dangerous than rural living. Crime rates for violence, sexual offences, robbery, burglary, vehicle offences, theft, and criminal damage, were found 50 – 80% less in rural areas than in urban areas of England (DEFRA. *Crime*. 2022). Greater vigilance is needed for living in towns. It needs to be continuous and an insensible background form of stress.

Social deprivation increases mortality. Mortality is highest in densely populated areas like Merseyside and the North-East of England. In Norfolk, a rural county, it is lowest (Eames et al. 1993). Problems with privacy, living space, noise, overcrowding and pol-lution, are more likely in urban areas. In rural areas, however, there are fewer chances for employment – an increasing, major stress for many.

In towns, residents will often have to contend with crowds, and round-the-clock activities. Many town dwellers come to prefer this to the quiet of the countryside. Add to this, over-crowded travel on buses and trains, and the unreliability of overburdened transport systems, and even more energy needs to be spent on an urban existence. Urban drivers have much more to negotiate than rural drivers, and more often express anger, road rage, and other stress-induced behaviours. If traffic density increases further, urban drivers will experience even more frustration from lengthening journey times.

Town planning is a balancing act. It provides an opportunity for minor bureaucrats to exercise their power. In the UK, new towns and suburbia have come to share the same predictable, boring design features. The economics of uniformity makes it so, providing homes that are more affordable, and much more profitable for construction companies. There is hidden danger in the boredom of uniformity: it can create the feeling of environmental imprisonment and dissatisfaction. Although the character of many old towns can seem enriching, their reduced traffic flow and increase human density, can increase stress.

Many town dwellers think of rural life as boring, but cultural differences exist. The French and Russians prefer urban life (as reflected by property prices); many British people crave the peace of a rural cottage. British high-net-worth individuals frequently possess homes in both areas. They can reject the stress of urban living, as and when they desire. They have the choice – to walk through fields and forests or crowded shopping centres. In the country, the low human density, fresh air, and the individuality of many ancient dwellings, can be refreshing. Urban dwellers often remark, 'I don't know how you stand living in the countryside. There is nothing going on!' A false, but reasonable impression.

The current uniformity of flat and house designs in towns can be de-personalising, making the expression of individuality more challenging. One can only personalise them with internal fixtures, fittings, and personal effects. Otherwise, most must be content with all the possible variations of a shoebox.

In UK villages, many residents know others by their first name, although, social intimacy is not seen as an advantage by everyone. In towns, most inhabitants know few others, apart from their immediate neighbours. Valuing anonymity helps one live in an urban space.

For the health divide to reduce (especially in the USA), perhaps modern, socially-oriented new town planning, should simulate village living – each area having its character, perhaps with its own sporting teams, centralised shopping and other amenities nearby. Health promotional considerations should be embodied in every town planning scheme. What we are used to, what we find comfortable, and what we see as desirable, underlie some of the subliminal stresses affecting our health.

Nature, Nurture and Society

Are we all capable of becoming doctors, concert pianists or astronauts? Is our upbringing a big factor? Are slums like they are because of the types of people who live there? If so, would transplanting some middle-class people, transform them?

I well remember a conversation with my grandmother. Although she lived in a deprived area, she kept a clean and well-ordered home. I was only a medical student at the time but learned an invaluable lesson from her. The discussion concerned nature and nurture. She told me that soap was cheap! What she thought caused slums, was missing motivation, energy and soap. But might not those demoralised and depressed by living in a slum, find it too difficult to change? My grandmother didn't buy that excuse. Her view was that not everyone was inclined to cleanliness, hence the existence of both slums and uncared for mansions.

Whether the personality, outlook, behaviour, IQ., temperament and other characteristics required for success in life are the result of nature (genes) or nurture (upbringing), remains a hotly debated academic subject. Those with a measure of street wisdom, might see these characteristics as largely inherited, fostered by a privileged background – the effect of being 'born with a silver spoon in their mouth'.

Although the social and educational policies of governments should depend on the answer, politicians would shoot themselves in the foot if they didn't favour the nurture hypothesis. To believe in the nature hypothesis, is to remove any hope of change. Since that seems too cruel to contemplate, many will opt for a bit of both – trying to satisfy everyone. Will the controversy outlast the discoveries of the genome project? I doubt it, but we must wait and see.

Joan was a mother of three but felt under-loaded. After her hysterectomy, she and her husband decided to adopt two more children. Thereafter she fostered another three!

"I gave them all the same home, yet two of them turned out bad. They were undisciplined and were in trouble with the police very early on. None of my own children ever behaved like that. Those two were just no good from the start. I was so disappointed. I really thought you could make people turn out right by giving them

love, care, and attention. That's why I took on so many
children. I was wrong, and I've paid for it!"

Our chromosomal DNA determines how our minds and bodies are constructed, although, nurture can modify it. Grow the same seeds in different soil, and variations in plant size and health will result. For two of Joan's adopted and fostered children, nature won over their nurture. For the others, at least their nature and nurture were sufficient to allow a happy co-existence within the family. The mother and father of every child, each has their own genetic profile (equivalent to a hand of cards). Which cards each of their children gets at conception is a matter of chance. So, to some extent, it is luck that decides whether a genetic strangeling will be affable and compatible or not easy to live with!

Joan's natural children had to share their parents. All must have benefitted from experiencing her generosity of spirit, tolerance and understanding of others, different from themselves. Maybe the energy Joan spent on the anxiety and aggravation involved, was worth it after all!

Media Editing

As well as shaping our expectations and helping us to handle the events that may befall us, the media have a history of bringing images and experiences to our door, some of which we can do without. For some, knowledge in graphic detail could disturb their mental health. What they expose us to is a media editors job. Anonymous editing can deliver a version of the truth most of us will accept without further thought.

Media outlets exist to profit from informing us, yet bear a considerable health-related responsibility. They need to protect their consumers from unnecessary, disturbing information. After Donald Trump's many bold proclamations of press fakery, the public is now more aware of them subjecting the news to spin, exaggeration, bias, and falsity. As consumers, we need to be aware of the framing bias:

> *Showing pictures of emaciated Gazan children (July 2025) (for which there are many causes other than famine), was used to infer – but not prove – that Gazans were all suffering from starvation. Those blamed for causing universal, unverified emaciation (based on pictures supplied by Hamas), were cast as devils; those suffering it, became martyrs. Few enquired further.*

The framing bias is all important. Information can be presented with a point and cutting edge, as deadly as any bayonet. Information can be made acceptable or unacceptable; it all depends on what editors and reporters *choose* to convey. Getting to the truth, presented in its proper context is not easy. Even after hundreds of years, the truth about what really happened can remain obscure, especially if the motives, political biases, context, and need for gain at the time are not known.

A Place for Generalisation?

It is human nature, and a special function of the human brain, to generalise. Over evolutionary time, it is most likely to have represented a survival factor. Generalisations are useful when facing danger, helping to reduce the burden of information overload. Since generalisations ignore detail, and often dismiss exceptions, how reliable can they be?

Generalisations that result from repeated observation can be accurate, especially when trained and experienced observers are aware of their biases. Generalisations become inaccurate and misleading, when too many observations are deleted, cherry-picked or falsified. It is then that some political purpose may be involved.

Statistics provide a numerical version of generalisation. Measure or observe the same or similar thing, one hundred times or more, and two-thirds (68%) of the observations will lie near to the calculated mean (how near or far from it, being calculated as a standard deviation). This implies that any generalisation, based on repeatedly confirmed observation, can be of use. But how sure can we be, given most of us hold strong biases, and want recognition for being right?

Take the generalisation: 'smelling food before you eat it, prevents gastroenteritis'. One sniff can define whether milk or meat is 'off'. One sniff of an uncooked turkey will usually help you decide whether to cook it for Christmas lunch or Thanksgiving. Although not based on statistical appraisal (from many observations), such an observation based on a generalisation, could be life-saving.

We use generalisation to form many conclusions. But are they valid and worthwhile to continue with? Testing them for scientific validity requires an experiment to be set up. So, try this. Blindfold one hundred medical students; get them each to smell five prepared turkeys (some condemned as bacteriologically unsafe, others not); note their observations; compare smell reports to bacterial content. OK. Perhaps not! I think I'll just carry on using my experience and trusting my nose!

Some generalisations can be characterised as 'BLOB' – **BL**indingly **OB**vious. For instance: no elephant gives birth to a giraffe; no apple grows on a pear tree, and few will survive jumping out of an aircraft without a parachute. These are all generalisations, obviously true; none in need of qualification.

On the 12th June 2025, Vishwash Kumar Ramesh sitting in seat 11A of the Air India flight Al-171 from Ahmedabad to London, was the only survivor after his aeroplane, a Boeing 878-8 Dreamliner, lost power and crashed soon after take-off.

When flying, should we always ask to sit in seat 11A? Of course not. Our request would be based on only one observation, on only one type of airplane. Generalisation, extrapolated from only one incident, is very unlikely to be true. An observation, repeatedly confirmed to be true over a whole lifetime, is likely to be correct. Such is the basis of what used to be called 'Old Wives' Tales'.

The observation that foxglove extract could help those with heart failure and swollen feet (once called dropsy), was found to be true by William Withering in 1785. It led him to develop a pharmaceutical still in use today – digitalis for the heart.

Even though we live in a world suffused with the need for evidence (in science and evidence-based legal determinations), it is strange that nobody has yet felt the need to study the benefits of parachutes. The further one gets from experience and reality (typical of many bureaucrats), the less 'BLOB' is appreciated.

In the academic world, using generalisation alone has been totally outlawed. Although churlish and pedantic, few can now resist asking: '*What is your evidence for that?' 'How certain are you of your facts?' 'How can you be sure you are not fooling yourself?'* All valid questions, of course.

Humanity has arrived at a point where there is an obsessive need for certainty. I understand why. Many of us are easily capable of fooling ourselves. Many CEOs of companies, and those with political power, have no direct knowledge of what they are doing; their approach will often lack the common sense that comes with experience. Corporations stuffed with rule-based bureaucrats, can take years to make sense of something many street-wise, experienced observers, have known for years. Too many politicians and NHS executives, function at too great a distance from the action. In the latter case, too few have any first-hand understanding of patients or medical practice, yet they have the power to make health provision changes; making as many ill-informed decisions as their committees choose to make.

The same sort of functioning once applied to the British army. In the First World War, some high-ranking officers had never experienced action, yet they were charged with making life and death decisions for front-line soldiers. They should have asked the front-line observers first, but there-in lies a problem. There are big differences in the reliability of individual observers, and the biases they each have. Some are trained and experienced, but many are not.

> *When Monty (Field Marshall Bernard Montgomery), visited his front-line troops during the Second World War, North African campaign, my uncle Charlie was there – as a front-line soldier. Monty asked one of his fellow soldiers what he thought of the situation. 'I'm worried', said the soldier. 'We've had no bullets for ages. If the enemy comes over that hill, Sir, we will have to throw our guns at 'em!'*

> *Only a little imagination is needed to guess what Monty did next.*

Generalisations can be formed using fair and unfair bias. Politicos, those seeking power, and those seeking attention, can use generalisation perversely to draw attention to themselves.

In her remarkable book, *The Whole Woman* (1999 and 2007), Germaine Greer, generalises about men:

> *"Men are freaks of nature, fragile, fantastic, bizarre. To be male is to be a kind of idiot savant, full of queer obsessions about fetishistic activities and fantasy goals, single-minded in pursuit of arbitrary objectives, doomed to competition and injustice not merely towards females, but towards children, animals and other men."*

Who was she is generalising about, I wonder? How many personal biases were in play when she wrote this? Is her description pervaded by any essence of maleness? After seven decades of observing men, I fail to recognise much in her stereotype. Was she referring to her father, perhaps? Many women are strong and admirable, but feminism will hardly be strengthened by exaggerated anti-male bias. Using such obvious bias, discredits generalisation. I wonder if she consulted her father before writing it?

Abuse

The National Society for the protection of children, once ran an advert featuring eavesdropping – on a parent who was screaming and threatening her child. Interpretation of the observations present some problems. The advert should have prompted the question, 'who is being abused', the child or the adult? The NSPPC thought it was the child. But don't some children abuse their parents? Immaturity and a lack of understanding may be at fault, but abuse can work both ways.

The elderly, incapable of doing things for themselves, are easily deemed useless and worthless by their partners and carers. With no respect for what they may have achieved in life, younger people (more often from a western culture) may come to favour their demoralisation, rather than respect. At all ages, fear and conflict will burn energy. The risk changes with age. Fragile older people, burning lots of unnecessary energy through anger and frustration, might more quickly meet their end.

Conflict & Dilemma

People seek resolution. The reason people enjoy reading Jack Reacher novels is they get to experience someone capable of re-solving life's problems. So said their famous author, James Dover Grant, alias Lee Child, at a book festival in the UK. (2025).

Where there is a conflict of conviction or when a difficult choice between many attractive options arises, our feeling of personal energy can disappear fast. Over a long period, living with a difficult to resolve dilemma (especially if potentially life-shaping), can burn our energy in the background. Any pre-occupation with finding a solution, will disturb sleep. Many will wake at 4AM trying to solve the problem.

Chaos theory suggests that even the smallest of decisions, holds the potential to affect our fate. The healthy option would be to avoid all encounters, rather than run the risk of creating a dilemma. Such a life would be emotionally featureless, suiting best those without much adventurous spirit.

One can always solve a dilemma by tossing a coin. Getting as much information as possible before deciding is, however, the more rational option. Expecting someone else to make the first move, is one possibility. In this way, the decision is made by another person. Discussing decisions with those we trust, and those wiser and more experienced than ourselves, is always a sensible option.

Only the energetic should contemplate living with uncomfortable compromise. Those without the energy to spare, risk being demeaned mentally or physically.

Impersonal Energy Spending

We are told to rely on governments. Their duty is to arrange support services for our society, providing care from birth to death, in return for work and taxes. They are also supposed to provide security, equal rights and opportunities for all, while providing a safe environment. We are sold on the idea that without them, anarchy would be just around the corner.

The machinery of society is driven unseen, not by any government, but by those working for self-worth and personal happiness. A sense of fulfilment is gained, not from any government, but from the affection of friends, family, work mates, colleagues – and sometimes from complete strangers – friends we have yet to make!

Advertising and communications media are capable of biasing the reality we are allowed to see. By what they choose to report, and how they choose to edit it, they can affect our sense of security, opinions and happiness. Donald Trump's anti-media campaign has highlighted their capabilities and has questioned the power they think they have.

For a growing number of people, social media outlets can incite anarchy and insurrection. One job of government is to keep these influences at bay. Reading news output will help many to opt out of forming their own opinions. At the moment, reporters, editors and influencers, still have the opinions of the majority on a tight leash. This will remain so, while independent thinking is discouraged and in decline. Thinking can seem tiresome, and an energy consuming task for many. Being guided by media output is so much simpler.

BBC News (2025) in the UK, put itself in a vanguard position. "The fight for truth is on", said one newscaster, expecting us to believe that they, at least, should be trusted unconditionally.

Altruism and Profit

In any town like London, with many culturally diverse people who are less than integrated, achieving camaraderie can be challenging. During the Second World War, when this was not the case, Londoners came together in a collective, meaningful way, to expand the war effort.

From their literature, it seems that the citizens of ancient Greece and Rome, were worried and exhilarated by the same trials of life as we are today. Personal interaction remains unchanged, accept for its rapidity and technical diversity of means. While we might now save time, we have more to do. We are also free as ever to waste it. Human motivation still has the same origins –becoming noticed, gaining influence, making a profit and achieving safety and financial security. If these have not changed, what need do we have for so many, so called 'advances'?

There is now much worthy discussion about AI. It will benefit many individuals, but what about mankind? This is something for the young to worry about – their future security. Will there be jobs for them in the future? AI cannot perform carpentry, mechanical engineering or plumbing, so perhaps fewer will need to attend university, and more might need to get their hands dirty.

The communications business has succeeded in making even the most innocent of us, addicted to speed, even though very few actually need speedy communication. Only the super-rich and powerful can afford the luxury of communication-free zones –

they employ their subordinate minions to handle that for them. For the rest of us, staying connected might offer opportunities. Few are able to escape it for more than a week or so!

Is profit a dirty word? After all, someone, somewhere, will be gaining an advantage (financially, morally or spiritually). Is buying an apple for a dime, and selling it to a friend for two dimes, reasonable? Cultures are partly defined, by their attitude towards profit. From its malevolent root, comes one purpose – to take advantage of another person. Profiting from a service, with the purpose of helping others, has some moral justification; selling apples for an excessive profit, can sour our feelings towards vendors, and those who allow them to get away with it.

Most businessmen are not where they are to-day, because they gave away their goods and services: their art is a simple one – always buy things for less than the sale price. They will make a profit, only if they consistently sell the goods they have purchased. This is the risk they take, and one reason they deserve some profit. We justify our relationship with businessmen by feeling happy to pay for the convenience they offer. Nevertheless, there is an implicit distrust which can be measured, by how much profit is being made. Yes, I know, trading makes the world go around, but it leans heavily on customer disadvantage: the disadvantage of not having enough information to know where to buy the goods cheaper. AI promises to change all that and rebalance business.

The price we pay for making a profit is significant. We lose the pleasure of helping others – without a financial gain. Do good deeds deserve brownie points? Those with a religious conviction will usually think so.

One justification for a business making large profits is that they can use the money to do some good, thereby gaining a spiritual reward. The reward might get tarnished by know that charitable giving has another advantage – it is tax deductible. So, not quite the same as an altruistic pursuit. Purity and corruption of purpose, remain in opposition, possibly creating ambivalence. To maintain this balancing act, may require some subliminal energy expenditure.

Communication

In the beginning, the time taken for communication was at human speed – limited by the speed of brain neuronal transmission. The same time will always be necessary for the most appropriate, long-term deliberation, needed for sound judgement. Then came the marathon messenger, the carrier pigeon and the horse; warning beacons, the heliograph, postal services; the telephone, radio, and e-mail, all improving the speed of communication.

We are now presented with evermore bits of information, regardless of need. The lag-time between news formation and its transmission, is becoming shorter, with the amount of information available per second, getting greater. Many are now anxious not to 'miss out'; not to be 'left behind' or thought 'ill-informed' (which often means, we have not yet ingested the opinions of others). We are thus, evermore induced to spend energy needlessly. Nobody can avail themselves of every opportunity; most of us simply have too little time, money or energy for it. Frustration and disappointment are at hand, especially for those would-be winners of the life game, whose object in life is to make themselves happy.

So thick is the forest of available data, there is not enough time for anyone to assimilate it all. Hooked on the communications and profit game, the objectives are proving ever distant, illusive, and ill-defined. There is one dull side to the growth of information technology – it is replacing personal interaction. We now spend more time viewing and analysing irrelevant data than we ever did.

Men have always travelled and communicated, but never before at the current speed. While rapid information acquisition facilitates decision making, a surfeit of information, irrelevant or otherwise, will slow every decision-making process. Despite this, many are being asked to make decisions faster. We no longer seem to have surplus time to deliberate. The greater the speed you travel in a car, the more petrol per mile you will burn. Adding acceleration burns more. The same applies to making decisions. The more challenging they are, the more energy needed.

Every aspect of accurate communication is important for survival. The teaching of foreign languages, as extensions of one's own mother tongue, can reduce friction with others. It can smooth our path through life in a world, where language and culture still matter. Speaking well is only half the problem. Listening is critical, and a willingness to comprehend indispensable. Minimising energy expenditure through good communication is not only fulfilling, it also maximises our chances of healthy survival. It is never too late to improve our clarity of thought and communication skills. Life might become easier if these subjects were taught at school.

Sometimes one can be credited with good communication or linguistic skills, without them being deserved.

I had been living in Amsterdam for nine months. I was able to speak rudimentary Dutch, when outside the Concertgebouw in Amsterdam, I was stopped by an American tourist family. In a deliberately slow, pointed way, they asked me – "do you know the way – to – the – Rijksmuseum?" Pointing the way, and using BBC English, I said: "Cross here, go straight to the top of this road. There you will see a large building – about a quarter of a mile on your left. That's the Rijksmuseum". They thanked me, and as I walked away, I heard one say: "Gee, these Dutch, they speak such good English!"

Poor understanding or worse - an unwillingness to understand – will often lead to an unsatisfactory relationship. Estrangement, dispassionate relationships, diverging objectives, divorce and even premature death can result.

Insist on understanding. Don't be shy. Ask for clarification. Look up the meaning of words and colloquial expressions. Better not to fear technology and jargon; it may only be short-hand for something you already know. Improving your understanding fosters healthy survival. Recognise your need to understand.

> *I have a solicitor friend with an infallible technique for communicating with clients. He stops often, and says, "Now let's see if I've got this right. When you die, you want half of all your property to go to an animal refuge; the other half to the taxman?" By reiterating and confirming his understanding, he is never confused and always able to correctly prepare the required legal documents. He thus saves himself and his clients, unnecessary energy expenditure.*

I have noticed that British people are often reluctant to ask for clarification. The Americans I have worked with, are more intent on confirming their understanding. Cultures clearly differ in this respect. Some are shy or worried by the possibility of embarrassment. Some are concerned about losing face – perhaps the most dangerous of all communication traits. Other dangerous traits are arrogance and ignorance, with those afflicted carrying on regardless of their lack of understanding. These are of no consequence when trying to find a location address but are life and death issues for airline pilots and surgeons, responsible for the lives of others.

Life as a Struggle

Imagine trying to walk up a down escalator. Even though you work hard to ascend, you stay in the same place. Such a lot of energy spent without gain. The same feeling of drudgery happens in the early days of paying a mortgage. You work hard, pay lots of money to the mortgage company each month, but pay very little off the capital sum. I previously coined the word 'mateosis' to describe this active phenomenon of fruitless activity (from the Greek word μάταιος). Sisyphus experienced the same with his boulder. Every time he neared the top of a hill, it rolled back. He was doomed to repeat it for ever. His crime was to reveal one of Zeus's secrets.

Struggle burns energy. The poor struggle to get money; the rich struggle to put their money to profitable use. The educated struggle to get intellectual satisfaction and recognition; the uneducated struggle to find a job. Where lies peace? Can one find true peace without attaining that state of grace where there is no pressing need for choice, no cause for neuroticism, just acceptance, composure, happiness and contentment. This will describe a living hell for some; for others, their unattainable goal. I find it a tragedy that so few in modern life, will ever glimpse this state of being. Most will toil, trying to afford to 'get away from it all'. When they get there, they will mostly meet others struggling to escape in other directions!

Mistrust Drains Energy

I have a friend whose principle outlook is to mistrust everyone. He mistrusts his wife, his neighbours, and anyone in authority. The energy he spends on distrust is considerable. His personal situation could be better, but because he trusts nobody, non-one wants to help him. Distrust maybe a safe initial position to adopt in business dealings, but it will inhibit successful progress.

Distrust of others can be seen as self-protective. Since power corrupts, it is wise to be cautious when dealing with those with resources, status, and valuable information.

> *"The love of liberty is the love of others; the love of power is the love of ourselves."*

> William Hazlitt. (1819)

The energy and money it takes to shop around on the internet or otherwise, might make department stores seem worthwhile, even if their prices are exorbitant. What we lose financially, we can gain in convenience and energy.

In sexual relationships, there are two poles of trust possible. The one-night-stand requires none; gratification is short-term, and long-term trust is not an issue. Long-term relationships only become long-term, once mutual trust develops. If a loving partnership is to be successful, mutual trust must be its foundation. Supportive partners save energy for one another. From a biological and evolutionary perspective (essential considerations when survival is at risk), it is the mutual saving of energy, that marks all worthwhile relationships.

Simple energy considerations apply to the policies of institutions, like the armed forces, the police, banks, and large companies. Ultimately, mutual support is what all institutions should be designed for – like a good marriage, they save us energy, even though much hard work may be needed to keep them alive.

Failing Public Duty

From Richard Doll's first scientific reports on the medical dangers of smoking in 1950, it took fifty-seven years for successive UK governments to ban smoking indoors. Sanctioning tobacco smoking, authorised the culling of citizens.

The tax produced from selling tobacco, has remained considerable. This government profit monster is smart. It trades on metaphysical paradigms like 'in the public interest' and 'freedom of choice'; in this case, to smoke or not to smoke, as we choose. Most smokers are not told that their chance of reaching 65-years-of-age, is halved by smoking. A caring, benevolent society would surely remove smoking completely, but that would disallow ill-informed choice, and abuse freedom. The move will thus be suppressed for the sake of the system, and until the tobacco companies find profitable alternatives, like vapes. Tobacco companies are smart. Many years ago, they started investing in health insurance!

We have lost cotton and sugar slavery, but now many of us are slaves to society. As victims of fashion and usury, and servants of those wealthy enough to control our behaviour, our lives are all but completely controlled. Human energy is harnessed as much now, as it ever was. We all carry on regardless, hooked by the system, yet still believing we are free. Because most of us want to own our own home, we will resign our freedom to become a mortgage slave, at the same time despising human slavery. The only difference – plantation slaves had no choice; we have some choice, but only rarely free of some commitment to others. Also ironic, is our willingness to accept conflict and duplicity, as long as we find them expedient. Duplicity and conflict both burn loads of energy.

Even with any overstatement subtracted, there remain unpalatable truths: western society drains our energy, controls our will and thereby affects our health. We have unwittingly chosen life paths that lead to ill-health. This is nothing new, except we must now pay for the tools of our own destruction. Regardless of all this, most are living longer in western societies. Without the energy constraints listed here, perhaps we might live longer or have a better quality of life; perhaps both.

Some of us never need be victims. The rich and advantaged can opt out of every social system. They have no need for State schooling, the NHS or mortgage companies. They can buy houses in peaceful areas, with privacy, minimal noise and pollution. They can afford to eat high-protein diets, travel widely, and consult experienced professionals. In hospital, they can be nursed in quiet single rooms, with their dignity and privacy remaining intact. They can lead a healthier life. They live longer and suffer less disease than the disadvantaged. At least the introduction of the NHS in 1948, meant that the disadvantaged in the UK, no longer needed to suffer without treatment.

Confucius once asked a man who had been swimming in an unsafe river, how he stayed afloat.

> *"I enter the inflow, and emerge with the outflow, follow the Way of the water, and do not impose my selfishness upon it. This is how I stay afloat in it."*

Chuang-Tzu

Education and Energy Efficiency

An adequate education should help us understand one another, ourselves, and our duties to society. For this, we need to learn practical psychology and social science. Education should help us to know our place in our universe. For this we must study the arts, philosophy and science. Education should clarify the errors in our thinking and in our way of life – like favouring 'having', rather than 'being', as a main aim. For this we need to study religion and philosophy and try to discern good from bad. For this we need to understand and practise judgement – learning not to fool ourselves, becoming aware of both our own biases and those that run throughout the information we are fed. We might come to avoid false conclusions.

Does education to-day meet these needs? Must we remain content with the idea that these matters are only for intellectuals?

Parents have an essential educative role to play. For their children, they could promote relaxation and adequate sleep; something most children try to resist. Parents should encourage personal discipline, with timetables for study, for hobbies, and for time spent watching the TV or social media. Parents could promote the realisation that 'doing nothing' is not always idleness; it can be an achievement in itself, balancing the energy we spend on activity.

Parents could promote insight into relationships. This might serve to lessen the pain of rejection or inappropriate attachments. Children could be encouraged to conserve their valuable energy, investing in achieving maximal self-esteem. A lack of insight can make the aim of our ambition too high or too low for our talents. Both are dangerous.

One can easily underestimate the potential of a young person, before they are gripped by a passion. As parents, we might help them find that passion. If they reject that help, however, repeated trying can alienate them. All we can do, is to expose our children to as many safe life experiences as possible, through travel, education, and social endeavour. Through curiosity, they might find a captivating pursuit to follow. Befriending someone with passionate curiosity can help. For the lucky ones, that person will be a parent or grandparent.

Instead of regarding our children as potential professors of English, physics or maths, as so many parent and teachers seem to want, perhaps we should address what they are more likely to become

– parents, workers, employees and citizens. We might then educate them accordingly. There will always be a few scholarly nerds who excel at examinations and compete for prizes. Even parrots, can be proficient at repeating what they are told. Merit can lie elsewhere. I would give prizes to creative, independent thinkers, whose non-conformity will often block their path within every establishment formed to maintain fixed values.

As ever, Shakespeare has a succinct opinion.

> *"These earthly godfathers of Heaven's lights*
>
> *That give a name to every fixed star,*
>
> *Have no more profit of their shining nights*
>
> *Than those that walk and wot not what they are."*

Love's Labour's Lost

William Shakespeare

Scholars deserve their self-esteem, but not at the expense of relegating others to a life of intellectual inferiority. Far too many adults go through life feeling inadequate, having been unable to forget or accept the judgement of their teachers and peers. Teachers may now be more aware of this, but it still happens. Many adults have found success in life, after being thought non-contenders by teachers. For some, it is their striving to overcome unfair criticism that led to their success. For many, success came from independent thinking and its positive encouragement.

An analysis of the skills we need most in life, such as simply getting on with people, suggests the necessity to radically re-think what we teach children. This is not to say that we shouldn't continue to improve education for those capable of academia.

There is one basic priority required of all biological entities – to survive. The second is procreation, and the survival of further generations. Whatever extra endeavour we choose to undertake, be it education or otherwise, it will suit survival to minimise our energy expenditure. This can be done by learning the most efficient means of survival. Instead of trigonometry, many more would benefit from understanding relationships, personal finances, car and household maintenance. Before learning about the wonders of the universe, would it not be better to know how to change a light bulb or a car tyre? History, drama and literature, because they give examples of what has happened in the past, what is happening now, and what can and might happen in the future, should these be given precedence?

One fundamental aim of education must be to promote a less energy wasteful lifestyle. For example, how to earn or make money in the simplest way possible. Young people are now doing this by mastering on-line techniques, even before they have left school. They are selling digital products and are involved in digital affiliation and marketing. The impetuous and profligate will always spend more money and energy than they have, but the consequences need to be taught.

Schools should set up their own small businesses to give pupils first-hand experience of being a boss or an employee. If a healthy life rests on good judgement, the process should be taught.

Since many doctors fail to manage patients efficiently, with faulty timing and judgment (feedback from many patients in the UK), I have undertaken in many books to teach them how I came to build and run a private patient practice. Rather than have patients allocated to me, as in the NHS, I eventually attracted 20,000 private patients (some were refugees from the

NHS); none of whom complained about my practise during the 53-years the GMC allowed me a UK licence. Doctors may have the technical knowledge, but what about nous, communication skills and executive functioning? I am not sure whether these can be taught. For those interested, I have tried. Read the relevant chapters in my book, The Art and Science of Medical Practice.

The best learning aides are those that allow penalty-free experiences. Computer games and virtual reality can be used to simulate flying, driving, decision making, even being a doctor. From these we can learn what natural skills we have and improve them.

Youth may be wasted on the young, but knowledge never is. While there is no reason to withhold discovering Shakespeare, real experiences that help them develop maturity might help them more. Shakespeare's unparalleled understanding of human beings, their predicaments and behaviour, are the most succinct for learning about life and people. One never needs to stop learning, simply because there is such a lot that is fascinating. So why not introduce degree courses for the mature and elderly? Many would love to have improved engagement with others, without any need for a qualifying certificate.

I had an uncle (Alfred known as Alf), who did much to give me an appreciation of knowledge, before I went to primary school. The joy he had discovering obscure pieces of knowledge, inspired me. His memory stays with me. So does his message – discovering new things is fun – at any age.

Most societies benefit from providing an education system. Education, like health provision, consumes lots of energy and resources. But is there a better way to influence a nation's future?

Having to learn is tiring, but essential if we are to avoid making and repeating mistakes. If not a natural ability, learning to communicate can be difficult, but empowering. The ability to learn, to communicate and make connections, are all features of intelligence.

Maintaining Boundaries

As societies become ever more centrifugal, more individuals now feel they are playing less of a role. Individuals will now be more inclined to switch from a duty to society, to being recipients. No longer are pyramids being built, with direct community involvement. Instead, we need projects that enable individuals to become fully functioning, involved human beings. There are now so many people alive, a decreasing percentage need be involved in society. In the UK, immigrant groups are now so large, they have formed their own distinct societies. In the UK, this can now be seen among those of Asian origin. Might they soon insist on Urdu and Hindu being used to teach in schools, rather than English and EU languages? That would certainly challenge most white Caucasians, used to English being the *lingua franca*.

For a growing older majority, the societal trend is towards uselessness. Many people move to small communities – condos and retirement homes – there to rekindle older forms of lifestyle. The aim is to revive mutual respect and find self-respect.

All organised systems, including every society, must impose boundaries in order to function efficiently. A society with boundaries, however, acts as a prison, with its need for regulation and policing. As Jean-Jacques Rousseau said in the eighteenth century, 'Man is born free, and everywhere he is in chains' (*The Social Contract*). Happy are those older citizens, comfortable with imposed conformity; comfortable with being fenced in; happy to pay for services they never use. Many have done their duty and deserve the rewards society has to offer. The spoilt, self-oriented and egotistical, might wonder why they should accept these boundaries. If you are a dutiful, unspoilt, generous citizen, acceptance will be in your nature. We all exist someplace between these extremes; it is simply a matter of defining our place. Those self-aware enough to know they cannot fit in, must feign compliance or live outside the system. The dissident and courageous enough, will attempt to create their own system.

Collective Energy

Arresting oratory, pop concerts, shared religious experiences, 'being there' when history is made, can energise every participant to act and feel as one. Oratory is particularly unifying, focussing the whole audience together, intellectually and emotionally. Before battle, indigenous North American Indians used war dances and songs to build collective courage. They also used it for healing. The at-one-ness of these occasions can be a special experience.

> *"A speech is poetry: cadence, rhythm, imagery, sweep!*
>
> *A speech reminds us that words,*
>
> *like children, have the power*
>
> *to make dance the dullest beanbag of a heart."*

Peg Noon. U.S. Presidential Speech Writer.

When a psychotherapy group shares or reveals previously hidden secrets, its members sometimes develop a special bond. Those who exercise, or fight battles together, often become bonded as a group. They may feel what they describe as collective energy. This enables some to run further than is usual for them. It is especially useful for the members of a rowing crew or music group who have to work in unison. A music group and a boat crew and coxswain are all trying to perform as one.

In 1966, Robert Kennedy referred to the collective energy that can build to a point where it overcomes great obstacles. This force was later thought to bring down the Berlin Wall (November 1989).

"Each time a man stands up for an ideal, or acts to improve the lot of others, or strikes out against injustice, he sends forth a tiny ripple of hope. And crossing each other from a million

different centres of energy and daring, those ripples build a current that can sweep down the mightiest walls of oppression and resistance."

Robert Kennedy. June 7th, 1966. Cape Town. S.A.

One of my most energising personal experiences as an amateur musician, was playing in a modern jazz group. My colleagues and I were average performers at best, until we were joined one evening by three professional musicians. They joined us to 'jam', after their evening of professional playing for the Royal Shakespeare Company. One played bass, another played the drums and the remaining fellow played our vibraphone (electrified xylophone). They lifted our performance into the realm of expertise. It was their collective timing, vitality and energy that did it. We could have played all night. Our playing was never quite the same again, but it was an edifying experience.

Witnessing a catastrophe can quickly de-energise onlookers, leaving some stunned and drained of energy. Members of the public who witness road traffic accidents often feel 'shocked' and depleted. Many are easily startled and get fixed to the spot, unable to take any action.

The mechanisms by which these energising and de-energising re-actions occur in the body, are well known. They result from the action of the autonomic nervous system, a combination of various hormones (cortisol, adrenaline), and the release of brain neuro-transmitters like dopamine and serotonin.

Teilhard de Chardin, a Jesuit priest writing in the 1950s, expressed the concept of a 'noosphere': that collective sphere of intellec-tual or spiritual human energy, which influences the way ahead. Together we evolve constructively and continuously, rather than disintegrating. Some might argue that the direction the world is now taking is negative, and we have already sown the seeds of our own destruction. As people whose minds are confined to a box (society), with no windows, how can we know?

Father Pierre Teilhard de Chardin was a Jesuit priest who was a renowned geologist and palaeontologist. He combined a scientific life with a religious and mystical one. He provided us with visions of the future, based on both. He spoke of himself as 'a pilgrim of the future'. He believed that evolution had hardly begun for humans, and that the future would be essentially spiritual. He thought that Ultra-humans would have equal love for God and the world, and that this fusion of love would spread.

After writing a paper on the recent discoveries about the origin of man, he was exiled by the Church to China. He wrote 'inside me, there's something like real agony, a real storm'.

Barred from publishing it by the Roman Catholic Church, his philosophical work remained unpublished until his death. He wanted to convey to the supreme authority of the Church, 'the weakness, and also the strength of Christianity to-day'. He died from a heart attack in 1955. He was then an exile in New York.

It is possible to feel collectiveness without music, words or action. It can be inspired by special places – beneath the pyramids at Giza or sitting next the Trevi Fountains in Rome, and often present among those attending places of religious worship.

Hope

Governments and all societies must aim to maintain public hope. Without it, widespread dejection and demoralisation could bring economic ruin.

Hope is a major energising force, be it realistic, exaggerated or false. It has a biological purpose – making our energy available. The same can be said for religious faith. Even without any logical support (so said the logician, Bertrand Russell), faith can be galvanising, and can help survival. Those who limit themselves to logic alone, and become sanctimonious about it, will limit their survival potential.

Optimism, faith, self-esteem and hope are all energising, making energy seem available. Depression, despondency, negativity, and despair, limit energy availability, and make the escape from a survival situation less likely. They will need the help of others.

Following bouts of depression (some like Winston Churchill), will sense elation and energy (manic depression). They may have been given an unusual gift. During what Churchill called his 'Black

Dog' (depression), he saw the world the way it was. During the overactive, optimistic phases that followed, he would set about putting it right.

Much of what doctors, faith-healers, acupuncturists, physiotherapists, homeopaths, and osteopaths do for people, benefits from being laced with moderated faith and hope for the future. Re-assurance, and the sharing of a problem, go a long way to making a patient feel better, whether their condition is curable or not. The dispersion of worry and distress will lead to a reduction in energy expenditure – a real health benefit. In addition, confession, sharing problems, and disclosure, can all have a healing effect. A patient with breast cancer who genuinely believes they will beat it, will on average, survive three times longer than those who remain despondent and give in to hopelessness.

Statistics

The statistics used to define a society, have ancient origins in Babylon and Egypt. The figures can provide a measure of many things, including property dimensions and numbers of people, useful for economic and taxation purposes. The English and Welsh Doomsday records (1086) are an early systematised example. In the eighteenth century, the modern idea of *statistik* was attributed to the German philosopher Gottfried Achenwall. At about the same time, Sweden established annual population surveys (*tabellverket*); they were concerned about their population and their ability to defend themselves.

The concept of calculating future probability from statistics, perhaps originated with Cardano in the sixteenth century, but later developed by Pascal, Laplace and others. Its incorporation into statistical method was formalised by R.A. Fisher in 1925, illustrated in his book on statistical methods for research workers.

"Probability is a weaker notion than truth."

Gödel (Douglas R.Hofstadter, Gödel, Escher, Bach)

Statistics provide abstracted estimates of reality. A 'mean value' for instance, does not exist other than as a theoretical concept. Adding a range to the mean, creates context. If the average temperature in Anchorage, Alaska, is 5°C, what will the temperature be when you visit? In winter it could be as low as -8°C (-16°C with wind-chill factor). At least, knowing the mean temperature and range, might help you choose the most appropriate clothing.

Fourteen to twenty-five people out of 70 million, die each year on railway crossings in the UK. Our perception of catastrophe, however, ranges from an even chance of an event happening (50:50), to no chance at all of it happening. For the self-assured person with no anxiety about level-crossings, fourteen to twenty-five people dying each year out of 70 million, might well sound irrelevant. Even if the statistics are accurate, their relevance needs to be decided, but that will always remain a matter of judgement.

No human brain is objective. It will weight some bits of information more heavily than others, depending on any bias we have, like our fondness, disinterest or attitude to the subject. Many have a personal fondness for certain numbers, so when they are asked to choose numbers at random, as for a lottery ticket, most will use one or two of their favourite numbers. National lottery successes around the world, are a testament to how little the average person believes in statistics, and the calculations of chance. Many convinced they will win the Lottery, will spend their money on a 40-million to one chance each week. But who cares about the odds? Someone will usually win it; so why not me?

In many scenarios (weather, stock prices), what is sold as 'informed opinion' about the future, will always be part fallacy. Mostly, the future cannot be predicted - only guessed using extrapolation or induction (it's always hot here, so it will be hot tomorrow). But then there is well-informed guesswork, and ill-informed guess-work. The aim of science is to find out how things work, and to make the future more predictable – at least, for laboratory experiments.

Anxiety can influence numerical bias. In the case of railway crossings, a fear of trains might exaggerate the perceived risk; sometimes to the point of total avoidance. The less anxious are more likely to read statistics correctly. I had a patient who couldn't drive, but instructed her husband, never to drive under bridges or cross railway crossings.

Statistics are always retrospective. It's a good thing that the future mostly rests on the past or at least an extension of it. For the anxious, however, this reasoning may not suffice to calm their fears.

Organisational Neuroticism

Like individuals, organisations can also be neurotic. In response to their insecurities, some unhealthy companies will create high levels of tension among their employees. Some believe this will promote better results. Others engender a relaxed working environment, allowing employees to work at their own pace. Both produce results, as long as each employee has an attitude that fits the company ethos. Some employees will not be pushed, preferring time to think and develop; others need stringent rule-based controls to produce any results.

A non-neurotic organisation best suits non-obsessive, relaxed employees. The archetype of this organisation is Virgin, headed by Richard Branson. He has proven that the creation of self-empowerment, causes his employees to remain loyal and to commit to group success, even if they could earn more elsewhere.

Some organisations are obsessional. This can be found in legal and medical practices, where every small point can count. Every obsessive employee will be a boon to them.

Some job situations require safety consciousness. Airline pilots and public vehicle drivers have little latitude to act beyond rule-based checklists. This type of work provides safety and security for some workers, and a prison for others.

It is important for every individual to be aware about their choice of organisation; it will have energy expenditure implications. The organisation we work for should have characteristics that complement our own. The self-employed are free to create the style of system that suits them, although there is a high price to pay for the energy needed to create a business.

Organisations get the long-term employees they deserve, but energy equilibrium applies. Some businesses will survive only if the workers chosen to run it, supply the energy needed. Square pegs do not last long in round holes.

Most employees find their level within an organisation. This is the Peter principle. It depends on at least three main factors: luck, competence, and self-image. There are lucky and unlucky people, experiencing lucky and unlucky times. For those with good luck, good timing or both, advancement in life can come effortlessly (with minimal energy expenditure). For the unlucky, life can be a struggle. Energy expenditure can be high, their health compromised, and social advancement retarded. Many who fail, will blame poor luck, not incompetence. They could have blamed ignorant job selectors, who in the first place, were unable to fit the best candidate for the job.

Public Bias

Many people are snobs; even about the newspaper they read. The message delivered by them may be the same, but the style and words they use will be different. Educational level and self-image will help to promote choice.

> *"The Telegraph is read by people who **think** they run the country.*

> *The Guardian is read by people who **would like** to run the country.*

> *The Times is read by people who **do** run the country.*

> *The Mail is read by the wives of the people who run the country.*

> *The Sun is read by people who don't care who runs the country, as long as she has big t*ts!"*

Jim Hacker as Prime Minister. TV. Series: *Yes, Prime Minister.*

Most people on earth live in an urban minefield, struggling for an existence of variable quality; one dependent on their expectations, not on the likelihood of realisation. Our expectations can be fed by avarice and media exposure. Many simply have a need to keep up with their neighbours. These are just a few ways in which we spend our energy on everyday background issues.

Survival in any minefield depends on reconnaissance: finding out where to look; and what to look for; how to avoid any dangers, how to treat yourself when injured; where to find help, and how to put survival knowledge into daily practice. Most important of all is to locate the mines. As in any minefield, many of us living in the western world, face many unseen dangers. Having a map could help.

There are many whose only exposure to the complexities of life, are learned from watching television and films. This is not 'living', it is living by proxy. It can, however, conserve energy if we come to know how to avoid real-life dramas; learning about the dangers that lie outside our front door. True wisdom, however, comes only from knowledge tempered by experience.

Governments try to remove some of the naturally occurring pitfalls by providing sewage and waste disposal, safe means of travel, availability of food and clean water. In the western world, we take these for granted and do not often see them as a concern.

Tolerance and Power

Because most citizens respect power, most tolerate it. As organisations and societies become more liberal, they tend to become lazy and inefficient. Solicitors can take weeks to do what could done in hours. Some doctors will find it easier to be unhelpful – blaming the system they work for – even when patients are fast deteriorating. So much for 'patient first'!

Many of us tolerate substandard services; even paying for restaurant meals at ridiculous prices – all without objecting. To tolerate inefficiency is to allow the disintegration of standards. The frustration it leads to, will spend lots of our energy. Might it not be better to spend a small amount of energy on outspoken intolerance? Tolerating the substandard is a weakness, and weaknesses are not often survival traits.

Comedy can express the truth amusingly. Ronnie Corbett and Ronnie Barker once succinctly made a point about tolerance:

> *"Love makes the world go around, you know." "So does a punch on the nose old boy!"*

                    The Two Ronnies. BBC TV. 10.12.83.

Deprived Lives

Some are stuck with a daily routine they cannot vary or easily escape. A key feature is having little or no control over their circumstances. Few have any hope of change, unless they win the lottery or become a professional footballer or boxer.

By watching media output, they can indulge in how 'the other half' lives. They are not always, but quite often seen as deprived. Some societies will supplement their low income – one mark of a modern 'civilised' society. They are typically patriotic, but in the UK, have many environmental factors to tolerate, one of which is inequality.

Many deprived people are the working-class progeny of those who fought for Great Britain in two world wars. Because of unregulated immigration into the UK, they must now tolerate those who come but refuse to speak their language and are committed elsewhere. Even as they try to accept others, their children are being completely outnumbered at school by foreign children. At least children have little reluctance to assimilation and integration. Instead of enjoying and learning from the obvious differences between cultures – in my experience British people have always been accepting of others – they are now becoming more inclined to consider their own culture as dismissed, eroded and overwhelmed. These are emotive cultural issues, not primarily racist ones. Something else is magnifying working-class anger – they are unable to escape and must live together, whereas politicians and the rich can live where they choose.

The sexual mixing of different racial and cultural groups is thought advantageous from both biological and evolutionary points of view. It will happen progressively in the UK, whatever we think or do. Unfortunately, not many people find this an attractive reason for fostering cultural integration.

Deprived people survive less well than the wealthy. They are much more likely to smoke and drink alcohol, however, and are five times more likely to have a heart attack or develop cancer than the rich. If unskilled, they are twice as likely to smoke as 'professionals' (38% versus 18%) and will have double or treble the number of days off work due to 'restricted activity' (General Household Survey in Great Britain: OPCS 1994).

People in deprived groups are aware of smoking risks, but carry on through illness and pregnancy. Smoking is powerfully addictive, which partly explains why so many continue with the habit. I have heard many times – 'you have to die of something, so why not smoke?'

Good ideas can arise from both those who seem to know everything, and those who obviously know very little. Their thought processes will, however, be different. Some give no thought to smoking – their friends do it, so why not them? Those with advanced lung or heart disease might finally get the point but giving up then would be pointless. Some will not give up, even after their legs have been amputated and their heart has been scarred – the effects of artery narrowing, strongly promoted by smoking in those with an inherited tendency.

My friend Kenny Nicholls, while in his seventies, found himself in the above medical state. After my advice that he should give up smoking, he pronounced what he thought of medical professionals. He told me, 'You are all intent on removing the only pleasures I have left!'

For the deprived, everyday survival consumes their energy. Many try to gain some quality of life by reducing frustration. What energy they have left, might be spent on dreaming – that one day they will be rich and famous. Hope not reality, will help offset the depressing effect of a numbing life routine with too little pay.

Many lead their lives as low-paid workers. How many applied themselves at school, enough to escape a low-paid future? Some university graduates, however, are now in the same position, with too few high-paid jobs available. Working-class peer group loyalty, and group identity are common factors partially replacing their personal identity. Their support for football teams and sporting heroes is evidence enough of that. Imitation designer brands can become important identifiers – many will get self-esteem from the labels they wear.

Adherence to strong views, strongly held, can also come to define personal identity – often rigorously defended. Loose thinking promoted the 'Alf Garnett' school of philosophy. The TV series, 'Till Death Us Do Part', once evoked laughter, through displaying the anger and bitter resentment of a fictionalised, working-class head of a London, East End family, Alf Garnett (June 1966).

The financially deprived, need to spend a lot of energy on coping with uncertainty. The constant juggling of small amounts of money is necessary to make ends meet. High unemployment is common. The contrast between what they have, and what they might have, is projected in every advert; in the clothes others wear, and the cars they drive. For some it is dispiriting, even depressing. Some will feel there is no way out, unless providence intervenes.

Noisy, crowded surroundings, and the pressure to provide for a growing family, will further extract their energy. The only solace to be found might be in the commiseration of friends and the relaxation afforded by smoking, drinking, and drugs.

As for other groups, energy gets released by camaraderie, close family ties, living for their children, pride related to acquisitions (and those of their close friends), and displaced warrior virtues (pride in their chosen football teams' performance).

Worry for the deprived, often comes from wondering how to pay bills. 'Something will turn up', many will say. And so, it might. As my grandfather often said to my grandmother, "While I have my health, I can roll up my sleeves, get off my arse, and do some work!" My paternal grandfather who lived and died in Bethnal Green in the East End of London, died young and rich in 1922. He never abandoned his poorer friends. Behind the scenes, he would buy them drinks in pubs and paid butchers to supply fillet steak to his poorer neighbours, many of whom were too poor to eat every day.

The deprived have some advantages over others. There is selfless pride and real honour to be found here. Pride in doing a hard days' work; pride in patriotism, and honour between friends, family members, and colleagues, all of which surface once the 'chips are down' – with the country at war or with a friend in need. In this, I am describing those I have lived among from a young age. With first-hand experience, these are the attributes of those I am qualified to call 'true Brits'. I am sure that many similar qualities exist among those living in many other nations.

The 'true traditional Brit' is a kindly soul, but nevertheless a warrior. When the Argentines invaded the Falkland Islands, they faced British warriors who would have gone anywhere, at anytime, for their country, and regardless of any opposition. The same spirit created the British Empire; a flame that still burns bright in many British hearts, especially among the working classes. Their bravery and courage made their officers, traditionally drawn from richer more educated classes, proud to serve with them. Many are now frustrated by being under used; unfortunately expressed sometimes as football hooliganism. Many are heir to the untapped pride of having unused warrior virtues. Their country being sold off to foreign conglomerates, was never likely to endear them.

Inter-cultural and inter-racial strife, like inter-personal strife, is everywhere calling on our energy consumption, diminishing the health of some groups and individuals.

> *"Between the two poles of impulse and control, an ethic by which men can live happily must find a middle point."*

Bertrand Russell. *Human Society in Ethics and Politics* (1954)

Environments Ugly and Beautiful

I once walked along a London street and stopped to look at my surroundings. Like every battle-conditioned civilian who no longer hear bombs explode, the dilapidated condition of the street had been invisible to me. Those who can see, can perceive in different modes. Using an artist's eye, I saw a hotchpotch of colour, and a slowly moving mass of different vehicles. Windows ranged from filthy to clean, and curtains from tidy to torn. Ugliness can be dispiriting, bringing no prospect of aesthetic joy, except for renaming it euphemistically – 'local character' or typical of 'cosmopolitan life'; something that will attract tourists and those with no intention of living there. Ugliness needs to be blanked from our conscious perception – as if to hide the unpleasant truth from the inhabitants who must endure it. Without an alternative, they must adapt or move on.

Compare this street to one in Saffron Walden, an ancient Essex market town. There are ugly corners, but mostly one sees period properties, all easy on the eye. The common land is broad, green and litter free. The cottages, three hundred years old, are carefully tended by their attentive owners, many of whom have spent lots of time on their upkeep. With no need for adaptation, inhabitants can enjoy stability – something that can induce a longing to get back, when away. Comfort is to be found in the stability of the dated and historic. It is safe, unchanging and reliable – a low-energy consuming environment.

Unnecessary background music in shops; unwanted noise from personal stereos, and overheard folderol mobile telephone conversations, can all strike some as ugliness. A constant subliminal effort is required to ward off any depressing or frustrating effects they might have. We are demeaned if we accept the unacceptable; our self-esteem reduced by our unspoken intolerance. Visual and noise pollution are everywhere; unchosen and unavoidable. We can be left angered, left tolerating it, romanticising it, blocking it out or simply running away from it. All cost us in subliminal energy expenditure, unless we can 'chill-out' and accept it or ignore it. How much better to spend energy on viewing a beautiful sunset, an autumnal forest, majestic mountains or a garden tended to perfection on a summer's evening? We all have the choice, even if we must walk there!

Then there is people pollution: crowds so thick, one cannot avoid bumping into others; queuing and being squashed into trains, conflicting with our need for personal space. Crowding and queuing has become the new norm. Biologically, both are energy draining.

Because the rich and poor live in different environments, their different health and disease patterns are perhaps predictably different. The energy expenditure required to cope with an unsatisfactory environment is great, and probably contributes directly to the difference in mortality and morbidity experienced between the rich and poor – the health divide. The only respite for the poor, might come from escape – either to work more or go on holiday. Unfortunately, the underprivileged cannot often afford escape. When they try, it may be no more calming than an alternative nightmare.

If this argument is correct, clean-up programs should affect the health of urban dwellers. Creating places which bring joy and pleasure, might reduce queues in A&E. I suspect that the total effect on quality and quantity of life, would add up to more than the contribution of medical bureaucracy.

Governments will doubtless continue to scapegoat the medical profession and try to avoid responsibility. The Health of the Nation targets have made the medical profession responsible for reducing the mortality of chest disease, cancer, and heart disease, when a much larger impact might be had by the Department of the Environment.

An Energy Spending Society

Capitalism invites us to work harder and harder for improved future security. The obvious insecurities that surround us all, drive us to this end. The result is higher energy spending, just to gain a sense of control.

Care, kindliness, and love from others, can save us energy. The traditional family provided an island of peace, quiet, and comfort; a place for energy recoupment. The partial dissolution of supportive family life in the west, puts our societies at risk of depleted energy, diminishing our drive to evolve. If dissolution of family support progresses, the result could be a fatigued society, tired of the constant energy spending required to maintain well-being and health. Diseases increase as the feeling of control diminishes. With it, mostly comes a reduced resistance to infection. Tiredness, fatigue and exhaustion, will also exacerbate cardiovascular and other diseases.

The animal kingdom provides many examples of family group activity, sustaining healthy existence by minimising energy expenditure. Acting together in packs, animals hunt successfully and more easily provide for their young and old. Altruistic behaviour is not exclusively human. Old and toothless wild dogs in the Serengeti, are guarded by young braves as they suck nourishment from the bones of a carcass.

The strength of human families pulling together is more evident in some ethnic minority groups. Jewish, Muslim, Sikh and Gujarati families can be seen running family businesses in Great Britain; each able to profit from mutual co-operation and low labour costs. The support of a family group can provide individuals with unparalleled support – much more than any government-based, social system. This support is a central tenet of Islam, Judaism, and many other faiths with strict laws of observance. Jewish and Muslim women assume the role of the most important member of the family home. It is to them that falls the important task of providing succour for family members and cultivating a cohesive environment to which all members willingly return.

Relationship problems and family politics consume energy – where there is rancour, there is wasted energy. For 'healthily' functioning families, there is a net gain to be had. The psychodynamics of family units are factors to be taken seriously when trying to determine health. Happy families, where children are respected, loved, and sympathetically mothered and fathered, provide a more certain path to physical and emotional health than dysfunctional families.

All governments govern on behalf of citizens. A cynical view might be – all they do is tinker with the economy and provide us with rights and services by enforcing punitive laws – in exchange for vast sums of money obtained from taxation, most of which they use to maintain their power. It would, of course, be cheaper to be self-sufficient, but then we might have anarchy and fear to contend with. Another view could be summarised as – 'where would we be without them?' They provide the support services, caring for us from birth to death. They allow equal rights and opportunities and make the environment safe – all for the modest sums we pay in taxes.

The machinery of society is driven not by government, but by the people, powered by energy derived from self-worth and happiness. This comes from the fulfilment gained from friends, family, work mates, colleagues, and sometimes complete strangers.

Television, advertising, and media communications, can easily subvert the majority (especially the have-nots) by introducing dis-content. Governments, all of whom fear anarchy and the wrath of the people, as well as the opinions of businesses and the press, are left to balance the controls of society. They need to supply just the right amount of money and energy to support the structure of society, respecting that citizens will burn their personal energy struggling to survive. The same energy, redirected, could easily lead to anarchy and insurrection.

Inequality

Western society preferentially rewards entrepreneurs; the skilled or educated, will mostly take second place. The privileged – the rich and educated – are preferentially rewarded with better health. The reasons are many – some obvious; others not. It follows that teachers, who advise pupils to pursue higher education, may help them to gain a health advantage.

Most citizens will find their lives ruled by those with money and little education. Teachers meanwhile are often paid less than those who spurn their advice. Inequalities can inflame anger and resentment.

Who can reasonably support these differentials by turning a blind eye to merit? The system seems stable, except for a few dissidents who have no realistic hope of shaking loose the greed on which the system is based. While vast economic differentials exist, undercurrents of dissatisfaction burn much personal energy in the background. The drive many have for personal advancement, makes them blind to the cost. Like the earth turning in space, nobody is aware of it.

The most powerful substrate for ill-health – the health divide – can go unnoticed or be denied. It is denied by doctors, too busy with trivial cases, to deal with the underlying issues; in any case, powerless to help. Many are distracted, too desperate as modern hunter gatherers to acquire things, and – to become 'as rich as . . . '; 'to have as many holidays as . . . ' ; or 'to have a nice car like . . . ' to think about the reasons for their discontent and subsequent dis-ease. There is a commonly voiced solution – 'Someone should do something about this (the way things are).'

The situation is simultaneously denied by politicians – mostly addressing problems in the light of whose fault it was (usually the opposite party), rather than any underlying structural defect of society. They are tinkerers, and only do the bidding of their public majority to keep in power. They have little other choice if they want to keep their seat in parliament. The public wants to enjoy the benefits of self-interest and will vote for any party promising them lower taxes, cheaper beer, petrol and cigarettes.

As public content fights discontent, this unresolved situation is bound to swing between good and bad times. All empires have their day. Caught in a time-trap – few will live long enough to see much fundamental change; many pointless changes, improvements and deteriorations, there to be seen in a life 70-years long. The only way to cope with modern western society is to accept it and make use of it. One can move away from it as one who has benefited – to the isolation of an island or the countryside – or as a loser, move to the isolation of a prison cell or the exposure of a cardboard box. Choosing to stay and work is to battle against an unforgiving system, constructed to maintain the established *status quo*, many paying with their diminished health or their lives.

As an alternative, some seek the peace and solitude of a devotional life, in monasteries or academic institutions. A pious life of prayer, study or research, is a minority pursuit. For the religious, the devotional life is less an escape, than a duty to their God or idol. Any pressure to conform to the mores of society at large, will be rejected in favour of a more rigid set of disciplined duties which will seem onerous to anyone living only by the law of the land. The monastic life is an introspective one – minding one's own business, and aspiring to the higher virtues and ideals of Christianity. Freedom from a neurotic ego (nirvana) is sought by Buddhists. Because such a life is mostly predictable (being strictly timetabled), and unstressed (with few external demands), it easily becomes second-nature. Each individual's energy expenditure will be minimised. Although very few will choose it, this is the most energy efficient, healthy state for human existence – as far derived from the western way of life and death as it is possible to get.

CHAPTER EIGHTEEN

Factors of Consequence for Health Professionals

My interest in patients' emotional reactions to circumstances as aetiological factors in disease, began at Charing Cross Hospital, London, while working with Dr. Peter Nixon in 1973. I thought a better appreciation of emotional and circumstantial factors in relationship to disease would have been included in medical and cardiac practise by now. Not so, it seems!

In a recent British Medical Journal (BMJ) publication (October 2025), Helen Watkins describes the chest pain she developed soon after returning to the UK from Australia, and how she was handled in A&E. She was tired and jet-lagged when she first noticed chest pain (eventually thought due to acid regurgitation, not cardiac ischaemia or infarction), having left behind some of her family (for her, the emotional equivalent of a divorce or bereavement).

She thought that both her physical and emotional pain should have been valued. She wrote "I had become a checklist rather than an individual." Her recommendations to readers of the BMJ:

- "Actively listen to possible emotional causes for physical symptoms."

- "Do not focus only on physical signs and symptoms which you can easily measure and assess."

- Briefly acknowledge any emotional distress that a patient shares with you."

If the personal emotional and energy problems of patients are to be fully considered, a considerable change in UK medical practice organisation will need to take place. Because the NHS has remained inimical, it hasn't happened in the last 50-years, so why change? The principle requirement is to put patients first; not doctors, nurses or the bureaucratic machinery that overburdens many public health systems.

The 'patients first' principle has always been the *sine qua non* of UK private practice. It has to be, if patients are to be satisfied enough to want to return. Maintaining this principle will not endear a doctor to his colleagues. In my case it came before a 'colleagues first' principle and any prioritisation of the GMC's metaphysical guideline – "promoting and maintaining public confidence in the medical professions" (Good Medical Practice. GMC 2024). This is beyond the remit of any individual doctor.

I always acted to supervise everything my colleagues advised. Most of my colleagues had NHS ties so they had their own tight network of affiliation. It was simply financially expedient for them to deal with me. I chose them as suitable if they had the appropriate qualifications, experience (as in books and published papers) and reputation. If necessary, I would make referrals to places other than local UK facilities (mainly the US).

In private practice I had to satisfy every discerning patient without pandering to them. The doctor-patient relationship had to be adult to adult, not adult to child. My patients were mostly used to first-class hotels and travel and ran their own efficient and profitable businesses. They expected the same from me –

and they got it! They dealt directly with me, with no detached compliance-driven bureaucrat interfering at any stage. I was always available on the telephone, and they could trust me and my staff to sort out their problems – I provided a one-stop shop. This is how I practised for more than 50-years with no reliance on the NHS or other government entities to support me.

Before a doctor can practise in this 'patient-first' way, some essential features of their practice style and behaviour need to be introduced and maintained:

- Affability – it costs nothing for all staff to be approachable and helpful. Never to be of the obsequiousness, spoiling or pandering sort.

- Always face-to-face first for consultations, and as much as possible thereafter.

- Available: always contactable.

- Have no computer on your desk. During consultation, concentrate entirely on your patient having fully briefed yourself beforehand. AI recording could help.

- Trust is fundamentally important. In my case this developed slowly as I accumulated patients who preferred an ongoing doctor-patient relationship with me. It must be based on a reputation for diagnosing correctly and acting straight away to investigate and treat them. Personal trust is confirmed by a doctor being able to say to any patient "If I were you . . ."

- NO commercial intent. My patients were all in business. They would have known instantly if I tried to sell them some new unproven test; an unnecessary expensive test or had a business arrangement with another doctor.

- Always pass common-sense tests. When dealing with intelligent sentient beings one must deliver plain common sense, even in explaining technical issues. Urgent things must be dealt with urgently and efficiently. All advice given must always pass the common-sense test.

- Only very short waiting lists are acceptable. In the UK, patients die on waiting lists or have to suffer unacceptably. For diagnosis, getting test results or treatment, everyone benefits from prompt action. All my VIP patients insisted on it.

- Long-term commitment. I had a long-established, stable clinic-based practice. Patients would knock on my door or would turn up impromptu when the situation called for it. I most always accommodated them. My replacement by other doctors was never going to happen. Nothing beats continuity for building trusting relationships with patients, their friends and family. Early diagnosis is made easier, with knowledge of each patient's circumstances known or easy to define.

- Become a solver of medical problems, especially for last resort cases.

Few of these basic requirements are now given by NHS providers, although this was not the case for the first few decades after the inception of the NHS in 1948. It was State control and depersonalisation that doctors feared would happen; and happen it did.

Private hospital staff did what I requested them to do, not what any bureaucrat member of their office staff dictated. I had no bureaucrats to deal with (until the CQC first arrived in 2009). In the private hospitals I used, my patients dealt with me alone as the attending consultant.

> *A CQC inspector once asked me how I was going to keep my practice standards up to those of the NHS. I described a hypothetical case. In the NHS, a patient has chest pain. He gets a GP appointment in 48-hours or refers him to A&E. The GP recognises his need to see a cardiologist and arranges an appointment in 3-weeks' time. The cardiologist sees the patient and orders an exercise ECG for 3-weeks later. The test proves positive, and he arranges a coronary angiogram for another 3-weeks' time. This shows extensive artery narrowing, and the patient obviously needs a coronary bypass. This is arranged – possibly for six weeks later (total time elapsed: 107 days).*

The CQC inspectors thought these time scales acceptable for NHS practice. I then said, 'Let me tell you what I do in my practice'.

> *I will see the patient on the same day of asking. I do the exercise test ECG directly after our consultation. I arrange to do his coronary angiogram myself, three days later. With the result in hand, I will speak directly to one of my surgical colleagues, and arrange for a coronary bypass, three days later. (total time elapsed: 7-days).*

I asked if I had made myself clear about how I intended to keep my standards up to those of the NHS.

If it can be done for private patients, why not for NHS patients? The answers are always the same – not enough funding; too many patients, and daft bureaucratic controls. Money is an issue, except that most older UK patients needing a bypass will have already paid for one through their National Insurance and tax contributions – ten times over in fact! And the British persist in thinking they have the best medical service in the world, with many NHS doctors and other staff carrying enough arrogance and hubris to tempt certain nemesis.

The CQC inspector, must have regretted asking me his question, but his sanctimony, like that of most other NHS officials, persists regardless. No business I know of, could possibly survive with these attitudes amounting to a distinct NHS culture. And yet it persists, with an ever-growing managerial and directorial staff to control it. Doctors and patients never needed to be so managed.

I often wonder what would Elon Musk do to improve the NHS? What would Warren Buffett, Bill Gates or Richard Branson do to manage it better?

Private Practice Differences

Early in my career, I was an NHS GP for two years. I insisted that the more complicated cases returned for further consideration, outside of normal consultation hours. Even then (late 1960s) it was frowned upon by my colleagues. It worked for patients, allowing them the in-depth consideration they needed. Given the current UK, GP workload, I doubt this has become common practice.

In my private practice, in which I accumulated 20,000 patients over fifty years, I allowed 30 to 90 minutes for each consultation – but then, I worked a full day, with no interruptions needed to satisfy any NHS audit or other patient management system. It would have been inefficient not to have solved each diagnostic problem at one sitting. I suspect that most NHS GPs spend half their week away from their consulting room, partly doing 'paperwork' (albeit, computer based).

It is time for the CQC and GMC to recognise the major differences that exist in the quality of services available. No private practitioner would survive handling patients like the NHS, so the assumptions and considerations applied by regulators to the NHS need to recognise its many serious deficiencies (as reported by many patients).

In my case with the GMC, the MPTS Tribunal thought I had recklessly prescribed drugs to a patient addicted to pain-killing drugs and sedatives. What they never considered was that I saw her twice every week to check on her progress. I was able to make many therapeutic adjustments, and counsel her through all her difficulties. She was undoubtedly a challenging patient. She knew that no NHS practice could safely cope with her.

I specialised in solving difficult cases, so she was just one of many. The availability and close attention I offered her, was completely unavailable in the NHS. In fact, the NHS GP on the tribunal, had no way of knowing how differently she had been managed from what his practice could have offered. Had I been a detached, anonymous physician, they would have been right to accuse me of inappropriate prescribing. Instead they had no idea of how my practise actually worked – open all day, and available at all times.

Should all NHS GPs now reconsider their NHS employment status? Many, I'm sure, would like to dictate their own style of practice. So, why not establish a new healthcare system based on the private practice requirements, or indeed a separate private system as I have outlined (as once it was before the NHS). One does exist in part already, but remains fragmented. It would need to be pulled together before being offered as a stand-alone service. It might also be appropriate to create completely independent medical schools, with entry restricted to those capable of the art of medicine.

Patients First

The NHS tries hard to make it look like as if 'patients first' is their guiding principle, but it fools no patient I have ever met. The NHS did once have 'patients first' as its guiding principle, but the introduction of government directed, market-based bureaucratic management systems, came to supersede it. If it is to satisfy most patients again, the NHS must return to the 'patient first' principle. The ears of bureaucratic juggernauts are always too far off the ground to hear anything said at ground level. Although obvious to most NHS doctors and nurses with experience, they carry on feeding the anonymous juggernaut as an accepted priority – their job will depend on it.

At the moment, patients in consultation with their general practitioner are allowed to discuss only one problem at a time, and for only ten minutes or so. GPs in the UK, faced with patients complaining of tiredness, fatigue or exhaustion, are likely to experience heart-sink. Many will know that making an accurate diagnosis, will either be quick and straightforward (a virus infection) or be too complicated to consider in a few minutes (to define relationship problems or stress at work). The resolution of such problems not only takes time, it requires a doctor to be interested in more than physical disease alone.

Every doctor must look for the disease-related causes of fatigue. This list is not too long but does require a full history to be taken and a physical examination and laboratory tests to be undertaken. This will be too involved for some GPs, so many will refer their patients to a consultant medical colleague. In the UK, general hospital physicians are shrinking in number, but they were once best equipped to investigate patients in detail, ruling out every debilitating condition – from an under-active thyroid to Weil's disease (Adolf Weil, German Physician, 1848-1916).

The non-medical, mostly MBA and legal degree holders, who inappropriately govern the NHS, made one major mistake, among a multitude of others. They decided to replace general physicians and surgeons, who once formed the backbone of NHS hospital medical services, with specialised doctors having no need for broad clinical competence.

Once a doctor has ruled out every conceivable clinical physical condition as a cause, they must tell the patient they have looked hard, but could find nothing wrong. That will mostly incite the question: 'then why am I so tired doctor?'

The patient, now in limbo, might seek another opinion that makes sense. The GP will now have a few options to keep the patient 'in-play'. He could refer the patient to a psychiatrist or social worker – to anyone, in fact, who might help. Most doctors at this stage, have a 'management problem' – one that is not going to be resolved easily.

Issues of trust and competence might now arise. Whose responsibility is it to make a diagnosis? Who is best placed to make a diagnosis? And for the patient – who should they trust?

If the patient does not trust their doctor, they must find a sympathetic practitioner. They will need some luck or help from a friend, to find an interested doctor. Frustrated, some will accept the advice of a friend to see a counsellor, psycho-therapist, pharmacist, an adviser on food supplements or their hairdresser. Someone, somewhere, is likely to know someone somewhere, who might help.

Most of those who proffer advice, will know that the more one knows about a patient, the more appropriate will be the forthcoming advice. Only by fully understanding a client, his present and past situation, background, attitudes, ambitions and values, can any expert give meaningful advice. Previous exposure to the patient; continuity with them, and genuine empathy, are often the keys needed to arrive at a correct diagnosis, and thus to give successful advice. Obvious? Of course, but not now intrinsic to many NHS consultations.

With the UK medical profession now in free-fall from regaining patient trust, and hell bent on creating more anonymous, arms-length approaches to patients, patients are being exposed to more risk. A major part of the problem stems from using lesser trained staff and computer interfaces. Patients have noticed – for decades, doctors have looked more at their computer screens than at their patient. The UK medical profession has unwittingly configured itself to fail doctor-patient relationships. The evidence for this is now on the street. Patients are seeking advice from more approachable, personable professionals – pharmacists, nurses, chiropractors – even their hairdressers, whose record for issuing sensible advice has at last been recognised.

Doctors and Sleep Problems

At present, few doctors are interested in sleep, let alone its clinical relevance. It should be mentioned to medical students as part of their undergraduate curriculum. This audience might be too young to appreciate worldly stress and any connection to sleep. Why should they? Having led a charmed life thus far, many medical students will carry on with a privileged life, with little chance of encountering the same life stresses as their patients.

Insomnia can be thought of as a state of inappropriate hyper-arousal (Riemann, D. 2020). It has been defined by the American Academy of Sleep Medicine as:

> "*a perceived difficulty with sleep initiation, consolidation, duration or quality, despite an adequate opportunity to sleep, coupled with subsequent daytime*

impairment, and as chronic when lasting at least 3 months" (Edinger, J.D., et al. 2004).

There is a vast amount of evidence linking sleep disorders, poor sleep quality and physical health, to cardiovascular health, high blood pressure, obesity, diabetes; depression, anxiety, suicidal behaviour and all-cause mortality. The impact of sleep problems extends beyond personal matters – to workplace productivity, healthcare costs and public safety. At the same time, sedative drugs have been criminalised as addictive and unnecessary, but without much to replace their efficacy.

The Scale of the Problem

Over the last few decades, many questionnaire surveys of sleep have been undertaken. The results have not varied much.

In a sleep survey of adults in Finland (Hublin et al. 1996), 11% of women and 6.7% of men, noticed daytime sleepiness every day. Of those who were tired, 25% were thought to be depressed (with its attendant sleep problems – early morning waking, and poor-quality sleep); 9% had too little time for sleep, while 20.7% of women and 28.6% of men complained of insomnia, at least every other night. Sleep that was upset by breathing difficulties (due to lung disorders and obesity) with snoring and other forms of respiratory obstruction, was found in 19.5% of women and 42.3% of men.

In 2019, an Italian population survey found 14.2% of Italian adults dissatisfied with their sleep, and 29.5% with insufficient sleep duration (Varghese, N. E 2020).

In a more recent survey undertaken in South Tyrol, Italy, 4000 people were surveyed (mother tongue Italian and German). Poor sleep quality was reported by 17.8%, with 28.2% of participants reporting insufficient sleep (six hours or less). 12.7% had problems staying asleep (waking up to 3 to 4 times a week and unable to fall asleep again), with 8.7% finding it difficult to fall asleep in the first place. Sleep problems and poor sleep quality were associated with social and health-related factors, gender, age, mother tongue, chronic disease, and sleep hygiene (Ausserhofer, D. et al. 2025).

Poor night-time sleep does not always predict daytime sleepiness, as confirmed in the sleep laboratory (Lichstein et al. 1994). Perhaps this reflects the variance in energy available to different individuals, with natural differences in the effectiveness of their sleep.

The size of the tiredness problem is large. Its importance to the economy and personal health, cannot be ignored, but few doctors have the time or inclination to see it as a priority.

Sleep Disturbance and Health Risk

In 1989, it was found that sleep disturbance was often a forerunner to psychiatric problems. It was found to occur in 35 - 52% of cases with anxiety, obsessional complaints, depression, phobias, and panic attacks (Ford and Kamerow. 1989). Daytime tiredness caused by insomnia or sleeping too much, both led to depression and other problems within one year. In the fatigued, unskilled workers, heart attacks are the commoner problem. In this group, insomnia, but not over-sleeping (hypersomnia), was commonest (13.4% compared to 8% in executives).

In another study, a higher prevalence of heart attacks was found in those who slept more than 9-hours on average; angina was more common than expected in those who slept less than six hours (Partinen, M. et al. 1982). Long sleep (hypersomnia) is associated with more REM sleep, and heart and circulation problems. Those with additional respiratory disorders are more often tired, sleep longer, and have a higher prevalence of heart attacks during sleep.

In a review of studies linking insomnia with short sleep duration and cardiovascular problems, an increased risk of hypertension, acute coronary syndrome, and heart failure has been found (Java-heri, S. Redline, S. 2017).

Insomnia has also been associated with inflammatory conditions, greater artery 'furring' (atherosclerosis), increased cortisol and adrenaline levels, and increased insulin resistance (diabetes more difficult to control).

The Significance of Disturbed Sleep

One-third of our life is spent asleep.

Between 50 and 70 million Americans, report some sleep diffi-culty. Lack of sleep affects both our memory and our ability to think. Sleep deprivation can lead to a poorer quality of life, and reduced well-being; to neurological dysfunction, mood swings, hallucinations, and poor executive functioning. Those who do not get enough sleep have a greater risk of accidents, and of developing obesity, diabetes, and cardiovascular disease (Institute of Medi-cine, US. 2006).

Difficulty falling asleep or staying asleep (insomnia), despite an opportunity for sleep, causes impaired daytime functioning in 10% of people. Many treatments have been used to combat this. They include sleep hygiene measures (reducing light and noise), cogni-tive behavioural therapy (CBT), and pharmacological therapies: benzodiazepines, melatonin receptor agonists, selective histamine antagonists, antidepressants, antipsychotics, anticonvulsants, and non-selective antihistamines.

Alcohol and benzodiazepines can decrease REM sleep, even though benzodiazepines (Valium or diazepam, etc.) are a signifi-cant class of drugs used for insomnia. They can decrease the overall time spent in refreshing slow wave and REM sleep. They are useful, however, in reducing night terrors and sleepwalking. At least, highly stressed patients will get some form of sleep. In practice, I found these theoretical considerations to be insignificant – many hundreds of my patients reported an obvious benefit from taking them, some intermittently for many years.

The more severe the fatigue, the greater the inability to sleep – the sleep paradox. This drives the progression of tiredness, through fatigue to exhaustion; a frequent forerunner of ill-health, and the progression of some medical conditions.

In my clinical experience, few cope well with daytime problems, without sufficient untroubled sleep. Those who seem immune to daytime, stressful problems, may lack anxiety or any commitment to their situation. They can escape the sleep paradox and are less distressed by life's problems.

The body adapts to de-stabilising influences like dehydration, heat, cold, acidic and salty food, etc. It was propounded by the French physiologist, Claude Bernard (1813-1878). He proposed that adaptive bodily processes attempt to keep the *status quo* (*milieu interior*) – a process called homeostasis that can fail if disturbing factors become too strong. We now know that sleep holds an important place in the maintenance of this essential process.

Bernard was one of the first to propose experimental medicine. At the end of the 20th century, the acronym OPHERIC was given to his approach.

- **O**bservation. This then poses . . .

- **P**roblems (questions). So, formulate a . . .

- **H**ypothesis that claims to solve the problem. Then, design and carry out an . . .

- **E**xperiment, to invalidate or confirm the hypothesis.

- **R**esults of this experiment are collected, then

- **I**nterpreted, to draw a . . .

- **C**onclusion. Of course, every discovery opens up new questions; *'this is how medical science always progresses today'*. (Habert, R. 2022).

Without sleep, daytime tiredness will progress through fatigue to exhaustion, and the risk of catastrophic clinical events will increase. Like all cliff-edge, catastrophic phenomena, only a small nudge is required to bring about major change (Thom, René, 1972. Mathematical topologist). Such situations are bi-stable: from an intact body while above the cliff – to one fractured, lying at the bottom; from having a stable arterial narrowing, to one occluded by clot formation (leading to possible infarction).

Sleep Management

Humans do not cope well without sleep. Restful sleep refreshes those who become tired of toiling with life. While some sleep is recuperative, disturbed sleep often results in daytime tiredness. Fast heart rates, high blood pressure, and daytime levels of physiological activity can accompany REM, dreaming sleep. REM sleep – the active dreaming state, is not restful.

Freud believed that dreams allow glimpses into our sub-conscious. The significance of dreams has always been controversial, with no means to verify any theory. Some believe that dreams help to anticipate coping with future events. They may need repeating if they find no solution. Jung thought dreams represented a conversation between our self and ego. Freud believed dreams to be based on fantasy, lies and distortions of the truth. A more modern view is that dreaming consolidates our daily formed memories.

In 1953, Hall suggested that dreams express relationships with those in our environment (Hall, C. 1971). More recently, Erik Hoel suggested that dreams are disruptive enough to cause our reasoning to come unstuck. In fictional narratives we might find solutions to difficult problems. He links dreaming to creativity. This might explain why we can go to sleep with a problem, and wake with a solution. Birds and mammals also dream. They go through a learning process with the rumination of dreaming helping their survival (Hoel, E. 2021).

Getting to sleep (sleep induction) works best if we control the prevailing conditions. Repetitive motion or a boring environment can help. A slow relaxing experience, under conditions of reduced light and noise, will usually aide sleep induction. Disturbing and challenging entertainment or arguments before sleep, can inhibit falling asleep. Sleep induction disorders occur in those troubled by pain, restlessness, and psychiatric conditions. Optimal sleep conditions vary between those who can sleep anywhere, to those who have strict requirements.

Optimal sleep induction can benefit from time-clock considerations, especially after long-haul flights. Circadian rhythm and the production of melatonin are important, although no official recommendation yet exists for melatonin use.

The Biological Clock

Throughout each 24-hour cycle of sleep and wakefulness, hormones, body temperature, alertness, and sleepiness, follow our internal body clock, driven by the pineal gland and the hormone melatonin. This 'clock' is daylight driven. Without light exposure, and no knowledge of whether it is day or night, the cycle length will vary between 25 and 27-hours, with peaks and troughs that are different for each of us (Mills, J.N. et al. 1974). For most, alertness and executive efficiency, is maximal in the morning. This is when most people transact their business. For those rarer individuals who are 'evening people', alertness comes at the end of what is the usual working day for most others: between 5 to 9 pm. So called 'night people', peak between 12 midnight to 4 am; they are rarer still. In over 50-years of medical practice, I encountered only two. Both found work at times when others were asleep – one became a croupière in Las Vegas.

Alcohol, Food, and Sleep

Only a minority believe that a meal before sleep will cause wakefulness; most find that food is soporific and promotes sleep. Raised blood fat levels, lowered hormone levels, the induction of cerebral slow waves or foods containing melatonin, can be responsible. Meals can induce palpitation, indigestion from a peptic ulcer, acid regurgitation and heartburn from a hiatus hernia (on lying down). They will benefit from early meals and medication.

Alcohol can disturb sleep and influence mental and physical functioning. Although for millennia it has been advised as beneficial for sleep, alcohol affects sleep in complicated and perverse ways. Many depend on it for sedation. While small amounts can create an optimum level of sedation, too much can cause agitation and less effective sleep. Alcohol both stimulates and suppresses the brain. It is responsible for more REM sleep, and can reduce slow-wave, refreshing sleep. Alcohol can affect the brain longer than a few hours. From a disturbing mixture of stimulation and sedation, it can disturb mental arousal and impair well-being and performance. All this has important economic consequences.

In the City of London, a few decades ago, a significant number of office managers accomplished too little work after lunch – such was the effect of their alcohol and food intake. Alcohol can impair the performance of drivers and pilots, from slowed reaction times and alcohol induced sleep deprivation. Tiredness from debilitating illness produces similar effects.

For moderate drinkers, a revelation awaits. Abstinence from alcohol allows more restful sleep and improved daytime energy. In times of stress, however, drinking alcohol will seem to improve relaxation, and help one cope. Excessive alcohol intake always deteriorates performance, but this is not always appreciated. It can be mis-perceived as therapeutic.

Sleep Surrogates

Resting in a semi-sleeping state, lying on a beach and meditating, can temporarily reduce the energy we spend on cognition and emotion. It is assumed (throughout the whole canon of world literature) that sleep, relaxation, and talking less are beneficial.

Many and various scientistic views about preserving our energy abound in the media. For instance:

> 'Every time we open our mouths we release a powerful energy. If we could learn to hold on to that energy, it could be used to nurture our dreams, heal our bodies and fuel our minds.' Also,

> 'Talking is something we must learn to use, not something we must always do. There is a power in silence that energises the mind, body and soul.' 'When we perfect the art of silence, chances are we will get a lot more done.'

Vazant, I. 1995.

While not talking or thinking (reducing neuronal traffic), we allow brain neuronal pathways to unblock and to refresh our brain. Nobody has yet proven that those who talk less, live longer or suffer fewer illnesses. Talking less and silence is but one minor ripple, superimposed on something of much greater significance – the tsunami of strong genetic influences that more strongly affect both morbidity and mortality.

Few physicians with experience of dealing with the sick, doubt that sleep aids recovery. That sleep aids healing was fostered by the Spartans, and observed by Florence Nightingale, during the Crimean War. She saw benefits for wounded soldiers. The science of immunity has been slow to explain her undoubtedly correct observations.

By denying the need for personal ego and avarice, Buddhist meditation, reduces energy expenditure. It prescribes removing energy waste, to achieve harmony, contentment, and peace within. Living for the moment, with no need for over-thinking, worrying analysis, decision making, planning or prediction, will also reduce mental energy expenditure. The life consequences of taking life as-it-comes, and mindless reactive behaviour, are another matter.

Westerners find it easy to criticise Buddhist attitudes. While meditating beneath a bodhi tree has its benefits, westerners used to treadmill living conditions, will find it difficult to achieve composure in their workplaces or during inter-personal conflict. I suspect, however, that few religious Buddhists opt to work in offices or engage in conflicting relationships.

Sleep Hygiene

Simple strategies can help some get to sleep: wearing eye patches for disturbing light conditions or using earplugs in a noisy environment, for instance. Although these can help with external annoyances, more disturbing still are recurring thoughts of stresses, perhaps later to be rehearsed during REM sleep.

The benefits of a comfortable bed and a pleasant place to sleep need no challenge. Although some can sleep anywhere, others might want a choice – between a hammock, a waterbed, a king-sized bed with a well-made mattress, or a rolled-up towel for a pillow on a beach. Some prefer a certain ambient temperature, from icy – windows fully open in winter (or with air-conditioning) – to tropical heat and high humidity. The adaptable are more easily satisfied, although fatigue or exhaustion, by increasing agitation and irritability, will reduce adaptability. Obsessive patients, and those who are fatigued are more easily annoyed by distractions and could demand specific sleeping arrangements. Like Goldilocks, everything may have to be 'just right' before they can sleep.

Falling Asleep – Sleep Induction

In the early days of commercial television, some adverts depicted a family before bedtime, peacefully gathered around a fireplace, each holding and sipping a warm milky drink. The picture was that of an ideal sleep induction scenario – the gradual, relaxed decline of arousal – rather than sudden immersion. Watching a disturbing film, engaging in arguments before sleep, trying to sleep with adverse physical conditions (light, heat, noise) or drinking alcohol or caffeine-loaded drinks beforehand, can cause agitation and delayed sleep induction.

The same principle applies in anaesthetic practice. The smooth induction of anaesthesia is best after some sedation, given in a sub-dued environment. A patient brought frightened and screaming into an operating theatre, will need much more anaesthetic than usual to render them unconscious.

Many people have their favourite sleep induction methods. Some will listen to music, read a book, eat or first have sexual intercourse

– some will be disbelieved, claiming they are too tired for it! Many stressed people *will* be too tired. Fetishes that require a special time and place, and a special format, are inadvisable.

Drugged Sleep

Taking sedatives is now deprecated by UK medical regulators, most of whom are not medical experts, and certainly not experienced physicians. Their policies show more concern for addiction and accountability, than fatigue management. The risk of addiction is real enough, but so are the potential risks of increasing fatigue and exhaustion. To use them wisely, demands proficiency with the art of medicine. As many older UK patients now recognise, this is a fast diminishing medical skill. It has been side-lined by prioritising science to form anonymous, non-specific regulations, rather than to improve individualised patient care.

There is no doubt about the efficacy of benzodiazepines (drugs like Valium) in relieving anxiety and acquiring sleep. Anti-depressants are now more commonly used (non-addictive), but few match the efficacy of diazepam or lorazepam. Cognitive Behavioural Therapy (CBT) works well, but is time-consuming, and does not suit everyone. In the appropriate dose, I never met anyone who resisted the sedative effect of a benzodiazepine, for sleep or anaesthetic premedication. Hangover effects would sometimes occur but presented no problem to those with chronic anxiety. For the relief of anxiety and agitation that induces calm without side-effects (albeit addictive), I never found their match for uncomplicated general use. Again, the same question arises. Should patients and doctors trust experienced physicians or regulators with law degrees and MBA's, to decide clinical management?

The prescription of all drugs needs to be personalised. With benzodiazepine use, it is most important to recognise addiction-prone and addiction-resistant individuals. Typically, addiction resistant subjects dislike medication of all sorts, and are often anxious about the possible side-effects. The addiction-prone worry less, and will more readily embrace an experimental, therapeutic trial. All those with experience of life, as well as medical practice, will know to recognise the importance of one old principle – horses for courses!

Self-discipline is an important patient variable; it relates to how readily a patient will become addicted. The assumption that every-one will get addicted to sedative drugs is incorrect. Doctors need to rely on their clinical judgement of individual patients and the risk and benefit balance, to make their therapeutic decisions. They are now more likely to follow rules made by anonymous regulators (scared witless by the possibility of certifying another Dr. Harold Shipman) than to use their personal experience and judgement. Whether to the detriment of their patients or not, the strategy doctors must now employ, will at least help them avoid bureaucratic investigation.

Many experienced doctors concur. It is substance abusers, not the substances themselves, that are the problem.

Benzodiazepines are chemically harmless; at least as safe as the water flowing through the taps of London, UK. The adverse side-effects of liberally used alcohol and tobacco are significantly greater. Taking an adverse view, one must at least recognise that diazepam (Valium), will sometimes uncover depression and can induce hangovers and addiction. Despite its addictive nature, I have witnessed it freeing patients from chronic over-anxiety, en-abling them to live a normal life without side effects. I never en-countered a toxic chemical side-effect. Because some people have used benzodiazepines for suicide, their general use has remained controversial. Few can deny their efficacy for relaxation, effective sleep induction and restful sleep. These benefits (as referenced here) far outweigh their injudicious use, especially when they are prescribed by experienced, informed physicians, who by virtue of long continuity, know their patients well.

This issue arose at my GMC tribunal. Those on the tribunal – a lawyer, a biologist and a GP from Birmingham, could hardly offer as much experience as I had in deciding the propriety of benzodiazepam drug use for patients so well-known to me. They thought my prescribing excessive, and not for one moment considered my particular patient population (rich, educated, executives) or my experience over many decades, handling these drugs safely (no complications or complaints in over fifty-years). Their thoughts concerned the general case – that no doctor, no matter how experienced, should be allowed to decide about patient safety when it comes to drug use. They had to side with current opinion, which offered no evidence for the safety of long-term benzodiazepine use. They used guidelines as rigid rules, without enough clinical acumen to know more. This is how doctors are now regulated in the UK. After experiencing the clinical ineptitude of medical regulators, I happily resigned my license to practice in the UK, and also my membership of the Royal College of Physicians. They, and most of my colleagues kept quiet – no doubt fearing retribution; some, without doubt, agreeing with the GMC. Read all about it at the end of my book. The NHS. Our Sick Sacred Cow. 2023).

Withdrawal from an addictive drug, given to promote sleep, rarely presents a problem; especially when the most suitable patients are selected in the first place, and the timing of withdrawal is planned. Benzodiazepine withdrawal can be troublesome, but the only price to pay for the patients who have needed them. The withdrawal effects are not as alarming as the heart attack and strokes they can prevent – occurrences made more likely by disturbed sleep and exhaustion (in those at risk).

I always allowed patients to withdraw from their benzodiazepines while on holiday, when a few sleepless nights and anxious days would be easily tolerated – a small price to pay for years of improved sleep, albeit not quite 'normal' sleep quality, but with improved relaxation and composure throughout troublesome times. One important proviso pertains to the management of all addictive drugs: their success and safety is most easily achieved when they are taken by intelligent, compliant patients, concerned about addiction and with no wish to perpetuate it. Even though their prevailing stress may continue, all my private patients, most of whom ran businesses, knew that their early withdrawal would be encouraged.

There is a useful strategy for managing addictive drugs. That is to prescribe three separate drugs, each to be used in rotation; alternating each over a one to three-week period. Intractable addiction to one drug then has less time to develop. This simple technique is especially useful for doctors dealing with high-risk patients, like those with severe ischaemic heart disease (deteriorating angina, recent cardiac infarction), resistant hypertension or a recent transient TIA, where avoiding progressive fatigue and exhaustion might be of paramount importance. Doctors must balance the risk of addiction with that of medical catastrophe.

Managing Bereavement

After the problems causing a patient's fatigue have been resolved, quitting their sedative drugs is usually easy. When the disturbing factors remain, such as with bereavement, psychological adjustment may take six to twelve months. Taking a safe drug for this period, combined with counselling, can reduce the time needed for adaptation. Unlike bereavement, some other ongoing stresses have finite solutions. After finding an acceptable solution, successful drug withdrawal may only take a few days.

In the UK, doctors are limited to what they can prescribe, regardless of the patient's situation. For instance, they will prescribe only ten tablets of diazepam at a time, even to those who are bereaved. I take this as evidence of how more concerned they are about regulatory retribution than patient care. It also suggests that addiction and regulation concern them more than the risks of fatigue. They might take time to compare the risk of bereavement to that of sedative drug addiction. There are, of course, alternatives. They could prescribe a much less addictive drug which is less effective than a benzodiazepine. Antihistamines, antidepressants, herbal medications (like valerian) and CBT, can all be considered.

The associated risks of bereavement are surprising. Using data derived from a Medicare-based cohort of married couples (aged 67 to 98-years at baseline; survey number: 373,189, in the US between 1993 and 2002), all-cause mortality increased by 18% for men, and 16% for women, after the death of their spouse.

A wife's death increased the risk of the spouse's death by more than 20%. The major causes were: chronic pulmonary disease, diabetes, accidents or serious fractures, infections or sepsis, cancer and all other known causes. The effect exceeds 10% for seven more causes of death: colon cancer, ischemic heart disease, congestive heart failure, nephritis or kidney disease, cerebral vascular accident or stroke, other heart and vascular diseases, and other cancers (Elwert, F., & Christakis, N.A. 2008).

Bereavement in those of average age 55-years, increased the likelihood of death by 40%, mostly in the second year after the death of their spouse. Not only the remaining spouse suffers. Many other close relatives (mean age 71-years) also die, in the four years following the death (seven times more than in control subjects). The subsequent death of relatives is highest if the death took place

distant from their home. It was also more frequent when the
death occurred in hospital (Rees, W.D., Lutkins, S.G. 1967).

The Siesta

Afternoon napping is an important strategy for overcoming fatigue and its avoidance. Common misconceptions exist about
short-term sleep. Many believe an afternoon nap will reduce
their ability to sleep at night. In fact, the relaxation that ensues
from napping, often allows for better night-time sleep induction.
Some think napping is a waste of time. I have heard it said, 'I've
paid a lot of money for this holiday. I'll not waste it in bed!'
Perhaps they are more concerned about getting value for money
than their health.

Those who choose to treat fatigue by taking a holiday, may
need five consecutive days of siesta to get any improvement in
their well-being. The holiday effect – the promise of pleasurable
'down-time' and reduced arousal – can make the idea of a siesta
attractive to some, but not to all. Many will give in to the prevailing group social pressure, pursuing activity rather than rest.

Attitudes to Fatigue

I was trained by doctors with Second World War practise experience. Doctors taking time off for tiredness alone, was thought
of as a weakness. Being unable to cope under pressure was seen
as a serious weakness. Keeping calm and carrying on, was a basic
requirement. At the time (1960s), many junior doctors went sick,
unable to cope. The rest of us, quite often worked day and night,
with few breaks. Those who survived, enjoyed every minute of it,
and would happily return to it. Those who might say 'that was no
life', might not fully understand the full meaning of a vocation.
If being anachronistic would suit patients' clinical welfare better,
perhaps we should resurrect some of the older values.

Knowing the difficulty of making a diagnosis, some doctors have come to prefer limiting their scope of reference to laboratory data. Hospital doctors, whose theatre of operation is the out-patient clinic, the cardiac laboratory or the operating theatre, will often choose to leave social factors and psychology to G.P's and social workers. Doctors specialising in the heart, brain, liver or kidneys, can easily justify this – modern medical bureaucracy no longer favours general medicine and doctors with a broad-based medical knowledge. Their divide and conquer strategies have worked well – the UK medical profession has been forced by regulation to lose its interest in the holistic approach and the art of medicine, both of which are necessary for technically proficient, optimal patient care.

To ignore the patient as one whole sentient being, favours a re-stricted scientific view, denying any consideration of the multiple interactions typical of every biological system. Unfortunately, we no longer have Hippocrates around to guide and correct us – isn't the whole point of medical practice to make each patient feel as whole and healthy as possible – or is that now, old hat?

Businesses survive longer when they ask customers for their opin-ion, and feedback about their services. It is not often that patients are asked what they think of medical practice management in the UK. Few occupying medical ivory towers would want to go there! Perhaps they fear what they might learn about their fitness for purpose.

The heart specialist needs to know that fatigued and exhausted people are more liable to angina, clotting, and heart attacks. Liver and kidney specialists need to know that exhausted people can have reduced resistance to infection. Like their heart disease col-leagues, they also need to know that their exhausted patients (many of whom have taken alcohol and drugs for years to offset their stresses) will also have disturbed clotting functions, promoting dangerous clotting in both their veins and arteries. So, can they afford to ignore patient tiredness, fatigue and exhaustion?

Optimal recovery from any illness requires certain conditions. Sharing a noisy hospital ward isn't one of them. Hospital wards can be noisy and uncomfortable places, lacking privacy – hardly conducive to refreshing sleep and recovery. To tarry there, could induce complications such as thrombosis and delayed healing. The modern trend to discharge patients from hospital as soon as possible, can also have adverse effects. Early discharge to a home situation where rest is easily possible should be advised; discharge to an unsuitable home could lead to a prolonged recovery phase; at worst, to re-admission with complications. Clearly this is a short-sighted policy.

Since the time of Hippocrates, good patient management has depended not only on knowing the patient, but his family and both his home and work circumstances. Since humans have not evolved over the intervening millennia, has their general care needed to change – from the rest, relaxation, the good food and exercise he once prescribed? Doctors may now be proud of their quick turnaround of beds as an indicator of their efficiency, but at what cost to discharged patients? All this is too important to be left to financially oriented hospital managers, whose job is to demonstrate an efficient use of resources.

Politicians who believe in an effective welfare state and NHS, should take note. Patients should never have to suffer the modern equivalent of being accosted by a highway robber like Dick Turpin. His usual demand was "Your money or your life!" Without the money and facilities necessary to preserve life, the loss of life is inevitable. Without dedicated, experienced and able medical staff who put their patient's lives first, patients will need to go elsewhere to survive.

Medical Causes, Effects, and Associations

Migraine, irritable bowel syndrome, colitis, peptic ulcer, high blood pressure, angina, palpitation, anxiety and depression are among the commonest conditions with symptoms associated with all causes of fatigue. These symptoms can wear patients down with worry and concern, guaranteeing their further persistence. An adverse change of life circumstances, constant fear, excessive anxiety, and a wasteful obsessional trait can all deplete our perceived energy. Perhaps they can cause a more permanent and extensive form of neuronal channel blocking. If so they can also unblock fairly rapidly.

When in 2025. the tired, chronically stressed, sleep-deprived Israeli families were reunited with their released hostage family members, they slept well for the first time in two years. Relief from fatigue will likely have followed within days.

A Medical Paperchase

Fatigue left untreated can lead to a well-known medical paper chase. After drug '1' has failed, give drug '2'; after that consider drug '3'. Many doctors will get exasperated if asked: "What are you going to try next, doctor?" The doctor, knowing of no alternative, might reply: "I've done all I can. There is nothing more I can do for you."

At this point, the patient must consider seeking a second opinion. In the UK, for NHS patients, this can only be had by asking their GPs permission. Even private consultants require a referral letter. In most other countries, this would be laughable, given that the patient should take priority, not the medical system or insurance companies who pay and thereby control doctors. In the UK, a patient requesting a second opinion is likely to disgruntle their doctor – the implication – a lack of continuing trust. The total collapse of their doctor-patient relationship could follow. There is no free movement of patients allowed between GPs in the UK, so what is the patient to do? That question is now being answered by private GP practices.

A Need for Change

Tragedies of all sorts – redundancy, gross injustice, extreme frustration, loss of respect, indignity, divorce, and many other upsetting life circumstances, quickly cause fatigue and exhaustion.

Those with excellent coping skills will solve their problems, then go on holiday. Others, bogged down in a fixed situation, might slip down a spiral of ever-increasing fatigue; fatigue that can lead to psychological, medical or social catastrophe, in those prone to respond adversely.

Early recognition of this tendency allows preventative intervention, but first:

- Doctors must learn to recognise the early symptoms of demise and appreciate their possible clinical significance.

- Second, the disease-oriented medical professional, would have to re-learn an appreciation of holistic patient appraisal. It could save a life, as effectively as insulin or penicillin.

There are, however, disincentives for doctors:

- Doctors are not paid more for such services.

- They have not been trained for social intervention.

- There is no joined-up social care system in the UK for referral.

- Investigating the causes of tiredness, fatigue and exhaustion takes much longer than prescribing a pill, and under the present time-restricted GP system, it is not feasible.

Applied psychology should have an important place in every medical school curriculum, but this will have to await the re-humanisation of UK medical practice. We must await a reincarnation – the admission to medical schools of those students with an understanding of humanity beyond the physical sciences. Although Hippocrates was one of the first to proclaim medicine as a science, he also discussed the compassion, discretion, and selflessness needed by doctors. (Introduction: Hippocratic Writings, Penguin Classics, 1978).

Alternative Medicine

In the UK, King Charles started a weighty ball rolling when – he invited the medical profession to consider 'alternative medicine', representing as it does the holistic, humane approach to patients. 'Alternative' is of course the wrong word. 'Traditional' or 'historic' would be more apt. The medical bureaucrats serving orthodox medicine have an aim – to replace all humane medical approaches to patients, with a strictly 'evidence-based', so called scientific approach. They can then more easily control and regulate it. There was no need. The holistic approach complements the scientific one. Unfortunately, we mostly select as medical students, those who find science more attractive and exciting than humanity. Learning the art of medicine will thus become impossible for some, requiring as it does, an apprenticeship to someone who knows the value of customary practice, even in the absence of scientific (statistical) proof. Resorting to binary thinking – it is less energy consuming – many doctors will choose one and abandoned the other.

If patients prefer it (as do private patients in the UK), physicians and scientists will be forced to find the humanistic approach acceptable, once again having to respect the influence of our minds, emotions and circumstances on all medical conditions. Being paid for their service (as in the NHS), rather than having to accumulate patients by merit (as in many countries), means that doctors have been able to ignore this. As a result, they have become less personal, with many becoming anonymous.

In society, fashion always foregoes proof. In science, the reverse is true. While the medical profession has been ever mindful of this, it remains the duty of the scientific professions to safeguard the gullible from the follies of fashion, maintaining the highest standards of objective evidence through dependable scientific methodology. Being alert to fooling ourselves, does not preclude accepting the complexities of human nature and the art of knowing how to manage human beings reacting to their circumstances.

Governments want the medical profession to help reduce population morbidity and mortality. We must thus promote 'healthy diets', weight loss, reduction in alcohol consumption, and smoking cessation. But since the machine of society feeds on personal desire, governments must be duplicitous. The diseases we face are as much the fault of an ill-educated and unaware public, as they are of governments allowing tobacco and alcohol consumption for tax gain. The streetwise will not be fooled – they are fully aware of political duplicity, and the impotence of the medical profession to force any difference.

A Stressed Cardiologist

A senior cardiologist colleague of mine was always disinterested in the effects of stress on the heart. That was until he received his first inspection by HMRC tax investigators. He had earned large cash sums consulting in the Arab world. Many times, he was jetted off to the Middle East in an emergency. Innocent of the tax implications, he returned to spend his money freely. He collected oil paintings, Persian carpets, a large house with a swimming pool and tennis courts. The final Inland revenue judgement was estimated – HMRC said he owed £500,000 in tax (a lot of money in the early 1970s), payable over ten years. He then admitted to me that, for the first time in his life, he appreciated the full meaning and significance of personal stress. It can be difficult for those who have led sheltered, secure lives (like many doctors), used to harnessing dependable scientific knowledge, to begin to appreciate those whose lives are made fearful or anxious by stress.

Appreciation of Patient Stress

Even now, in the medical profession, there is little widespread appreciation of the significance of stress and its relationship to disease and ill-health. The concept is easily understood, but its relevance to ill-health and disease is often ignored.

Many doctors still live in metaphorical ivory towers, having been born into safe and sensible middle-class families, where any thought of the toils and strife suffered by the average man, can be overlooked with their sense of privilege and entitlement. Coming mostly from the fortunate, rather than the deprived, doctors have little reason to be empathetic, either to businessmen and their troubles, or to deprived families. There are some rare, notable doctors, who have broken this mould, and have devoted their lives to the deprived. They have come to fully understand the dynamics of an impoverished existence. Meanwhile, the entitled majority, need only pay lip service to their strife. The intake to medical schools of students from more varied social backgrounds, has done much to change this over the last twenty years. The ruling medical establishment, however, remains staunchly middle-class and detached. To paraphrase Hippocrates – it is necessary to understand the patient and all their intimate details, before one can treat them adequately.

Unprofessional?

Within the medical profession, questions that might expose the personal details of any patient, are still thought 'unprofessional' by many; even though, hidden circumstances can be potent causes for patient demise – often marked by progressive fatigue, ill-health, and exhaustion. While fatigue will nearly always affect health, it more rarely affects disease. Only those pre-disposed to 'fur' their arteries, might suffer a clinical problem once fatigued. Those liable to generate arterial clot under stress, might then die from cardiac infarction, a stroke or pulmonary embolism. While widely accepted as important by patients (and their families), disturbing psychosocial aetiological factors, may fail to excite cardiologists and other physicians, whose focus will be condoned should it remain solely on clinical intervention.

Rest and Convalescence

Before the advent of 'scientific medicine', rest, relaxation, sleep, recuperation and convalescence were known to be of value. The ancient Greeks and Spartans certainly recognised the significance. In sleep, the Greeks thought that the God Æsculapius visited their mind to perform healing and restorative work. Allowing restful sleep in UK NHS hospitals, has never been a practicable possibility. Hospital wards and ICU units are not designed to cater for it. Also, the concept of convalescence – rest in a restful place that aided recovery – was discarded by the NHS. Taking time to recover under medical supervision, was seen as too expensive for medical bureaucrats to condone. By the early 1970s, few convalescent homes remained open in the UK.

Throughout my career of over fifty years, I observed both anonymity and economic priorities gradually prioritised over the provision of personal care. To spend enough time with each patient, to take their history and examine them, is basic to accurate and effective diagnosis, but nevertheless, NHS medical bureaucrats decided that this was wasted time and too expensive – medical practice decided on by largely untrained committees, no doubt.

As new technologies spare our time, we have
less time to spare.

As the illusion of life becoming ever more complex grows, we will need more time to understand our predicament, and even more time to aid those defeated by it. With correct political planning, we might again provide as much time for one another, as once we did – before the advances of medical technology, and before we were forced into a world that allowed human disinterest and anonymity.

The Health Divide

Solving the medical and lifestyle problems of those leading deprived existences, is unquestionably difficult. There are several reasons for this. First, the control deprived people have over their circumstances, is limited. Second, when the level of educational achievement is low, understanding will be restricted and emotional reactions can take precedence. These impact medical practice, and any outcomes achievable. Where strong belief, but no evidence exists, effective doctor - patient communication may not be achievable.

Traditional working-class fatalism ('we've all got to die of something'), has a lot to answer for. It allows smoking and its associated diseases to be ignored or overridden with streetwise logic, such as – 'what's the point in extending the life I lead?' Smoking may even be seen as a good way to end an impoverished stressful existence. As a result, the deprived smoke much more than the privileged. Although depressing, it is not an attitude always associated with depression – it can be pragmatic – coming from the recognition and acceptance of an inescapable fate.

So why not spend more, educating the poor? One academic treatise concluded that this was a waste of educational resources. Herrnstein and Murray (authors of '*The Bell Curve*'), found that the poor in the US made much less use of educational facilities than those already advantaged – pupils in the best private schools. This dismal conclusion should not inhibit those dedicated to helping others, even if their initial enthusiasm is soon to evaporate. In my experience, succeeding medically with the deprived – those referred to me in desperation as a last resort – was mostly disappointing. A beneficial outcome was so difficult to get, it seemed a 'waste of time'. Without middle-class resources, many were unable to achieve the best for themselves (as could private patients in the UK). Many existed without being able to access adequate medical facilities; some were destined to die on a UK, NHS waiting list. I reluctantly came to the view, as a doctor whose patients were mostly wealthy and advantaged, that real medical help for anyone deprived of motivation, money or education, would take even more money, energy and coercion than was needed to treat the privileged.

From whatever viewpoint, few can doubt that the inequalities in most societies are profound, depressing, and inescapable. The provision of better housing, schools, job security, and an environment worthy of pride are no longer affordable in many countries. Without such advantages, the job of every physician to improve the health of the nation, must remain hampered. Obviously, the social changes necessary rest with the power of the State, not with the medical profession. Despite this, the medical profession is easily made a political scapegoat.

What incentive do governments have to help? Which Government for instance, will ban smoking altogether, while the tax revenues are so lucrative? Which government will improve inner-city schooling and living conditions, while the voice of the deprived is so easily ignored (until just before an election, that is)? Which government will provide the milieu to motivate its citizens to do their duty to their fellows and to their country. Meanwhile the deprived become further deprived by smoking, while more of their middle-class compatriots have given it up. While the deprived continue to squander their limited resources on impossible odds, like the National Lottery, the middle classes are spending theirs on medical check-ups, private education, private healthcare and healthier food.

If everyone became middle class, with incomes that allowed saving, and a desire to live a longer, healthier life, would national survival and quality of life improve? Although possibly true, it remains a socialist fantasy. Another socialist fallacy is that if all poor performing pupils at school worked harder, they would all become above average. Unfortunately, there is a natural order to all things – there will always be a bottom, a top and an average – the Poisson or normal distribution never goes away. We might, however, raise the average standard.

Scientific Medicine

Doctors now practise in the investigation-oriented, data-driven era of scientific medicine. Experience and learning from observing the customary practice of experienced professionals, has been waning for decades. Unfortunately for doctors, patients prefer to be treated as sentient human beings, not as guinea pigs or experimental subjects.

Hospital doctors, whose theatre of operation is the hospital ward and out-patient clinic, the cardiac laboratory or the operating theatre, have no need to bother seeing patients as human entities; that is something they can leave to G.Ps or social workers. Those doctors who prefer it this way, will likely choose to become heart, liver, brain or kidney specialists. Because this attitude lacks human perspective and context, such an attitude will come at a cost. Ignoring patients' circumstances and personality characteristics, will exclude their personal energy considerations. That is unscientific, simply because energy, as the most basic stuff of the universe, can never be ignored without a loss of understanding.

Heart specialists need to know about patient energy, because exhausted people are more liable to angina, arterial clotting, and heart attacks. The liver and kidney specialists need to know about exhausted people because their resistance to infection is often reduced, and the toxic effects of alcohol – often taken to relieve stress – can disturb clotting function. The neurologist needs to know about tiredness and fatigue, simply because it can increase the frequency of migraine, raise blood pressure and cause haemorrhagic stroke. Those stresses patients might like to hide, can initiate therapeutic grand tours of drug treatments, diverting attention from the real cause of their exacerbations of angina or migraine. Many neurologists, cardiologists and nephrologists, however, might correctly see themselves as inappropriate to deal with their patient's relationship problems or their legal or financial stresses. This lack of humane band-width, can follow from their upbringing, personality and desire for anonymity (for more, see my book, *Doctors, Nurses and Patients*, 2024).

Many older patients now ask – where are those wise GPs who once knew their patients personally, together with their families and circumstances, through dedication, loyalty and continuity? Patients could rely on them for pastoral care; for their understanding of the human predicament, with a complete picture that allowed for wise and practical advice.

Doctors Dealing with Tiredness

John Cleese once had a problem. In his introduction to *Families, and How to Survive Them*, he describes how he felt when tired, and how the medical profession handled him:

"... I had suffered for at least two years, from low-grade 'flu symptoms which my doctor wasn't able to cure. Eventually, after three full check-ups, he advised me that the cause was probably psychosomatic, and suggested that a psychological approach to the problem might prove fruitful."

A medical check-up, incapable of the discovering that his tiredness was caused by the increased energy expenditure of a relationship problem, was of no value except to exclude 'organic' disease. Many doctors, by refusing to ask 'personal' questions, will miss the wood for the trees, their brief being focussed on the discover and treatment of 'disease', while ignoring the whole, functioning person.

Most doctors love diagnosing interesting conditions. It can provide interest, and kudos among colleagues. As physicians, we all have a duty not to miss organic disease. No doctor would be worth much if he thought every patient complaining of tiredness and fatigue, had only relevant psychosocial problems. He would risk missing Addison's disease or an underactive thyroid.

If for convenience, the medical profession continues to deny the existence of a sentient being within each body, we will reduce our chances of preventing medical catastrophes – especially when they are linked to the patient's 'way of life' and the stresses they cope with. Every person has feelings, attitudes, beliefs and policies, adopted to cope with their life. Because their relationships and circumstances can physically affect their functioning, a diagnosis of 'psychosomatic' can be too trite. It can deny the recognition of serious pathophysiology and be used as a 'put-down' or 'cop-out' by doctors who prefer to treat only 'organic' disease.

Disease, Hospitals and Energy Depletion

When an urgent medical condition, like rapidly deteriorating angina occurs, doctors and nurses must focus on the physical needs of their patient: matters of blood coagulation, artery narrowing, and any electrical problems of the heart. Focussing on the patient's fatigue must take second place, despite the fact that it can precede artery clotting (the cause of heart attacks), heart electrical instability or both. They should, of course, give some thought to their patient's anxiety and fear, while wheeling him wide awake and frightened, into a ward full of monitors, bright lights, and other people having cardiac arrests. Although disturbing when fully conscious, an intensive 'care' or a coronary care unit may be the safest place for him, although, much more attention to how patients might react, can be worthwhile.

At such times, its peace and tranquillity with finessed technical expertise that is required, not fear and disquiet. The very last place an exhausted person needs to be is a thirty-bedded hospital ward. For those having a heart attack, such conditions could hardly be more adverse. Any disquiet will cause unnecessary sympathetic drive; any resulting increases in nor-adrenaline could precipitate heart rhythm disorders, deep vein thrombosis or heart failure in some cases. The sooner they get home the better, but only if home is a place of peace and caring.

In private hospitals, individual rooms are usual. As a result, recovery is often less stormy. This could be because the cases admitted are less serious; it could be that the internal hospital architecture and patient staff ratios, contribute significantly to recovery. A quiet, calm, optimistic, and comfortable environment works best. It is not known how many complications occurring in hospitals, result from the hospital architecture and environment. My guess is that the proportion is large.

Politically, no constructive changes in the NHS are likely to happen, with UK patients mostly grateful for what they have received – partly a hangover from the charity they once received in hospital. My paternal grandfather was rich enough to make donations to the London Hospital, Whitechapel, in which he met his demise. Meanwhile, patients continue to enter hospital for treatment and come out exhausted from the experience.

Depression or Fatigue?

Tiredness is a manifestation of depression, and depression a manifestation of tiredness. Both depression and fatigue can be associated with a lack of neurotransmitters (serotonin, etc.) in the brain, and the blocking of neuronal pathways. Tiredness can be depressing. Depression is associated with pathway inhibition and the perception of reduced energy.

Doctors find it convenient to categorise illness. Finding oneself in a high coping, critically important, emotional charged situation is typical of some with exogenous depression (the result of personal, external influences). In 'endogenous' depression (having an 'internal' origin), no external causes will be obvious. Doctors have for centuries been comfortable categorising some medical conditions as 'essential' (as with high blood pressure), 'endogenous', 'constitutional' (as with asthma) or 'idiopathic' (unknown cause). In all cases, an obvious cause is missing.

Such labelling can inhibit progress, because no further thought is deemed necessary. I lived with the term 'essential' hypertension for most of my professional life. Now, the same entity is referred to as 'primary' hypertension – a term that is no more informative. It might be better called arteriosclerotic hypertension since it is most often caused by small artery, muscle wall thickening, for which there is a strongly inherited component.

Freud and those who followed him, had much to say about the social and developmental origins of depression. It is now a more fashionable notion for depression to be considered metabolic – the result of altered brain chemistry. This shift has released doctors from considering the person within (holistic approach), and to consider their brain chemistry alone (using the culture of scientism).

Manic depression is an interesting sub-type. It involves extreme energy spending at times, with a withdrawn, tired and depressed state, seen at other times.

From a biological and evolutionary perspective, depression is important, because it limits energy expenditure and causes social and mental withdrawal. Depression thus makes survival less likely. The ability to adapt and cope with changing circumstances will be affected.

All levels of perceived mental energy affect physical performance. Physical activity can stimulate our perception of mental energy. Perceived mental and physical energy often occur together. Physical exhaustion, collapse and death, can occur in challenging environments or with extreme sporting activities. The death of Dr. Michael Mosley may have resulted from the unfortunate combination of arduous physical activity and a hot environment. He was found dead on the island of Symi, Greece, in June 2024, having walked for a long time in extreme heat.

Physical Causes of Fatigue

Here is a limited list:

    (a) Severe **Anaemia**.

        (All causes of hypoxia – low blood oxygen.)

    (c) **Endocrine Diseases**:

Diabetes (blood sugar too high)

Thyroid Disease.

Addison's Disease.

Growth hormone deficiency.

Menopause.

(d) All **Infectious Diseases** (TB, brucellosis, hepatitis, glandular fever, etc.).

(e) **Inflammatory Diseases** (autoimmune diseases like rheumatoid arthritis etc.).

(f) **Cancer** – usually, in the late stages only.

(iii) **Brain Conditions:**

Functional:

(a) Depression.

(b) Narcolepsy.

Pathological:

(a) Meningitis and encephalitis.

(b) Brain tumour and raised intracranial pressure.

(c) Cerebrovascular disease: too little blood flow (ischaemia) or brain damage   (infarction) from embolus or bleeding (haemorrhagic stroke).

(d) Cerebral degeneration/infiltration: Senile dementia – too few brain cells or infiltration with amyloid protein. Alzheimer's, etc.

(iv) **Therapeutic Causes**:

(a) As a side-effect of drugs: some antihistamines, beta-blockers, methyl-dopa, sedatives, antidepressants.

(b) **Iatrogenic** (doctor induced).

The Medical Profession and a Growing Loss of Trust

Patient satisfaction with the medical profession has been eroding for decades, so it is appropriate for the profession to look at methods which might restore some faith. If lay people can 'get to the bottom' of patient's problems, and can significantly help them, patients will more often choose them as a workable alternative. They may not be able to evaluate carotid artery stenosis or evaluate the need for heart valve surgery, but they will be able to handle 95% of all other medical issues. Traditionally trained physicians will retain their edge, but only if they can combine their subjective and objective skills.

The NHS executive wanted the NHS to function as a marketplace. Medicine is not a business; profit and loss are not issues. Medicine is a vocation, to be practised independently of all commercial considerations. To have done otherwise, has been to lose the respect of profitable business people. Now NHS executives and the politicians who direct them, will have to answer to savvy patients for their ignorance of both medical practice and business management.

Mind and Body

Since they are actually connected by many millions of nerve fibres, it is unsurprising that the mind and body work together. Despite revered physicians such as Hippocrates and William Harvey trying to impart the idea of humanity to their colleagues, professional apathy remains.

This current attitude is perpetuated by a lack of hard 'scientific' evidence for psychosomatic disorders. As a result, they are thought to be more apparent than real. The avidity of 'alternative' therapists for the mind-body template, and the interest many patients now have in them, has alienated many doctors who wish only to practice scientific medicine – with no need to consider or practise its art.

These are serious matters for fatigued patients, since even non-specific tiredness can affect the severity of symptoms, as well as morbidity and mortality. Leaving 'non-organic' fatigue untreated is not satisfactory, especially when it is constant tiredness that has motivated a consultation. In many cases one might say: help the tiredness, and the symptoms will look after themselves. This is a more useful dictum than many think, especially since it can influence the progress of organic disease.

Energy considerations are basic to the understanding of both biological and mechanical entities. Few physicians choose to address how the human body deals with energy. The same can be said of the stress concept, although this is not fundamental enough to provide a full understanding of how health, ill-health, and disease interrelate.

Tiredness and Healing

One remarkable nurse was rather more perceptive than any army doctor of her time. When Florence Nightingale observed injured soldiers in the Crimean War, she found them slow to recover from their wounds if exhausted. The wounds of those who had been in battle the longest, failed to heal; instead, they festered and became gangrenous. Injured, newly arrived soldiers, however, healed without delay. Her observations first made more than 170-years ago, have gradually gained experimental laboratory support – not that she needed it. Nightingale had no need of laboratory support – she had the opportunity to observe the same phenomena, day after day, for two years. She had no need to know that tired rats, exposed to a virus, would succumb more readily than healthy, well-fed, rested ones. My guess is that she would have predicted the result with accuracy and without doubt. For experienced observers, observation is real, whereas statistics provide conjectures qualified only by probability, and many times removed from reality. For experimental scientists, observation and anecdote mean nothing without wads of data and statistical analysis to overcome any false belief and presumption. In the right hands, both custom and experiment have validity.

Energy, Diagnosis and Medical Practice

A quick five-minute consultation, appropriate for minor issues, has no place in clinical energy management. Most experienced doctors, will come to a reasonable presumptive organic diagnosis within a minute or two, but gaining a full understanding will take a lot longer. If it is true that some minor ailments provide clues to more significant ones, then further investigation will often be needed.

Some patients may not be receptive to an in-depth approach, even if their problems are chronic and have remained unchanged after many medical interventions. One may need to wait until the time is right. Doctor-patient continuity, trust and mutual respect, then become issues if a correct diagnosis and management plan are to be forthcoming. We were once there, but now, most of these invaluable entities are being lost. Although now clouded by money, politics and bureaucracy, making people better remains the primary object of medical practice. Outside of that, much is superfluous to any doctor with a vocational need to help others.

No longer can patients easily find doctors, trained sufficiently to extend their considerations to their family. Super-specialisation is denying patients general appraisal – a medical holistic approach, once common among those doctors who taught me medicine and best practice. Doctors will legitimately say: 'I'm not a social worker or psychiatrist. You must seek help elsewhere'. And patients are doing just that, consulting other therapists, pharmacists, healers and counsellors, many of whom have sprung up to meet the need.

Many doctors investigate their tired and fatigued patients and will find nothing abnormal. They will tell the patient 'nothing is wrong.' By this they mean 'nothing wrong physically that I can find'; some actually mean, 'nothing wrong with you that I care to take further'.

Patients who find themselves in this situation, need to think again and look elsewhere for answers. In one respect, hairdressers will sometimes undertake as much dedicated diagnostic counselling as medical professionals. They are often the first person to listen intently, and the first to offer experienced advice. Many will have 'heard it all before'. The alternative is to consult a psychotherapist, gain some insight, and make effective changes that reduce energy spending. With less energy expenditure, their energy needs could be reduced, and they might gain composure and sleep better. If they can get refreshing sleep or adequate relaxation, they could reverse their fatigue and ill-health, and relieve some medical risk. They might even enjoy life again.

In disease states, there are many other considerations. The problem doctors have, is deciding whether patients are responsible for their tiredness and fatigue; whether they have a well-defined disease entity or an ill-defined one. Every doctor has an unchanged primary duty – to ensure their patient does not have a treatable condition, like an underactive thyroid or adrenal glands; the menopause, a lack of testosterone, diabetes, TB or a virus infection. (see chapter 12).

In my own analysis of 1000 patients, presenting partly with tiredness and fatigue, only 15 had an organic cause that I could find. The other 985 had no obvious organic medical cause. Only by gaining access to their non-medical, meta-information – their work situation or family relationships – was I able to understand the likely cause and offer them help. I advised most of them myself, as someone they knew and trusted, and as someone known to their family and business associates. Those I could not help, I referred for CBT, psychotherapy or a psychiatric review.

CHAPTER NINETEEN

Restoring Health

REVERSING TIREDNESS, FATIGUE AND EXHAUSTION

To fully recover from the causes of fatigue and exhaustion, many sufferers will have to re-think their life priorities, and re-hash their attitudes and personal philosophy. New timetables and accepted disciplines may need to be put in place, to prevent the same things happening again. If we are to regain health and pursue further experiences, and make worthwhile enduring memories, we must counter tiredness and fatigue, have refreshing sleep and take personal control of our energy expenditure.

There are many strategies to help manage sleep. Some are simple, like wearing eye patches to exclude disturbing light, or using earplugs to combat noisy conditions. Some are more involved. But what is to be done about the most pernicious causes of sleep disturbance – the recurring thoughts that dominate a troubled mind?

Available Energy

If not mentally exhausted, nothing beats mindless physical toil to improve vitality: in a garden, digging up clumps of earth, filling wheelbarrows, building compost heaps; in a gymnasium, pumping iron or cycling – up a mountain, stationary or otherwise. For us to sense vitality – increased available energy – we have to refresh our brain. This occurs during slow-wave sleep, but also during 'switch-off'. Both are aided by exercise and furthered by becoming athletically fit.

Vitality is heightened by the exhilaration of success, and by worthy achievement. Although the exhausted are more in need of being mentally refreshed than others, they will find it more difficult to accomplish. Some are in the grasp of inertia; some will soon hit an energy barrier as they try to get started. The disappointment that such failure can bring, might then consume the remaining energy they have left. Unfortunately, these are body design faults – because they do not aide survival.

The more we need sleep, the less able we are to get it (the sleep paradox). The more energy we need, the less able we are to regain it (the energy paradox). In clinical medicine one phenomenon is well known. The sicker the patient, the more difficult it is to pull them back to health. It's as if there is a tipping point, beyond which medical intervention struggles to work. The lessons to be learned are –

- Aim to diagnose every condition as soon as possible,

- Treat any adverse condition actively and as soon as possible.

- Any medical system unable to accomplish these is to be avoided and not worth supporting.

The excitement of starting a new endeavour can sap our energy by the end of each day. Although the end of the first day of school term will be marked by some tiredness, it should also be tinged with excitement and expectation, undiminished by any yet to be revealed shortcomings.

An obsessional attitude will promote mental energy spending, and sleep that requires optimal conditions. Some obsessive characters harbour beliefs like: *'I can only sleep when it's quiet, and only when it's completely dark!'* – *'Only with my special pillow!'* or, *'Only with the windows open!'*

Since there is no equivalent to a battery in the brain (although one could argue that each neuronal cell works like a battery), the concept of being 'recharged' by sleep, is misleading. Because in health, the availability of high-energy chemical compounds in all cells is virtually infinite (the source of power in brain cells), fatigue must be caused by something other than a lack of power generation. Leave your car lights on for long enough, and your car battery will run flat, and an old car might not start next morning. For humans, the analogy of a flat battery to explain tiredness, fatigue or exhaustion, is compelling but false.

Fatigue might be caused by the rundown of chemical neurotransmitters, but these too, in an otherwise healthy person, are in infinite supply (failing to be delivered only in dementia and other brain diseases).

Traffic Analysis Theory of Tiredness

A concept that better explains mental fatigue, is the gradual blocking of millions of brain neuronal pathways by mental transactions – all that thinking, planning, deciding, and emoting that we do while we are awake. A more appropriate analogy to explain tiredness uses road traffic. Even though all twenty road routes from outside London to Marble Arch are blocked by 6PM (rush hour), by 3AM they will all be open again. The concepts of blocking and unblocking routes; or closing, opening or re-setting brain neuronal routes while asleep, are more apposite than the concept of 'recharging'. I know, few care to understand the reasons. Most of us want to be completely refreshed by sleep, then to have enough energy to lead our lives as we wish. To further understand tiredness and fatigue processes, however, doctors have a duty to understand the mechanisms involved.

Since the brain is always switched on – even when deeply unconscious – all we may need to do, is allow enough downtime for our refreshing processes to take place. This implies switching off all decision making, thinking, emoting and mind-talk. We might choose from a number of alternatives.

To treat tiredness, chronic fatigue, and exhaustion satisfactorily, we must:

- Remove all precipitating causes (adverse life circumstances draining our energy and treat disease).

- Reduce the adverse psychological responses to circumstances (anxiety, fear and depression).

- Use psychotropic drugs (sedatives and anti-depressants) or cognitive therapy when necessary.

- Implement measures which improve restorative, slow-wave sleep (non-REM sleep) and reduce REM dreaming sleep.

- Introduce lifestyle adjustments which foster relaxation and mental detachment from long-term, causative situations. These might include exercise, meditation, yoga, hypnosis, prayer, massage, holidays, distracting pursuits, hobbies, and sleep-related cognitive behavioural therapy (CBTi).

Brain Re-Setting

Several practices claim to switch-off our 'mind talk' (thinking to ourselves), and to reduce mental energy expenditure. Among them are thinking of nothing, hypnosis, meditation, yoga, prayer, and

Qigong (an ancient Chinese healing practice: meditation with controlled breathing and movement). All can aid relaxation and mental switch-off.

Yoga

Yoga can take several forms. It is powerful enough to have a modest clinical effect on blood pressure (with less medication needed thereafter). The long-term sustainability and effect of this modest advantage is another matter. At least, yoga can reduce blood pressure for some patients experiencing stress. The three most important components of yoga are:

- Adopting different postures.

- Breathing practice, and

- Meditation.

The five principles of yoga are:

- *Relaxation*: letting go of worries and fears; releasing tension in the muscles and resting.

- *Exercise*: yoga positions, stretching and toning muscles and ligaments.

- *Breathing*: rhythmic breathing exercises to control our mental state.

- *Diet*: one that is balanced and nourishing.

- *Positive thinking and meditation*: to remove negative thoughts, to still the mind and transcend thought.

Some who practice yoga attempt to achieve a 'higher state of consciousness', expressed as the degree to which they can detach themselves from reality. Some will thereby gain a state of greater composure.

Self-Management

There are other essential strategies for saving personal energy. By quickly resolving situations, one can switch off slow, smouldering indignation, resentment and feelings of injustice. All burn vast amounts of energy and can cause ill-health. Fear, anger and resentment hurt most.

There are many behavioural techniques that can help in conflict situations, like assertiveness training which uses simple phrases to focus the attention of others. Movies provide many examples. I rather like the phrase, repeatedly used by John Travolta while playing Chilli Palmer in 'Get Shorty'. To arrest the attention of those he is talking to, he prefaces his remarks with, "Now look at me . . ." In the film, at least, he never fails to get attention; in real life it may not be quite so easy or effective. Other strong film characters, portrayed by Humphrey Bogart, Lauren Bacall, Tom Cruise, Arnold Schwarzenegger, James Cagney, John Wayne, Sean Connery and the like, demonstrate the coolest of 'in control' demeanours. Others instantly recognise their power and charisma. This commands their attention. They are unapologetic, direct, and use only words that count.

As we progress through life and meet different challenges, we may have to act as a subordinate, taking commands from others, before acting as a leader later on. We may have to be the middle man, the manager, the 'meat in a human sandwich', to be devoured by our boss if things go wrong. We might also have to come to accept being despised by those over whom we have authority. It would be useful if we could all switch roles and outlook whenever needed, but we mostly see ourselves in one or other role.

To achieve vitality as an adult, we need to start early in life. One of the benefits of teaching drama to children is for them to experience different roles. One of the most important would be to act out parenthood, allowing an appreciation of childhood.

Self-Potential

No amount of practice-time and energy spent will make the untalented into a virtuoso. It takes almost no energy, however, for the talented to excel. The only proviso – they must have enough energy and commitment to achieve excellence. As a consequence, there are multitudes of talented people who will achieve nothing, either because they have no energy or have no wish to apply it.

Many spend enormous amounts of energy on an unfitting role in life. Instead, they should gain a foothold on the most appropriate ladder at an early age. If we only understood the talents and true aspirations of our children, we could better advise them and better direct their future. We could help them avoid wasting their energy on pursuing inappropriate paths. The happiness, contentment, and feeling of fulfilment each person achieves, may depend on such considerations. Unfortunately, not all parents can inspire their children. It often takes one special person.

Here are a few good examples: Robert Baden Powell who inspired young people to learn, achieve and survive life by founding the Boy Scout Association in 1907. The Robin Williams character – teacher in 'Dead Poets Society' (1989. Touchstone Pictures), and more recently, Freddy Flintoff, the retired England cricketer, who inspired groups of relatively deprived, disengaged young people in Preston, Lancashire, UK, to take up cricket (Field of Dreams. BBC iPlayer. 2025). One man helped several cricket teams of young people without much direction in life, to achieve self-worth and find joy in camaraderie.

The world abounds with those who feel incomplete. Many have not answered one fundamental question about themselves – 'What is it that truly makes me happy?' Putting fantasy aside, they need to know if they are truly loving and giving or are more in need of getting love and affection from others. Are they a controlling person or in need of being controlled? Are they naturally gregarious, sharing experiences with others or a happy loner? Are they truly academic? Are they practical? Are they altruistic, greedy for money or a manipulator and user of others? Such self-knowledge is fundamental to finding happiness at any age.

Reality insists that we must learn to compromise and rationalise our failure in achieving what would truly make us happy. So often, parents direct their children to professions that fulfil their own ambitions. Desperate for reflected glory, they push their children into becoming lawyers, priests and doctors, when all their child wants is to lay brick, act or sing.

Two Bubba's (Jewish grandmothers) meet pushing their prams in a park.

'What a lovely boy', one says to the other.

'Yes, this is David, he's going to be a doctor, you know!'

'Really. This is Yitzak, he's going to be a Rabbi.'

'A Rabbi!' says the other Bubba. 'Is that a good job for a Jewish boy?'

Most major cities have many main-line railway stations. We must first decide our destination, before choosing the correct station for departure.

Alpha-Rhythm and Meditation

When the brain is 'switched off' but awake, our brain waves (on an EEG) are slow – alpha-waves (7-13 cycles/second). This accompanies mental quiet when our eyes are closed. Some believe that time spent with a brain alpha-wave rhythm will improve their attention and academic learning. This has been disputed. Alpha-rhythm can accompany hypnosis, yoga, and meditation.

For centuries, a tranquil state of mind has been associated with 'pure awareness' (*samadhi*). Some associate it with enlightenment. This state of consciousness has long been the object of Vedic, Buddhist, and Taoist practices. Transcendental meditation (TM) represents a later, western addition. The body can change with this mental state. For instance, there can be increased cardiac output, increased brain blood flow, less carbon dioxide generated in muscles, and amplification of brain waves and their synchrony. (Jevning, R. 1992).

In parallel with general anaesthesia, meditation can be associated with various depths of consciousness. As brain waves slow, unconsciousness deepens. Executive processing, external monitoring, and attention are all reduced during meditation experiences.

Thinking of Nothing and Qigong

Some have compared 'thinking of nothing' to Qigong. With each, there is different brain activity. EEG alpha-waves in the right hemisphere were more active during Qigong. In the left hemisphere, slightly faster (beta-1) frequencies, were seen with 'thinking of nothing' (Faber, P.L., et al. 2012).

Meditation can improve executive functioning, mental health and blood pressure, although the EEG changes occurring during both meditation and hypnosis are unpredictable.

The unscientific rationale behind alternative therapies, is easily disputed, but the reality of their benefits cannot be so easily dismissed. Explanations for why, and how they work, often lack objectivity, and can be unverifiable and not reproducible. Those with no knowledge of the scientific method, might be more vulnerable to myths. Some imaginatively present their beliefs as stemming from a separate system of thought, inaccessible to non-believers.

Prayer and Composure

Anything that reduces energy output can help to improve our vitality – the perception of having energy. Prayer can have this satisfying and replenishing effect for worshippers of all religions. Conforming to a strict code of disciplined behaviour, like daily fasting, can raise one's sense of personal dignity, integrity and self-worth. Ramadan, Yom Kippur, attending midnight Mass, and reciting mantras are examples.

Based on personal circadian rhythm, there should be optimal times for meditation and relaxation. For contemplative meditation, a waking state is best. When trying to achieve a prominent alpha-rhythm state, choosing a low point in arousal might prove better.

A calm mind fosters purpose and decisiveness. Without sufficient personal energy, composure can be difficult to acquire. Instead of trying to achieve composure, many give up and revert to busying themselves with daily duties as displacement behaviour. Some will act out dramas in their life, because they have little resourcefulness.

In this aroused state, they must deal with life as it comes; planning for future events will be side-lined and left to serendipity.

Any lack of control now, will usually commit us to increased energy expenditure later. We will need extra energy to overcome any problems accumulated, and thus reverse any effects of entropy. Just 'getting back on track' or 'putting things right or back in place', takes a lot of energy. The same consequences await those, who ruled by their emotions, decide on impulse rather than after intelligent consideration.

Some consider that the only way to live is to rid oneself of all stress: going where life leads (analysis and judgement being suspended), free to enjoy the consequences. This is the hunter-gathering mind set. It is more common among employees. It stands in contrast to those whose wish is to fence-off fields, create a farm, build a farm house and live off the profits of their labour. This is the usual mindset of those who desire freedom from outside control and prefer to be self-employed.

Sleep Management

During daytime activity, getting things done effectively and efficiently (with excellent executive functioning) can depend a lot on prior sleep quality, although this dependency varies a lot between people. Some anticipate their need for sleep and plan it: choosing an early bedtime and avoiding prior alcohol and disturbing experiences (intense conversation, arguments and watching horror movies) before sleep. A quiet preliminary phase, an hour or so before sleep, makes falling asleep (sleep induction) smoother. An untroubled mind promotes refreshing sleep. Sleep hygiene can help – reducing ambient noise and light, a comfortable bed, and suitable pillows.

Insomnia affects the disadvantaged and some cultural subgroups more than others (Chen, X. et al. 2015). Sleep disturbance has a social dimension. The wealthy more often have control over their lives, with some able to sleep whenever they like. For the poorer members of any society, sleep will often be controlled by work schedules and adverse environments beyond their control. For the poor, insomnia can be inescapable.

Could these sleep issues help to explain the health divide? When considered as large groups (statistically), I suspect they might. Individually, there will be lots of variation; some people remaining completely unaffected.

Sleep Therapy

One ancient Greek suggestion was that wine could induce 'sweet' sleep. For Penelope, stressed by Odysseus' absence (Homer. *The Odyssey*), wine helped while awaiting his return. The ideal was to sleep like the god Zeus' or like Agamemnon, whose sleep was described as 'ambrosial'.

In 1942, during the Second World War, the English psychiatrist William Sargent, started to treat exhausted British soldiers returning from the Dunkirk rout. He prescribed three-weeks of drugged sleep, using amylobarbitone. In his memoir (*The Unquiet Mind*, 1967), he recounts using it *'for restoring the shattered nervous system of war casualties'*. Before that, Emelio Mira y López had used 'sleep therapy' for soldiers fighting the Spanish Civil War (1936-1939)(Mira y López, E. 1943).

While working with Dr. Peter Nixon in the 1970s, at the Charing Cross Hospital, London, I became involved with short-term sleep therapy. Peter Nixon designed it to last three to seven days for patients with fatigue, exhaustion, and potentially dangerous heart problems (he referred to this as pre-infarction syndrome). Patients with progressive heart pain (angina) and uncontrolled high blood pressure (hypertension) were sedated, and their progress observed. Both diazepam and the sedative anti-histamine promethazine, were used every night, every morning, and after lunch. Patients had three sleep periods and were mobilised in between, thus avoiding chest infection, muscle and joint stiffness, and deep vein thrombosis. We saw very few complications. To achieve low-risk sleep therapy is, however, not easily achieved. It required a nursing team capable of spotting patient agitation and distress, and capable of making observations that would allow the appropriate sedative doses to be given. Between some physical activities, the objective was to maintain a patient in a state of peaceful, refreshing sleep.

After two or three days of sedation, patients' restlessness would usually disappear; they awoke less often, and their breathing and heart patterns stabilised. This suggested they were spending less time in REM (dreaming) sleep, and more time in restful, slow-wave sleep. A slow pulse, quiet breathing, and low blood pressure became characteristic. Anaesthetists make the same sort of observations: the rate and regularity of breathing indicating the depth of anaesthesia. In deep anaesthesia, the patient has the same slow, regular breathing, typical of non-REM sleep. Some anaesthetists now use EEGs (spectral analysis) to confirm the level of brain activity, although Dr. Norman Eve, who taught me most about anaesthetics, would have smiled with incredulity.

Early on during sleep therapy, one would observe some physical activity while asleep, presumably while the patient was dreaming. Those with dogs as pets know the phenomenon. Sleeping dogs often make purposeful movements while asleep – as if they were galloping over fields, dreaming of chasing rabbits. Without being able to tap into their dreams, who can know?

Once they had recovered from sleep therapy, we would interview each patient in depth. The aim was to discover any psychosocial reason for their demise. Often with the involvement of the patient's family, friends and work colleagues, we attempted to discover and assess their problems, afterwards helping them to find solutions – should they wish. Unfortunately, not all wanted this. Despite the possible danger of a heart attack or stroke that might be incurred by carrying on in the same old way, some refused to listen. On a few occasions, a previously non-compliant patient would return after having had the heart attack we predicted. It would have been unprofessional to say, 'I told you so', but sometimes, the urge was strong.

Some patients required the professional help of psychotherapists and family therapists. Sometimes, just one simple suggestion solved a complicated problem.

Not all cases were simple to resolve. Sometimes, too many people were involved in the patient's demise. Quite often the patient regarded their situation as inescapable. Those with limited resources; those who lacked insight, and those whose outlook was based on ignorance and arrogance, were the most difficult to help. Dr. Peter Nixon named some of them, recalcitrant recidivists.

Drugged Sleep

There are many harmless sedatives like valerian (from health food shops) and chlophenhydramine (Piriton in the UK), that can help some sleep in the short-term, with no risk of addiction.

Tranquillisers like diazepam (Valium) and lorazepam (Ativan) – benzodiazepines – are addictive, with most doctors reluctant to prescribe them. They could, like me, be accused of risking or causing addiction – even though they are harmless and effectively relieve stress induced anxiety and insomnia.

Such attitudes, driven by inexperienced bureaucrats can interfere with experience-based medical practice. These drugs are immediately effective and pharmacologically harmless. Rather than natural sleep, they induce a drugged sleep. For short-term use, they have no equal. I prescribed them for decades, from a time when only unacceptable barbiturates (phenobarbitone) and drugs like chloral hydrate and Largactil (chlorpromazine) were in use. Because benzodiazepines are so effective, many patients demanded repeat prescriptions. To manage them safely, specific experience is invaluable. Having worked with Dr. Peter Nixon using sleep therapy, and having been an anaesthetist, I fitted the task.

I used benzodiazepines successfully for decades, with no complications occurring. The addiction that occurred in almost every case, was easily overcome. I suggested patients withdrew them on holiday, after having resolved their problems. I had no complaints from any patient, but after being reported by a pharmacist to the GMC for repeated use, I vowed to withdraw all my patients and prescribe them an alternative, none of which compared in efficacy or patient acceptability to a benzodiazepine. My patients posed a question. Is it better to suffer insomnia induced by stress (with a higher blood pressure and more angina or migraine) or take a harmless, albeit addictive drug, that allows me to sleep and cope with my problems? Not one of my patients saw any sense in what the GMC directed.

There is a superficial secret to share. Very few bureaucrats have any medical experience, so they must rely on the Nuremberg defence – 'I was only doing what I was told to do'. Regulators whose main concern is the obedience of doctors, have insufficient clinical wisdom to judge the actions of any experienced doctor who knows his patients well. I remain concerned about the interference of ill-inform and inexpert bureaucrats in medical matters. Even the doctors employed as bureaucrats will rarely have much appropriate experience or expertise; why else would they choose to become administrators?

The risk of addiction to benzodiazepines is real, but the consequences of fatigue and exhaustion can be worse.

Several anti-depressants have a sedative effect and are non-addictive. One such drug is prothiaden, although some patients will complain about its hangover effects. It is best suited to patients who are depressed as a result of their stress. It should then be used preferentially for sleep, especially if they have an addictive tendency.

Doctors need to know their patients well enough to appreciate their addiction-prone or addiction-resistant tendencies. Typically, the addiction-resistant subject dislikes all medication. They are often anxious about the possible side-effects. The addiction-prone individual rarely worries and will favour personal therapeutic trials. There is an obvious clinical link here between self-discipline and an addictive tendency.

To simply assume that everyone will become addicted to a sedative drug is naive. Guns are dangerous, but more dangerous in the hands of some than others. Judgement about individuals need to be made by all doctors and nurses. Unfortunately, medical bureaucrats have come to think that doctors are too inept to judge their patients, even if they have sixty-years of experience and no record of patient harm. Advocating the blind observance to rules is their fail-safe option. They have no place commenting on any acute medical scenarios, where context is crucial, and only free thinking and quick reactions to save potential tragedy are in use by experienced clinical experts. They are deluded when thinking they can possibly comment meaningfully, understand or know best. All they are capable of doing is to quote guidelines and rules, while unable to respect clinical context (as made clear by all NICE guidelines).

Reforming medical regulation is urgent. Lawyers and lay-people should not have the final say in the fate of any doctor's professional status, and guidelines should never be used as immutable laws of clinical practice.

Many doctors agree that the problem doesn't lie with drugs, but with those who take them.

Although some drugs (like benzodiazepines) are as safe chemically as water, dangerous drugs like alcohol and tobacco, remain freely available to the public. Diazepam can unlock depression and it is addictive, but has almost no adverse effect on any organ, including the heart, liver or kidneys. The same cannot be said of some other sedatives, anti-depressants, alcohol or street drugs.

An important consideration is the withdrawal of addictive drugs used for sleep. This is rarely a difficult problem, especially when the most suitable patients are chosen in the first place, and the timing for withdrawal is appropriate.

Withdrawing from benzodiazepines can be troublesome, but not as troublesome as a heart attack or stroke, caused by not treating increasing fatigue. I always suggested that patients should withdraw their sedative drugs while on holiday, since a few sleepless nights and anxious days will then be tolerated more easily. A short, sleepless withdrawal phase is a small price to pay for years of improved (albeit not 'normal') sleep, during periods of unavoidable stress. Many of my many patients, thought they held untold value.

Another technique is to replace benzodiazepines with other drugs that are easier to withdraw.

The alternative technique of progressively lowering the dose, patients can find too difficult.

It is much easier for patients to withdraw from addictive drugs, once their stressful problems have been resolved. In cases of bereavement, a period of six to eighteen months is often necessary, before a patient becomes resigned to their loss. Taking a safe drug for this period, combined with appropriate counselling, will allow most patients to regain control of their emotions. I still hear that

doctors are inclined to give only ten tablets of diazepam to bereaved persons. Not only does this lack experience and common
sense, it is also clear evidence that regulatory compliance and fear
of inducing addiction (and perhaps facing bureaucratic investigation), are greater than their appreciation of a patient's plight.

The fear doctors have of retribution from regulators, is not un-
founded. Doctors in the UK have been told that independent clinical thought is potentially dangerous; instead, they are required to
follow bureaucratic rules and guidelines, even if patients might suffer as a consequence. I am reminded of what the famous wartime
pilot Douglas Bader said about rules – "Rules are for the obedience
of fools and the guidance of wise men".

Unlike bereavement, business problems more often have a shorter,
finite solution. Once a solution is found, it is time to withdraw any
sedative use.

One strategy for handling the addictive qualities of sedative drugs
is to choose three separate ones, alternating each over two to three
weeks. Intractable addiction to one drug is then less likely to occur.
This technique is especially useful for doctors dealing with addiction-prone patients.

Some with severe ischaemic heart disease (angina, recent cardiac
infarction), and very high blood pressure, perhaps with a recent
transient ischaemic attack (mini-stroke or stroke), are in situations
where their control using standard cardiac medication is inadequate. If one reason is their fatigue, sleep deprivation or an over-
burdening stress, night sedation could be life-saving. In such situations, the risk of a medical catastrophe (heart attack or stroke) can
outweigh any know effect of addiction. The judgement required to
balance these risks, can only rest with those experienced enough to
handle them, and who are long acquainted with their patient. This
is not for bureaucrats, regulators or the medically inexperienced,
for whom obeying rules blindly is their only safe option.

Tactical Napping

A NASA study (1995), found that pilots who napped for 26-minutes, experienced a 54% increase in their average alertness, and a 34% increase in performance, compared to those who did not nap. The pilots who napped, experienced less sleepiness toward the end of their flights; those who did not, experienced twice as much daytime sleepiness (Rosekind, M. R., et al. 1995).

There are other benefits:

- Improved memory.

- Improved creativity.

- Decreased reaction time.

- Improved focus and concentration.

- Lower blood pressure.

Hypnosis

Hypnosis for sleep induction is variable and unreliable. A review of twenty-four studies, found 58.3% had improved sleep after hypnosis; 12.5% yielded mixed results, and 29.2% reported no benefit (Chamine, I. et al. 2018). The study did not select patients according to their hypnotic susceptibility.

Hypnosis has an advantage. Only a few short sessions are needed, and adverse effects are infrequent. It can also be used as an adjunct to psychotherapy. The place of self-hypnosis needs further exploration.

Distractions and Relaxation

Distractions aide relaxation, especially for productive people needing to switch-off. As counter-productive, distractions can act as displacement activity; the purpose being to shield the stressed person from coping with further challenges. Listening to the many twittering inanities broadcast on social media, radio and television, easily distract us from the problems we need to solve. Sometimes, distraction acts as a parallel activity. Thinking while driving, for instance. Also, repetitive exercise, with no need for active thought, can help generate new ideas and solutions to problems – allowing them more easily to spring from the sub-conscious.

Personal success and acknowledgement can result in exhilaration. With boosted self-esteem, happiness and contentment, one can feel a sense of fulfilment and satisfaction. Such feelings help re-laxation, effective sleep, and the perception of improved energy.

Exercise training has both physical and mental benefits: increased confidence, with improved sleep, libido, and vitality. Physical training can improve attention, concentration, and focus. Many who train regularly, accept these advantages as the norm. By producing various chemical changes in the brain, getting fit can produce a euphoric mental state, similar to that caused by some drugs. This experience can foster further activity and the desire to maintain fitness.

Many active families encourage their children to be active; sloth-ful ones might not. I suspect the inclination to be active or lazy, is mostly inherited.

The Yekuana tribe, living in the Venezuelan rain forest, view wake-fulness and sleep as equally valuable. They sometimes wake at night to share a joke, then return to sleep, with no feeling of any annoyance. Jean Liedloff, in her book *The Continuum Concept* (1975), describes how the Yekuana respect laziness (as viewed through western eyes) and activity, as being innate. The lazy are ac-cepted for what they are, while the inherently active, simply get on with mutually worthwhile activities. It is their acceptance of such differences that distinguishes their tribal attitudes and behaviour from modern western ones.

Cognitive Behavioural Therapy (CBT)

The primary focus of CBT (or CBT-i for insomnia) is to address the factors causing chronic insomnia. Some are predisposing ones, like emotional reactivity to situations. Then there are *precipitating factors,* like stressful life events. It is also important to discover *perpetuating factors*, like unacceptable living and work conditions; especially those that have created fears about future security and relationships.

To be effective, CBT may take up to five or six sessions. Each session will have a specific agenda, like evaluation, developing a treatment plan, intervention, checking adherence, and considering any relapses. The objective is to promote the natural sleep drive.

One technique used is sleep restriction. The aim is to restrict any extended time in bed – time taken to compensate for poor sleep. By prescribing a sleep schedule, sleep induction can get faster, with less time spent awake at night.

Part of the therapy is to remove stimuli that might disturb sleep induction: watching TV, reading, listening to the radio or scrolling through social media. It directs subjects to go to bed only when sleepy, and to get up rather than lie awake. It can involve introducing consistent wake-up times, with no naps.

Cognitive therapy attempts to create realistic expectations for sleep and tries to dispel any misguided thoughts preventing it. Maladaptive thoughts and reactions are examined, and replaced with realistic thoughts, explanations and expectations. The process is one of guided discovery. Exercise is also promoted, with alcohol and caffeine use discouraged.

CBT can reduce insomnia related symptoms by 50% to 80% (Morin, C.M. 1994, and 2009), with benefits that appear to be stable. Consistent improvement in daytime executive functioning is less certain. Because CBTi is at least as effective as pharmacological interventions, it is now recommended as the first-line treatment for insomnia (American College of Physicians).

Life Training

Roy Whitten developed methods that allow better self-understanding; methods that allow less energy to be spent, dealing with life issues. In particular, his training helps to identify reactionary behaviour – especially that which manifests as a personal drama. His methods require the self-questioning of beliefs, fears, judgements, expectations, and decisions. The aim is to achieve an understanding of how these might interfere with a purposeful, open, loving way of life.

This contrasts with an opposing, much older view of self-knowledge:

> *Ich kenne mich auch nicht, und Gott soll mich auch davor behuten!*

> *(I do not know myself, and God forbid that I should!)*

Johann Wolfgang
von Goethe (1739-1832).

For some, coming to know themselves might be a painful, even unbearable experience. Even when some personal insight is essential for their health, some patients will get stuck or fail to improve.

I used the principle of self-understanding in my book on weight loss (*Who Loses Wins*). There I describe what I learned from hundreds of overweight people. I named what I found – the 'Fat Mentality' (as opposed to a 'Fit Mentality'). While craving just one more cream cake (having given them up for ten days), their inner voice might say:

> *"Go on, have another one. You deserve it. You've worked so hard this week. You can handle just one more cake. Give them up next week, when things feel easier. You know it makes sense. You're not going to live forever anyway."*

This *'poor little me'* drama will undermine personal discipline. Undermining self-discipline is our ego trying to delay the achievement of self-esteem. If we act on this inner voice, we lose personal integrity. We might then give in and eat more cakes, regardless of the inevitable weight-gain. Many overweight people offered cakes while on a diet, will rationalise their lack of discipline. They are easily convinced that refusing hospitality is bad behaviour.

> *Prof. Kevin Gournay and Dr Richard Elliot of Oxford University's School of Management, found that one in ten compulsive shoppers, shop for revenge. Many are resentful about being ignored or are unhappy in their marriage, perhaps because their professional husband is always too busy working to pay them enough attention.*

> *Julie, a doctor's wife from the Midlands, said: "If I think I am being done out of weekend trips away because my husband is a self-confessed workaholic, shopping is a way of getting back at him."*

> *It is now thought of as a new middle-class disease, and as a 'revenge-control paradox'. When they are shopping, the person feels in control at a time when they are least in control.*

London Times. 16.12.96.

Using discipline, heightened awareness, and a step by step analytical process to examine our mental processes, it is sometimes possible to resolve long-held resentments, and to stop inappropriate responses to life events.

Life training can enable people to gain personal mastery in an ever-changing, challenging world. As far as human thought and feeling are concerned, the world is much the same as that contemplated by Plato, Marcus Aurelius, Shakespeare and Dickens. Events such as bereavement, love, marriage, birth, death, joy, and the agony and ecstasy of relationships, have all remained unchanged.

Mastery over our thoughts and feelings has always been thought desirable. What is new is the need to respond rapidly to a fast-changing external world, with its seductive technology, bent on making travel more rapid and communication ever faster. The basis for it all – greater profits. The rapidity of change creates as many problems as it solves, but that too is good for business. While all these changes are external to our being, the essence of our being remains unchanged.

The Journey

The conscious mind is often driven by doubt, guilt, and criticism, but these are just a few of the factors that give some a bad time. Somewhere along the way, during our formative years, we all learn to protect ourselves from pain; either by avoidance or reconnaissance. We doubt and distrust, in order to avoid further hurt. Instead of protecting us, our 'mind talk' discussions can make us miserable, often helping to perpetuate misunderstanding or resentment. Most of us can keep these voices anchored to reality, but those who cannot, might make their life impossible to bare. Constant self-analysis, self-criticism, suspicion, and doubt will drain vitality. As a result of being consumed by conscious deliberation, we risk failing to discover our true motives and feelings.

'The Journey' is another, complex analytic process, created by Brandon Bays from her personal experience. By breaking through our conscious barriers, we might be able to contact the feelings and emotions that lie beneath. The objective is to encounter the source – going down through various layers of feeling – to that state of mind that lies beneath any anger, pain, loss, depression or abandonment.

Once we arrive at this state of mind, one might be able to talk directly to the other players in our personal life drama, both as an adult and child. The ultimate purpose of the process is to understand and forgive them. Through such revelation and acceptance, some are relieved of their panic, depression, fear, and any anger previously inflicted upon them.

Along with such self-analytic learning methods, I would advocate the same as happens in France: the inclusion of philosophy as a key subject for study by all pupils at school. It can provide them with a framework for both religious and speculative thought. Many could benefit from a little French *esprit critique*. The publication of Jostein Gaarder's book, Sophie's World in 1991, advocates this important step. The book was originally bought by adolescents, searching for meaning in their lives.

Chapter Twenty

Some Case Histories

Bill J.

Bill is a business associate of mine. He has been tired all the time and gets breathless when he lays flat. He is now in his 50s and takes medication for high blood pressure. He had a small stroke in the past which affected his speech transiently. He was also said to have had a small heart attack, along with atrial fibrillation – an irregular heart beat that still persists. His medication relates to his cardiac condition only. He has been given nothing to aid sleep or relaxation. He is worried about having repeated strokes, heart attacks and perhaps heart failure, despite being on full preventative medication.

All his life, Bill has been nervous person. He has undertaken CBT and seen other therapists but recently he has become fearful and panicky again; so much so, he has been unable to travel on occasions, overwhelmed by anxiety. He refuses to drive on motorways in case he has a panic attack. He is also too frightened to fly, so some holidays during which he might relax are denied him.

Bill has always been physically fit and even now does regular weight training and some boxing practice – without getting breathless – a fact incompatible with a diagnosis of heart failure.

His life over the last few years has been clouded by constant business worry – an apartment building project went well to start with, but when sales slumped, the bank demanded their loan money back. For the last few years, these concerns have combined with worry about his wife. She has now been fighting lung cancer for several years.

He needs a siesta every afternoon - because he simply can't keep awake. At night he wakes worrying about his many problems - real and conjectured. So far, nobody has suggested night sedation to help him sleep or a tranquilliser for daytime use – his doctors refuse to prescribe them in case he gets addicted.

What he needs most is relief from fear and anxiety. Reassurance from a heart echocardiogram done recently, found him to have normal heart functioning.

Knowing this, helped to reassure him, but alone was not enough to allay his anxiety.

He needs refreshing sleep at night and a short form of sleep therapy would be most appropriate. The lesser alternative would be to leave him to manage his own sleep. An appropriate antidepressant or occasion diazepam at night would help or he could attend a sleep or cognitive therapist.

Cognitive therapy, combined with a drug like diazepam 2mgs for occasional daytime use – available in his pocket should he need it as an emergency – would help him greatly. It could certainly help him cope with his low-quality existence; potentially, a risk much higher than benzodiazepine addiction. No UK GP is sanctioned to prescribe long-term diazepam for him, even though his need is appreciable and the risk minimal in the hands of an attentive physician.

Fortunately, relief from his business problems is not far away. Knowing that he has adequate heart functioning, with all the preventative medication he needs, means that his prognosis could soon improve.

Mrs C.

I once admitted a 62-year-old woman to Loughton Clinic (my own medical nursing home at the time) with resistant hypertension. With her husband, she managed a small, family-run manufacturing company. Her claim was that her role required her to work six days every week. She regarded her role as 'essential'. Without her presence, she thought the company might not survive.

A different picture emerged from her husband. He had founded the company twenty-years before. When I discussed her 'essential status' with him, he smiled. He said they had plenty of staff to fulfil her role. Instead, he thought of her as interfering, rather than essential. She had, in fact, refused to retire many times, despite increasing tiredness, fatigue, irritability, and resistant hypertension. Pride and her need for self-esteem, made her continue.

The solution I suggested was that she should retire on medical grounds. This would preserve her dignity and could reduce the risk of her having a stroke, given her resistant hypertension (something also suffered by her mother). She agreed and retired with her self-esteem intact. On follow-up, her hypertension became easier to manage on much less medication.

Kathy's Case

Although originally referred for palpitations, I had been treating Kathy for long-term debility and neuralgia. She needed narcotics to control her pain. She had had breast cancer cured some fifteen years before. She then had early vaginal cancer diagnosed and removed with total success. My colleague, Sunit Ghatak did the surgery. Like myself, he also practised preventative medicine as a mission. I was aware that she was not too happy in her marriage and had for many years lived in a compromised state with her husband. In any case, she acknowledged him as a good man, even though not her ideal partner.

After knowing her for many years she unexpectedly said: "I suppose you would like to know what's really wrong with me?" She had a resigned look in her eye, as if to say, I think, after all these years, you deserve to know my secret.

I sat back and awaited her explanation. I had always wondered what the root cause of her ongoing debility might be. She then told me:

"When I was 23-years old, I fell hopelessly in love with a naval officer - a second lieutenant. We had a won-

derful time together. He seemed to be in love with me, but something indefinable was wrong. Anyway, to cut a long story short, he arrived at my home one day. He was dressed in his white, official tropical uniform. He announced that he was about to depart on a long tour of duty. He also told me, he had something special to tell me – that he was gay and thought it best if we didn't see one another again. This broke my heart, even though I fully understood. Since then, every time the telephone rang or there was a knock at the door, I hoped it might be him. If he did turn up and ask me to leave with him, I would – without a second thought."

She was living a dream with a broken heart. No wonder she was tired all the time. I was privileged to be the only person she had told about this in 45-years. Not even her husband knew – or did he?

Whether a secret is relevant or not, is a matter of judgement. Usually the revelation fills a gap in the narrative. To know it, can give one a sense of completeness and satisfaction – like finding a missing jigsaw puzzle piece. Quite often, one can sense something missing – but not know what it is. There is an interesting thing about secrets. Once revealed, most of them seem quite ordinary and unexciting, although, solving a mystery is always satisfying.

One implication for physicians is the need to provide an appropriate amount of time for each consultation. With patient continuity, a doctor can do better. Admittedly, this is no work for technocrats. It could follow that medical students, chosen primarily for their technological excellence, might lack enough natural empathy and communication skill to do the job. Given that most medical problems are simple, some students will have been sold a bad deal.

Choosing scientists to practise simple uncomplicated medicine, has created many disillusioned doctors. For most doctors, unlike the few who are locked away in the ivory towers of tertiary teaching hospitals, complicated and scientifically challenging cases will be few and far between. Every day, the majority of experienced doctors deal mostly with the common and unchallenging problems of humanity.

Many doctors are right to declare having no interest in psychiatry or psychosomatic and psycho-social matters. If capable, they can choose to specialise only in mechanistic disease processes. But therein lies a numbers problem. How many doctors should we allow to deviate from the commonest needs of patients?

Intractable Angina?

Joe was a long-term cardiac patient of mine; a 65-year-old widower. He had everything in life he wanted, except a partner. His wife had died from leukaemia some years earlier. His regular gardener had fallen ill and a young woman, forty-years his junior, had replaced him. They fell in love at first sight; not something either of them had expected.

He had sought my clinical advice many times over several decades, and we had a close doctor patient relationship. His last consultation concerned his angina. It was stable but occurring regularly on exercise. This time, he only sought my pastoral advice, given all I knew all about his family, personal circumstances and medical condition.

> *His question was: 'What should I do about this un-*
> *expected new relationship?' I replied with a rhetori-*
> *cal question: 'What have you got to lose?' With this he*
> *agreed. Not only had it relieved his bereavement and*
> *loneliness, it had unexpectedly improved his angina.*

> *Following a CABG many years before, we later failed*
> *to place a stent in Joe's extensively narrowed, distal*
> *anterior descending coronary artery bypass graft. I told*
> *him then, we could do no more for him other than*
> *try different medications. It was a surprise to observe,*
> *therefore, how his new relationship had improved his*
> *exercise tolerance.*

Joe's arteries could not have changed much over the short course of his new relationship, so how might his improvement be explained? Could it be that happiness, by reducing his catecholamine drive and myocardial oxygen demand, raised his angina-free exercise threshold? It is certainly worthy of some thought and further research. It is interesting to recall that Heberden's original description of chest tightness (angina), included emotion as a provocation factor.

There is another snippet of cardiovascular research history relating emotion to the heart. It has mostly escaped notice, but I found it while reading a translation of William Harvey's book, made famous after he described the circulation of blood (*de Motu Cordis*, 1628). Harvey's original interest was the connection between human emotion and the pulse rate, not just the circulation of the blood. After all his research, he failed to find any connection. This was because the autonomic nervous system, connecting the brain to the heart, had yet to be discovered. That would have to wait until the 19th century and the work of many, including Claude Bernard, A.V. Waller, and the Weber brothers. It was J.N. Langley FRS, who in 1901, coined the phrase 'autonomic nervous system' (Langley J. Observations on the physiological action of extracts of the supra-renal bodies. *J. Physiol. 1901; 27:237-256*).

Joanne's Story

I was once asked in passing, by a female office colleague of mine, about the rash she had on her hands. Her skin was rough, sore, and itchy – a common skin complaint called cheiropompholyx (something like eczema). This is well known to occur under stressful circumstances, especially those sufficient to disturb sleep and composure. Treatment mostly includes steroid creams but should also include an understanding of its development from a psycho-social point of view. She had tried steroid creams, given by a dermatologist, but they had only helped a little.

I briefly suggested a possible mechanism – the presence of some ongoing, stressing factor. What happened next, came as a surprise. This highly controlled, 'in-charge' office manager, burst into tears – standing at my desk, in the middle of an open office full of working colleagues.

The cause, I was later to find, related to a recent relationship she had. Against her better judgement, she

DR DAVID H. DIGHTON

had subjected herself to her boyfriend's sadistic sexual control. She felt forced, by his strong disapproving tendency, to sit naked while he ate his meals. Otherwise, he often made her stand naked at a window, enjoying her discomfort; knowing that strangers might see her and lust after her. There was more of his behaviour to be revealed (now called gas-lighting activity). While in a relationship with her, he had seduced her best friend, and then told her all about it. She finally dumped him. That was six weeks before our impromptu consultation.

Her control and self-respect had been suppressed for the sake of maintaining love. Her boyfriend had somehow persuaded her that his behaviour was 'perfectly normal' (which it is for sadomasochists). She subsequently found out that her boyfriend had had two previous girlfriends, both of whom had rejected him for similar reasons. His good looks, charm and persuasiveness, had seduced all of them into accepting his abuse.

Cheiropompholyx resulted from her relationship loss, from discovering duplicity, a previous liability to eczema as child, and her increasing disillusionment and discomfort with oppression. A steroid cream alone, was hardly going to effect a cure.

Joanne had already sought the advice of a dermatologist, pharmacist, an herbalist, an acupuncturist, and a homeopath, but had been embarrassed to tell them the full story – not that she had connected the two together.

Without a complete understanding of her condition, I would have risked the same therapeutic dance routine as her dermatologist – suggesting one dermatological cream after another, all of which would fail her.

It has now become a great strength of alternative or complementary therapists, that they give time enough to take a full personal history. They are often empathetic, and happy to take up the challenges discarded by medical professionals. In the absence of scientific plausibility, the confidence inspired by their understanding and sympathetic approach, can help patients more.

Joanne was ready for catharsis. Such revealing moments can be among the most special any doctor witnesses. It has physical equivalents, like the relief brought about by incising a painful abscess or the removal of a troublesome tooth.

If physicians delegate every consideration of their patient's emotional state to psychologists, psychiatrists and counsellors (GMC good practice advocates referrals only to certificated experts), many more mistakes will occur. A collegiate, interdisciplinary approach, works best for patients.

Eileen's Brush with the Law

Eileen and Dennis had been driving all day long, when at 4 o'clock one dark winter afternoon, they found their headlights defective; working only on full beam. A mechanic advised them to stick tape over the main beam to avoid blinding other motorists.

They went home, washed and changed and went out to a restaurant, driving the same car. They could easily have walked or taken a taxi but instead decided to drive.

Eileen, had a problem with high blood pressure, made worse by the 'white coat syndrome' – entering a doctor's consulting room usually increased her blood pressure. During the meal, she drank one and a half glasses of wine, but felt OK to drive. She had only been driving a few minutes when she was stopped by the police for defective headlights. She was given a roadside breath test which she failed. Since she failed on a second try, she was arrested, and taken to the police station, where five times she proved incapable of performing a blowing test correctly. She was then charged with failure to provide a specimen but was not offered a blood or urine test. Unfortunately, she omitted to advise the police that she had an asthmatic breathing problem. The police assumed that her failure to perform the tests was intentional.

In Court, I gave medical evidence based on an evaluation of her anxiety, using a standard questionnaire. Her neuroticism test results, showed her to have a high hysteria and perfectionism score – she was the sort of person who might react adversely to stressful, authoritarian situations, perhaps with hypertension and hyperventilation.

In court, the Magistrate told her it was serious not to provide an adequate specimen; more than to have a raised blood alcohol level. Despite being her first o-ffence, and despite the fact that she testified to having little more than one glass of wine, she was banned from driving for eighteen months and fined £750!

The indignation and feeling of injustice she felt, could easily have given her a stroke, with her blood systolic pressure often exceeding 200mms of mercury! Her ar-rest could not have happened at a worse time. She was experiencing some financial difficulties and was now unable to use her car. Her main concern was the con-tinuing care of her elderly parents. As their sole carer, they depended on her for shopping. They also enjoyed occasional trips together.

At the very least, the way she had been dealt with appeared to be insensitive and unappreciative of the wider social and medical aspects of her case. She came to believe it was the intention of the law to punish people, even before being brought to Court and being found guilty. She was perplexed by the absence of com-mon sense, and the complete absence of applied wisdom in defining an appropriate punishment. Legal process-es, however, are not obliged to demonstrate either.

Lilian's Chest Pain

Lilian had pains in her chest at rest. She had angina – heart pain (actually, tightness rather than pain), accompanied sometimes by difficulty in breathing while walking. Because this was worse on exercise, I decided to image her coronary (heart) arteries. This is done by injecting dye through a small catheter. Fortunately for her, her arteries were entirely normal – there were no narrowed areas restricting blood flow. This represented a mystery, since angina is mostly caused by poor blood flow through at least one narrowed coronary artery. How could she have classical angina of effort and no arterial narrowing?

To help her, I prescribed an adrenaline blocking drug (beta-blocker), hoping it would reduce the effects of any anxiety on her heart function. She gave me no clue at the time, why she might be anxious and tense, but the medication helped.

Some months later, it came to my notice that her daughter had marriage difficulties and was seeing a counsellor. She and her husband later separated. When I next saw Lilian with worsening discomfort, I asked her about any stress she might be experiencing. She thought not, although, after a brief listing of all her problems and a description of her situation, we agreed that she was living a stress-laden existence.

There were three areas in her life that drew on her coping ability. First, she and her husband were both upset by their daughter's marital separation; they saw the failure as partly theirs. Had they not let her marry too early? Because their daughter and son-in-law wanted to live apart, and because their son-in-law was unhappy living in the matrimonial home, Lilian agreed to have him live with her. Meanwhile, their daughter stayed in their marital home. Their son-in-law worked with her husband, so this was convenient for a while. That was until he made it known that he was seeing someone else!

Apart from the worry of her daughter's separation, Lilian now had mixed feelings about her son-in-law; tolerating his presence, his tales of a new romance represented disloyalty to her daughter. Not only was this keeping her awake at night, her tennis elbow and shoulder pain were also. Her chance of getting replenishing sleep was minimal.

Lilian's case posed a number of important questions. How could any heart tablet help her, given her background family stresses? Why do so few admit they are stressed, even when they have serious symptoms?

One medico-political point. Why do doctors persist in offering only 10-15-minute medical consultations – too short to reveal the pertinent details in a case like this? Doctors are thus encouraging their own failure when trying to diagnose, treat, and manage complicated patients appropriately. They can add another failure to this – sometimes trying to chase a cure – trying one drug after the other, while ignoring the underlying, albeit time-consuming, analysis of any possible psycho-social problems. Their reply to this is easily anticipated – they are not paid to be counsellors or social workers and also have too little time.

Afterword

"In the old days, you know, you were better off because nowadays, they (doctors) are all specialists, and getting better and better at less and less".

Kenneth Williams. Comedian. *You Tube: On his spastic colon. Aspel & Co. LWT. 1987.*

Unless a patient has a clear cut, disease-related cause, solving their fatigue conundrum has become more difficult for several reasons - most of them political.

During my working life of over five decades, I witnessed the UK medical profession becoming less engaged with patients and resigned to be managed by bureaucrats. Both have caused a decline in patient care; especially with the management of patients presenting with tiredness, fatigue and exhaustion – all of which can take more time than doctors are prepared to allow – abrogating the ancient, 'patient first' directive. Perhaps this explains why "The British public are deeply unhappy with the National Health Service – just 1 in 5 people (21%) in 2024 said they were satisfied with the way the NHS runs' (published by the Nuffield Trust and The

King's Fund. April 2025). This is a drop of 39% in satisfaction compared to before the pandemic. In 2024, only 63.4% had trust and confidence in UK GPs, whereas the figure was 80.2% for hospital doctors. (Nuffield Trust. Quality Watch. 19/12/2024).

To achieve long-term success with patients, doctors must regain an interest in their patient's lives, not just in their symptoms, signs and investigation findings. Doctors who base their medical practice on technology alone, reduce their chances of understanding the demise of human beings, whose basic components of mind, body, and soul, integrate to form one whole, sentient functioning being. In my private-only practise, I specialised in the diagnosis and management of difficult clinical cases – those who had been failed by the NHS. As a result, I accumulated 20,000 patients over a fifty-year period. Dr. Peter Nixon once called such patients, refugees from the health service.

Those doctors dealing with one-off accident cases, bone fractures and tumour removal as their primary function, can easily avoid in-depth patient consideration. They can easily retain anonymity. Their relationship to patients can remain limited to the functional. Should they wish, those who do not manage patients long-term, can try to avoid personal involvement, although this will rarely contribute to successful patient management.

Although doctors can easily succeed in identifying and controlling disease, this will hardly satisfy every fatigued patient. Doctors with a detached and anonymous attitude, who for millennia had to satisfy their patients in order to make a living, would fail to survive in private practice.

Are we recruiting doctors without a vocation to care for patients? Is UK medical practice losing its traditional caring role to alternative practitioners, many of whom wish to appraise the whole person? To pursue the type of medicine I learned from Dr. Peter Nixon, one would have to recruit not only cardiologists capable of implanting pacemakers, and passing technical examinations, but those with a talent for human understanding.

To solve their problem of tiredness, fatigue and exhaustion, it is essential for patients to play their part; to examine their own lives: their successes, failures and *raison d'être*. To improve their outlook, many will need some conviction to change, altering course to prevent further ill-health and medical catastrophe. Half-hearted conviction won't do. Some patients need a complete change of heart and mind, but that can happen only after gaining an understanding of just how they 'got their life wrong', before suffering illness. Only by truly admitting their mistakes and learning new strategies, will some be able to avoid further illness. Apart from asking doctors to help, they must come to know what part anxiety, obsession, fear, anger and chronic resentment might have played in causing their tiredness, fatigue and exhaustion. They must realise what they might have lost through induced blindness to the benefits of gratitude, magnanimity, acceptance, tolerance, forgiveness and failure – to better understand those they see as opponents.

Personal energy management is not only important to quality of life, but in some cases, to life and death. Too dramatic? Not from where I stood most of my life as a doctor! This is why it has been my mission to complete this book. Once a doctor, always a doctor – in my case my life's mission and vocation – with or without a licence to practise in the UK.

Glossary of Terms Used

Atherosclerosis: Cholesterol, calcified tissue and scarring, building up in the interior of arteries. It occurs in patches or plaques. When these rupture they attract clot, possibly blocking the artery.

Arteriosclerosis: Thickening of the middle, muscular layer of small arteries (arterioles). Causes some arterial narrowing – increased resistance to flow – and high blood pressure when it develops beyond normal (muscle hypertrophy).

EEG: Electroencephalogram. Recordings of brain activity.

Heart Attack: Damage of heart muscle cause by an arterial occlusion.

Insomnia: Difficulty with getting to sleep, maintaining sleep or quality of sleep.

Ions: Charged atoms. Sodium, potassium, calcium, chloride and magnesium are they common ones.

Neurones (neural, neuronal): Brain nerve cells.

REM: Rapid Eye-Movement Sleep occurs at the same time as dreaming.

Slow-Wave Sleep: Deep non-dreaming sleep with slow brain waves on EEG. Thought to be when tiredness is refreshed.

Stroke: Usually refers to brain damage from local haemorrhage, local clot formation or a small clot travelling to a brain artery (embolus), from somewhere else in the body (heart valve or neck arteries). Associated with more permanent loss of speech, limb paralysis etc.

T.I.A.: Transient Ischaemic Attack (in the brain). Sometimes referred to as a mini-stroke. Caused by either a small bleed or a small clot. Can be transiently associated with loss of speech, sight or limb paralysis.

Appendix 1

We all harbour biases. Since Kahneman and Tversky published their original work, others have added more (including my own. See later).

1. **Ambiguity Bias:** ambiguous information diminishes the probability of a correct decision.

2. **Anchoring (or Focussing) Bias:** becoming fixated by one bit of information. It can lead us astray. The diagnostician's curse is paying too much attention to the wrong clues.

3. **Attribution Error Bias:** inductive reasoning: my grandfather is bald, therefore, all grandfathers are bald.

4. **Automation Bias:** the belief that a computer / processing machine, or algorithm, is likely to be correct (an error revealed in 2020: 'A' level grade results were wrongly 'processed' by a standardising algorithm).

5. **Availability Bias:** giving preference to what is easily accessible.

6. **Availability Cascade Bias:** repeat something often enough, and it will seem true.

7.   **Backfire Bias:** after dismissive evidence for a theory becomes known, belief in the theory may strengthen.

8.   **Bandwagon Bias:** the tendency to believe the majority knows best.

9.   **Barnum (or Forer) Bias:** the tendency to overestimate the value of one's individuality as unique.

10. **Belief Bias:** the strength of an argument increases with the believability of its conclusion, even when the conclusion came from a series of doubtful assumptions. Doctors invested in their clinical opinion may see no need to seek confirmatory evidence. Arrogance has no place in the management of complicated, complex, or flummoxing clinical cases.

11. **Berkson's Paradox:** believing a statistical conclusion while ignoring the important conditionals applied.

12. **Blind-Spot Bias:** seeing oneself as less biased than others.

13. **Choice Support Bias:** seeing our choices as better than they are.

14. **Chronology Bias:** current information is more valid than older information.

15. **Cluster Illusion Bias:** over-rating the significance of clusters in data sets. When playing roulette, the belief that an unusually long run of REDs (rather than BLACKs), will continue.

16. **Confirmation Bias:** recognising only those examples that prove our point.

17. **Congruence Bias:** testing for only those diseases we think are likely.

18. **Conjunction Bias:** the 'out of the ordinary' is more likely than the ordinary.

19. **Conservatism Bias:** unwillingness to revise a view, despite fresh evidence.

20. **Control Bias:** the over-estimation of the control we have in various situations.

21. **Correlation Bias:** over-estimating the connectivity of facts and events.

22. **Courtesy Bias:** giving a socially acceptable version of the truth, rather than the actual truth (more common in some cultures than others).

23. **Curse of Knowledge Bias:** the tendency of knowledge-able people to not appreciate the thinking of those less educated.

24. **Declination Bias:** things ain't what they used to be. A tendency to view the past as more favourable.

25. **Decoy Bias:** a tough choice between A and B is easier if one chooses C.

26. **Distinction Bias:** A & B viewed together, seem less different from A & B viewed separately.

27. **Dunning Krüger Bias:** the unskilled tend to overate their ability; the skilled underrate their ability.

28. **Duration Bias:** the tendency to underrate the time something will last.

29. **Empathy Gap Bias:** a tendency to offer an inappropriate level of empathy (too little or a too much). Can lead to under-treating pain, and failing to recognise distress (or the reverse). *(Loewen-*

stein, G. Health Psychology (2005). *Hot-Cold empathy gaps and medical decision making).*

30. **Exposure Bias:** favouring what we are used to.

31. **Extrapolation Bias:** believing that trends will continue uninterrupted.

32. **Fading Bias:** the tendency to forget unpleasant events and remember only the pleasing ones.

33. **Flat-pack Bias:** while awaiting construction, we think structures are better than they are.

34. **Framing Bias:** belief follows the excellence of the presentation, rather than the value of the evidence.

35. **Frequency Illusion Bias:** once we have learned an unfamiliar word, it appears everywhere.

36. **Functional Fixity Bias:** the tendency to follow 'tried and tested' functions, and not to look for new ones.

37. **Gambler's Fallacy Bias:** the pattern of past events will reliably predict future events.

38. **Gap Bias:** with both ends of a spectrum recognised, what lies between (in the gap) gets dismissed.

39. **Google Bias:** Internet facts are easy to find and easily forgotten.

40. **Hindsight Bias:** 'I could have told you that would happen!' Belief in our ability to predict the future using our experience of past events.

41. **Hot Hand Bias:** an exemplary track record predicts winning in the future.

42. **Information Bias:** the more data, the more likely are we to make a significant discovery.

43. **Instrument Bias:** if all we have is a hammer, everything looks like a nail.

44. **Jess's Bias (added 2025):** a doctor who fails to except the possibility of a young person having cancer

45. **Loss Aversion Bias:** the value of something lost is greater than something gained.

46. **Naïve Cynicism Bias:** others are more egocentric than us.

47. **Naïve Realism Bias:** I alone can see things the way they really are – others cannot.

48. **Negativity Bias:** weighing losses more heavily than gains.

49. **Neglecting Probability Bias:** disregarding probability in uncertain situations.

50. **Normalising Bias:** refusing to recognise potential risks until they happen.

51. **Observer Expectancy Bias**: to see only what one expects to see.

52. **Omission Bias**: harmful actions are worse than harmful omissions.

53. **Optimism Bias**: a cup is half full, not half empty.

54. **Ostrich Bias**: ignoring the obvious.

55. **Outcome Bias**: the judgement was wise if the outcome was good.

56. **Overconfidence Bias**: of the 99% who are sure, only 40% are correct.

57. **Pareidolia Bias**: seeing patterns that are not there: A face on the moon.

58. **Progress Bias**: all progress leads to a better place (Utopia, perhaps?).

59. **Pro-innovation Bias:** new ideas are better than old ideas.

60. **Projection Bias:** the tendency to believe in projections and models.

61. **Pseudo-Certainty Bias:** taking more risks when the outlook is bad; taking fewer risks when the outlook is rosy.

62. **Reactance Bias:** the urge to do the opposite.

63. **Reactive Devaluation Bias:** to oppose anything suggested by an opponent.

64. **Retrospection Bias:** the past *was* rosier.

65. **Rhyming Bias:** giving credence to rhymes: 'If the gloves don't fit, you must acquit.'

66. **Risk Compensation Bias (Pelzman Effect):** the greater the perceived safety, the greater the risks taken.

67. **Selective Perception Bias:** seeing only what one wants to see.

68. **Self-Serving Bias:** feeling more responsible for success than failure.

69. **Semmelweis Bias:** rejecting the evidence that does not fit our paradigm.

70. **Social Compensation Bias:** choose only non-competitors to associate with.

71. **Social Desirability Bias:** the over-estimation of our social attributes and their acceptability.

72. **Spotlight Bias:** the need to be in the spotlight, or to avoid it.

73. **Status Quo Bias:** we are better as we are.

74. **Stereotyping Bias:** the assumption of group characteristics.

75. **Subjective Validation Bias:** the tendency to disbelieve what others believe.

76. **Survivorship Bias:** the virtue of survivors is greater than non-survivors.

77. **Time Saving Bias:** over-rating the time saved by speeding.

78. **Third Party Bias:** media messages influence others more than us.

79. **Trait Ascription Bias:** I am less predictable than others.

80. **Transparency Bias:** overestimating our insight into others.

81. **Travis Effect Bias:** the present is more credible than the past (see bias '56').

82. **Parkinson's Law (Bias):** the tendency to overvalue the importance of the trivial.

83. **Von Restoff Bias:** what stands out is better remembered.

84. **Weber-Fechner Bias:** wrongly valuing minor differences in large quantities.

85. **Zeigarnik Bias:** the incomplete is better remembered than the complete.

86. **Zero-Bias:** a preference to reduce quantities to zero.

87. **Zero Sum Bias:** the tendency to see actions as zero-sum: gains = loses.

Some of my own:

1.   **Anecdotal bias:** Belief in personal observation.

2.   **Assumption bias:** all my assumptions are valid.

3.   **Belief Transference bias:** *everyone* looks forward to a special event (Royal Wedding, etc).

4.   **Bunker Bias:** it is never safe to expose our ideas to others.

5.   **Consensus Bias:** committees make the best decisions.

6.   **Cultural Bias:** my culture is best (see Ex-Pat bias).

7.   **Dawkins' Bias:** the scientific method alone can reveal the truth.

8.   **Democracy Bias:** decisions are best made by public consensus.

9.   **Drug Bias:** life is sh*t, so life must be better on drugs.

10. **Epicurean Bias:** without Michelin starred restaurants, life would not be worth living.

11. **Equality Bias:** the notion that all humans are equal in ability and performance (or would be if they had equal opportunity).

12. Ex-Pat Bias: ex-pat culture is better than the local culture.

13. Fat & Carb Bias: all foods containing fat and carbs are bad for our health.

14. Fresh Air Bias: the secret of health and happiness lies in breathing fresh air.

15. Geography Bias: Things are better here than there or *vice versa*.

16. God Bias: all you need is to trust God (or someone famous).

17. Healthy Food Bias: health and the prevention of disease are diet dependent.

18. Hedonism Bias: if it isn't fun, what's the point?

19. Iceberg Bias: small clues lead to large discoveries.

20. Inamorata Bias: an inability to see those we love as they really are.

21. Incomprehensible Bias: that which is incomprehensible is too clever to be wrong.

22. Intervention Bias: Positive – doing something is better than doing nothing. **Negative** – doing nothing is better than doing something.

23. Mañana Bias: waiting until tomorrow will work well.

24. Manipulator Bias: believing yourself clever enough to get whatever you want from others.

25. NHS Bias: the belief that the NHS is a world-class medical service.

26. Overload Bias: more must be better than less.

27. **Peasant Bias:** Inferior breeding causes failure.

28. **Peter Pan Bias:** I appear younger than others of my age.

29. **Philistine Bias:** life is too short for intellectual pursuits. The price of something is more important than its wider value.

30. **Posthumous Bias:** the dead were wiser than us.

31. **Print (Publishing) Bias:** if it's in print, it must be true, and worth knowing.

32. **Profit Bias:** working without profit is a waste of time.

33. **Royalty Bias:** only superior breeding leads to success.

34. **Self-Esteem Bias:** only activities which bring self-esteem are worthwhile.

35. **Rumsfeld Bias:** many unimagined truths are yet to be discovered.

36. **Selfish Bias:** If it can't be mine, I'm not interested.

37. **Serendipity (Panglossian) Bias:** Everything will work out for the best in the end.

38. **Sports Bias:** The only way to be healthy, and live longer, is to exercise.

39. **Statistics Bias:** statistical truth is the only truth worth having.

40. **Status Bias:** only that which raises our status is worthwhile.

41. **Under-load Bias:** less is more.

42. **Unknown Information Bias:** what we don't know is more important than what we know.

43. Utopia Bias: only in Utopian can we achieve equality, fairness, and ultimate happiness.

44. Vanity Bias: only that which satisfies my vanity has value.

45. Wealth Bias: the only way to be happy is to get rich.

46. Wizard of Oz Bias: someone, somewhere, will know the answer.

47. Yonder Bias: better there than here.

Does all this mean that human impartiality is a myth?

Appendix 2

The object of this unverified, independent checklist, is to crudely assess liability to mental energy spending, and to help energy spending minimisation, for those who are constantly tired, fatigued or exhausted.

Several steps are essential:

- First, try to answer all the questions honestly.

- Second, get a close friend to answer them independently.

- Third, compare the two, and discuss the results between you.

The aim is to gain insight. There are no right or wrong answers.

1. **Your Personality:**

(a) Are you a dynamic character – always seeking to be involved, trying to be 'where it's all happening'?

(b) Do you like to be noticed; the centre of attention?

(c) Are you ambitious, with a 'nobody is going to stop me' attitude?

(d) Do you like to do things fast?

(e) Do you love challenges?

(f) Do you push your boundaries, trying things that might scare others?

(g) Would fishing be one of your preferred activities?

(h) Is lying on a beach something you love?

2. **Your Neuroticisms:**

(a) Are you often anxious about what is happening in your life?

(b) Are you worried about the future?

(c) Are you a perfectionist – or try to be?

(d) Is being 'on time', important to you?

(e) Do you like to check, and re-check things?

(f) Do you easily get emotional about things?

(g) Do you dislike heights, spiders, or being in enclosed spaces?

3. **Your Behaviour:**

(a) Are you always in a rush?

(b) Do you get anxious about arriving late?

(c) Are you known for your punctuality?

(d) Have you ever been late and missed an airplane or train?

(e) Would playing 18-holes of golf take too long for you to bear?

(f) Given the chance, will you always choose the quickest route?

(g) Are you an impatient person most of the time?

4. **Your Work & Life Circumstances:**

(a) Do you prefer to work under pressure?

(b) Do you dislike deadlines?

(c) Do you have debts that concern you?

(d) Are your work circumstances not to your liking?

(e) Would you change jobs if you could?

(f) Do you ever feel trapped, at home or at work?

(g) Do you feel that life is a struggle?

(h) Have you recently changed partners?

(i) Have you recently moved house?

(j) Do you often have vivid dreams (more than three times every week)?

(k) Can you sleep well, despite too much light or noise?

(l) Do you prefer living in the country rather than in town?

(m) Are you happy where you are living?

(n) Are you lonely a lot of the time?

(o) Are you tired by lunchtime?

(p) Are you tired by late afternoon.

(q) Are you too tired to consider any mental or physical work?

(r) Do you have more than one holiday every year?

(s) Do you earn more than you need for a comfortable life?

(t) Are you happy as an employee?

(u) Are you happy as an employer?

(v) Do you feel in control of your circumstances at home?

(w) Do you not feel in control of circumstances at work?

(x) Do you feel loved and supported by others?

(y) Are you living with any unsolved dilemmas?

5. Your Attitudes, Beliefs and Convictions:

(a) Do you observe religious practices?

(b) Do you have strong political views?

(c) Do you think the world is changing for the worst?

(d) Do you trust politicians?

(e) Do you have enjoyable family relationships?

(f) Do you have more than two close friends?

(g) Do you meet friends often?

(h) Have you experienced more than two broken relationships?

(i) Do you (or did you) get on well with your parents?

6. Your Abilities, Intelligence and Aptitude:

(a) Are you easily capable of the work you do?

(b) Are you bored by the work you do or the life you lead?

(c) Do you have a University degree?

(d) Is you job beneath your ability?

(e) Is your job beyond your ability?

(f) Would you like to change your life?

(g) Are you content with what you earn?

(h) Have you achieved some of your ambitions?

(i) Do you have time for hobbies?

(j) Do you regard yourself as intellectually superior to others?

(k) Have you ever felt downtrodden?

7. **Your abilities:**

(a) Are you a sports person?

(b) Do you sense the killer instinct when playing sports?

(c) Has winning always been important to you?

(d) Can you play a musical instrument sufficiently to entertain others?

(e) Can you speak another language other than your mother tongue?

(f) Do others regard you as a good communicator?

(g) Are you at ease in social settings.

8. **Sleep & Relaxation:**

(a) Do you sleep well?

(b) Do you wake more than once every night?

(c) Does stress keep you awake?

(d) Do you awake feeling tired?

(e) Are you able to siesta or nap when needed?

(f) Can you close your eyes and relax easily?

(g) Have you ever tried meditation during the day?

In answering these questions, focus on your own life equation – how much energy you are spending and how well you are minimising the energy you spend. I have made no attempt here to assess any disease processes; diagnosis is for your physician. However, a survey of 1000 of my patients found only 15 (1.5%) with a disease-related cause for their tiredness and fatigue.

Twenty key energy spending questions are: 1(a); 1(c); 1(d); 1(f); 2(a); 2(d); 2(e); 3(a); 3(b); 3(g); 4(a); 4(d); 4(f); 4(g); 4(h); 4(w) 4(y); 5(c); 6(b); 7(c).

Twenty key questions about minimising energy spending, to which the answer is YES, are: 1(g); 1(h); 4(k); 4(l); 4(m); 4(r); 4(s); 4(w); 5(e); 5(f); 5(i); 6(a); 6(g); 6(h); 6(i); 7(g); 8(a); 8(e); 8(f); 8(g).

How many apply to you (out of twenty)? Are there more 'YES's for energy spending than for energy minimising, or is it vice versa?

A person in healthy energy balance, will have more 'YES's among the energy minimising scores, than for energy spending. These are energy conservers. Those in balance, will have a similar number in each group. Those spending too much energy – the big energy spenders – will answer 'YES' to more of the energy spending questions.

References and Further Reading

'Assassins'. (1995). Film. Warner Brothers.

Ausserhofer, D., Piccoliori, G. et al. (2025). Sleep Problems and Sleep Quality in the general Adult population living in South Tyrol (Italy): A Cross-Sectional Survey Study. *Clocks. Sleep; 7 (2):23*

Balog, P., Falger. P., et al. (2017) Are vital exhaustion and depression independent risk factors for cardiovascular disease morbidity? Health Psychol.; 36, 740–748.

Beard, G. (1898). Neurasthenia or Nervous Exhaustion. *The Boston Medical and Surgical Journal 1869; 217-221.*

Bennet, Glin (1983). Beyond Endurance: Survival at the Extremes. *Martin Secker & Warburg.*

Berne, Eric (1964). The Games People Play. *Random House.*

Brunner,E., Smith,G., Marmot, M., Canner, R.L., Beksinska, M., O'Brien, John. (1996) Childhood social circumstances and psychosocial and behavioural factors as determinants of plasma fibrinogen. Lancet; **347**: 1008-13.

Buysse, D. J., et al. (1994) Clinical diagnoses in 216 insomnia patients using the International Classification of Sleep Disorders (ICSD), DSM-IV and ICD-10 categories: a report from the APA/NIMH DSM-IV Field Trial." *Sleep;* 17(7): 630-637.

Cartledge, S., Ryan, Joanne (editors).(1983) Sex and Love. *The Woman's Press Ltd.*

Chaganty, S.S., Abramov, D. et al. (2023, Aug 30). *Int J Cardiol Cardiovasc Risk Prev.*

Chamine, I., Atchley. R., Oken. B.S. (2018). Hypnosis intervention effects on sleep outcomes: a systematic review.*J Clin Sleep Med.;14(2): 271–283.*

Chuang-Tzu (2001). The Inner Chapters. *Hackett Classics.*

Chen, X., Wang. R., Zee. P., et al. (2015).Racial/ethnic differences in sleep disturbances: The Multi-Ethnic Study of Atherosclerosis (MESA). *Sleep; 38 (6): 877–888.*

Citri, A., Malenka, R.C. (2008). Synaptic Plasticity: Multiple Forms, Functions and Mechanisms. *Neuropsychopharmacology; 33: 18-41.*

Clare, Anthony. In the Psychiatrists Chair (1992). *William Heinemann.*

Kenneth Clark (1969): Civilisation. TV Series. *British Broadcasting Corporation.*

Kenneth Clark (1982) Civilisation. *Penguin Books .*

Dickens, Charles (1837). Pickwick Papers. *Chapman and Hall. London.*

Dighton. D.H. (2024). The Art and Science of Medical Practice. *MediCause.*

Dighton. D.H. (2024). Who Loses Wins. Winning Weight Loss Battles. A 'Fat Mentality' versus a 'Fit Mentality'. *MediCause. ISBN: 978-1-7385207-1-8*

Dighton. D.H. (2024). How to Become Heart-Smart. A User's Guide to Heart Health and Heart Disease Prevention. *MediCause.* ISBN: 978-1-7385207-0-1.

Dighton. D.H. (2024). Poems for Recycling Lives. *Medicause.* ISBN: 978-1-7385207-6-7.

Dighton, D.H. (2025). Tiredness, Chronic Fatigue and Exhaustion. Neurophysiology and Cardiovascular Risk. *MediCause.* Hardback ISBN: 978-1-0683597-3-6; e-book ISBN: 978-1-0683597-7-4.

Dighton, D.H. (2024). Doctors, Nurses and Patients. How to Survive Medical Practice. Medicause. ISBN:978-1-7385207-5-6.

Dixon, Norman F. (1976). The Psychology of Military Incompetence. *Jonathon Cape.*

Duranni, D., Idress, R., et al. (2022). Vitamin B6: A new approach to lowering anxiety, and depression? *Ann. Med. Surg. (Lond); 82:104663. doi: 10.1016/j.amsu.2022.104663).*

Edinger, J.D., Bonnet, M.H., Bootzin, R.R. (2024). Derivation of research diagnostic criteria for insomnia: report of an American Academy of Sleep Medicine Work Group. *Sleep.;27(8):1 567–1596.*

Edwards, Rex. (1964). A Coronary Case. *Faber & Faber.*

Elwert, F., and Christakis, N.A. (2008). The Effect of Widowhood on Mortality by the Causes of Death of Both Spouses. *Am. J. Public Health; 98(11): 2092-2098.*

ESC (European Society of Cardiology) Congress. August 2009. Heart Failure: More or Less Malignant than Cancer?

Eysenck.H.J., Nias.D.K.B. (1982). Astrology. Science or Superstition? *Morris Temple Smith.*

Faber, Adele, Elaine Mazlish, E. (2004): 'How to Talk So Kids Will Listen, and Listen So Kids Will Talk'. Avon Books.

Faber, P.L., Lehmann, D. et al. (2012). EEG source imaging during two Qigong meditations. *Cogn. Process: 13(3): 255-65).*

Feynman, Richard P. (1966). The Character of Physical Law. *Penguin Books.*

Ford, D.F., Kamerow,D.B.(1989). Epidemiology of sleep disorders and psychiatric disorders. JAMA.262:1479-84.

Friedman, M., Rosenman, R. (1959). Association of specific overt behaviour pattern with blood and cardiovascular findings. *Journal of the American Medical Association.* **169** *(12): 1286–1296.*

Friedman. M., Rosenman. R. (1974).Type-A Behaviour and Your Heart. *Wildwood House, London.*

Fromm, Erich (1978). To Have or To Be. *Abacus.*

Fromm, Erich (1993). The Art of Being. *Little, Brown.*

Gaarder, Jostein. (1991). Sophie's World. *Aschehoug.*

GMC. Good Medical Practice. 2024.

Good Schools Guide (The). *Lucas Publications.*

Good Will Hunting. (1997). *Miramax Films.*

Gray, John. (2005). Men are from Mars, Women are from Venus. *Harper Collins.*

Greer, Germaine (2007). The Whole Woman. *Black Swan.*

Gu-Seo, Myeong, Feldman, L.B. (2007). Being Emotional During Decision Msking – Good or Bad? An Empirical Investigation. *Acad. Manage J.; 50(4): 923–940.*

Habert, R., Claude Bernard. The Founder of Modern Medicine. *Cells (2022); 11(10):1702.*

Hall, Edward. (Prof. Antropology) (Jan. 1984). How to take Your Time. *Reader's Digest.*

Hall, Calvin. (1971). The Personality of a Child Molester. An Analysis of Dreams. *Routledge. ISBN: 9781315133805.*

Hanson, P. (1986) The Joy of Stress. *Pan Books.*

Hart, Carol T. (2025). Breastfeeding: Caring for New Mothers and Babies. MediCause.

Hazlitt,William (1819). Political Essays. Sketches of Public Characters. Printed for William Hone.

Herrnstein, R.J., Murray, C. (1994) The Bell Curve. Intelligence and Class Structure in American Life.*The Free Press.*

Hippocratic Writings. *Penguin Classics. 1978/1983*

Hlatky, M.A., Lam, L.C., Lee, K.L., et al. Job strain and the prevalence and outcome of CHD. *Circulation; 92:327-333.*

Hoel, Erik. (2021).The overfitted brain: dreams evolved to assist generalisation. *Patterns (n/Y); 2(5): 100244.*

Hofstadter, D.R. (1979). Gödel, Escher, Bach: An Eternal Golden Braid. *Penguin Books.*

Holmes, T. H., & Rahe, R. H. (1967). The Social Readjustment Rating Scale. *Journal of Psychosomatic Research, 11*(2), 213–218.

Homer. The Odyssey. *Book iv. Ryerson Univ. Toronto. 2022.*

Hope, Jane, Borin van Loon. Buddha for Beginners (1994). *Icon Books.*

Hublin. C., Kaprio, J., Partinen, M., Heikkila, K., Koskovuo, M. (1996) Daytime sleepiness in an adult Finnish population. *J.Int Med 239:417-423.*

Hume, David. Quoted by Bertrand Russell in *Human Society in Ethics and Politics.*

Hutton, Will (1996) The State We're In. *Vintage Books.*

Hwang, J-H., Lee, J-S. et al. (2023). Evaluation of viral infection as an etiology of ME/CFS: a systematic review and meta-analysis. *J. Transl. Med.; 21: 763.*

Illich, Ivan (1974) Energy and Equity. *Marion Boyars Publishers Ltd. London.* ISBN 0 7145 1058 0.

Jaušovec, M., Jaušovec, K. (2012). Working memory training: Improving intelligence – Changing brain activity. *Brain and Cognition; 79: 96-106.*

Javaheri, S., Redline, S. (2017). Insomnia and Risk of cardiovascular Disease. *Chest; 152(2): 435-444.*

Jevning, R., Wallace, R.K., et al. (1992). The physiology of meditation: a review. A wakeful hypometabolic integrated response. *Neuroscience and Biobehavioural Reviews; 16(3): 415-424.*

Jia, H., Zack, M.M. et al (2015). Impact of depression on quality-adjusted life expectancy (QALE) directly as well as indirectly through suicide. *Soc. Psychiatric Psychiatric Epidemiology; 50(6): 939-949.*

Johnson, Samuel Johnson and James Boswell (1775). A Journey to the Western Islands. *Penguin Books (1984). Edited by Peter Levi.*

Kahneman, Daniel. 2011. *Thinking, Fast and Slow.* Penguin. Random House.

Kaiser, R.G. (Sept. 1st. 1980). *Those Old Reaganisms May Be Brought Back to Haunt Him.* The Wahington Post.

Keller, L., Genoud, M. Extraordinary lifespans in ants: a test of evolutionary theories of ageing. *Nature* **389**, 958–960 (1997). h ttps://doi.org/10.1038/40130.

Kelly, E.L., Fiske, D.W. (1951) The Prediction of Performance in Clinical Psychology. *University of Chicago. Michigan University Press. Ann Arbor.*

Kipling, Rudyard (1901). 'Kim'. Macmillon. Later published by Wordsworth Classics (2009).

Kop, W. (2012) Somatic depressive symptoms, vital exhaustion, and fatigue: Divergent validity of overlapping constructs. Psychosom Med 74, 442–445.

Lesch, K.P., Bengal, D. et al.(1996) Association of anxiety-related traits with a polymorphism in the serotonin transporter gene regulatory region. *Science; 274(5292):1527-31.*

Lichstein, K.L., Wilson, N.M. et al. (1994). Daytime sleepiness in insomnia:Behavioural, Biological and Subjective Indices. *Sleep; 17(8):693-702.*

Lidell, Lucy. The Book of Yoga (1983). For the Sivananda Yoga Centre. *Ebury Press.*

Liedloff, Jean. (1975). The Continuum Concept. *Penguin Books. 1989.*

Luft.J., Ingham, H (1955). The Johari Window, a graphic model of interpersonal awareness. Proceedings of western training laboratory in group development. *University of California. Los Angeles.*

Maguire, E. A., Gadian, D.G., et al. (2000). Navigation-related structural change in the hippocampi of taxi drivers. *PNAS, 97, 4398–4403.*

Marmot, M.G., Smith. G.D. et al (1991). Health Inequalities among British civil servants: the Whitehall II study. *Lancet; 337(8754): 1387-93.*

Marmot, M.G., Smith, G.D. et al. (1997). Socio-economic Differentials in Health. *J. Health Psych; 2(3).*

Marmot, M.G., Bosma, H. et al (1997). Contribution of job control and other risk factors to social variations in coronary heart disease incidence. *Lancet; 350(9073):235-9).*

Mira López, E. (1943). Psychiatry in War. *Norton.*

Morin, C.M., Culbert, J.P., Schwartz, S.M. (1994). Nonpharmacological interventions for insomnia: a meta-analysis of treatment efficacy. *The American Journal of Psychiatry; 151(8):1172–1180.*

Morin, C.M., Vallières, A, et al. (2009) Cognitive behavioural therapy, singly and combined with medication, for persistent insomnia: a randomized controlled trial. *JAMA; 301 (19): 2005–2015.*

Morris, Dr. Desmond. (1996). *The Human Zoo: A Zoologist's Study of the Urban Animal* (Kodansha Globe) Paperback.

Nakamoto, R.K., Scanlon, J.A., Baylis, Al-Shawi, M.K. (2008). The Rotary Mechanism of the ATP Synthase. *Arch. Biochem. Biophys.; 476(1):43–50.*

Nixon, P.G. (1976). The Human Function Curve. With special reference to cardiovascular disorders. *Practitioner; 217(1302):935-44.*

Nesse.R.M., Williams. G.C. (1995), *Evolution and Healing: New Science of Darwinian Medicine.* J. Dent & Sons.

Pantev, C., Ross, B., et al. (2003). Music and learning-induced cortical plasticity. *Annals of the New York Academy of Sciences, 999, 438–450.*

Papillon. (1969). Henri Charrière. Robert Laffont.

Partinen, M., Putkonen, P.T.S., et al. (1982). Sleep disorders in relation to Coronary Heart Disease. *Acta Med. Scand.(Suppl). 660:69-83.*

Peck, M. Scott (1990). The Road Less Traveled. Section Two – Love. The Risk of Independence. *Arrow.*

Peggy Sue got Married (1987). Film. Director Francis Ford Coppola. *TriStar Pictures.*

Perls, Frederick.(1972). Gestalt Therapy. *Verbatim. Bantem Books.*

Plato. Phaedrus and Letters VII and VIII. (1973). *Penguin Classics.*

Plato. The Republic. Translated by Benjamin Jowett. *The World Publishing Company. 1946.*

Poulain, Michel (2012). The Longevity of Nuns and Monks. https://paa2012.populationassociation.org/papers/122836.

Rajabally, M. H. (1994). Florence Nightingale's Personality: A Psychoanalytic Profile. Int J Nurs Stud.:31(3):269-78.

Rees, W.D. & Lutkins, S.G. (1967). Mortality of Bereavement. *BMJ; 4: 13-16.*

Riemann, D. (2020). Hyperarousal and insomnia: state of the science. Sleep Med Rev. 2010;14(1):17.

Rosekind, M. R., Smith, R. M., et al. (1995). Alertness management: strategic naps in operational settings. *Journal of Sleep Research, 4(S2), 62–66.*

Russell, Bertrand (1954). Human Society in Ethics and Politics. George Allen and Unwin.

Sharpe, Robert, and David Lewis (1977). Thrive on Stress. How to Make it Work to Your Advantage. Souvenir Press.

Shootist, The. (1976). Film: *Paramount Pictures.*

Skynner, Robin, John Cleese (1983). Families and How to Survive Them. *Methuen. London.*

Solzhenitsyn, Alexandr I. (1973). The Gulag Archipelago. Harper and Row Publishers Inc. N.Y.

Quinlan, G., Mehmet Ali Döke, et al. (2023). Carbohydrate nutrition associated with health of overwintering honey bees. *Journal of Insect Science*; 23 (6): 16. doi: 10.1093/jisesa/iead084.

Rasheta, Noah. (2018). *No-Nonsense Buddhism for Beginners.* Calisto.

Sargent, W. (1967) The Unquiet Mind. *ISBN: 0 330 02635 6. Heinemann.*

Schultz, W. Fundamental Interpersonal Relations Orientation-Behaviour (FIRO-B). *British Psychological Society. DOI: https://doi.org/10.53841/bpstest.2018.firob.*

Searle, J., 1981, "Minds, Brains, and Programs," *Behavioral and Brain Sciences*, 3: 417–57.

Shakespeare, W. Julius Caesar. Brutus, Act 4, Scene 3.

Sharpe, Robert (1977). How to Thrive on Stress. How to make it work to your advantage. Profile Books Ltd.

Solantius, T., Rimpela, M. et al (1984). *The Threat of War in the minds of 12-18 year old in Finland. Lancet; 3232(8380): 784-785.*

Spartacus. (1966). Director: Stanley Kubrick. *Film: Universal International. Bryna Productions.*

Stratos Jets (2024): *https://www.stratosjets.com/blog/fear-of-fly ing-statistics-trends-facts/*

Stewart, J. (July 2022) Why are heart attack deaths 160% higher in some areas of England than others? Imperial News.

Tebecis, A.K. (1975). A controlled study of the EEG during transcendental meditation: comparison with hypnosis. *Folia Psychiatric Neurol. Japan; 29(4):305-313.*

Teilhard de Chardin, Pierre: Human Energy. *Collins 1969.*

Tolstoy, Leo. The Kreutzer Sonata and Other Stories. Penguin Classics(2008).

Turing, A., 1950, "Computing Machinery and Intelligence," *Mind*, 59 (236): 433–60.

Vanderbilt, William H. *New York Times, Oct 9, 1882, p. 1.*

Varghese N.E., Lugo A., et al. (2020) Sleep dissatisfaction and insufficient sleep duration in the Italian population. Sci. Rep .;10:17943. doi: 10.1038/s41598-020-72612-4.

Vazant, Iyanla. (1995). Acts of Faith: Daily Meditations for People of Colour. *Simon and Schuster.*

Watkins, Helen. (October 2025) When chest pain tells an emotional truth. BMJ; 391:r1898.

Wilde, Oscar (1891). Novella: The Picture of Dorian Grey.

Zukav, Gary. (1990). The Seat of the Soul. *Rider and Co. London.*

Index

B

C

deprived, 6, 129, 242, 274, 307, 360, 361, 370, 404, 405, 406, 407, 443, 447, 449, 450, 451, 469

deprived families, 447

deprived lives, 404

describe their true essence, 355

desensitisation, 181

deserters, 152

design, 7, 22, 52, 53, 61, 75, 77, 178, 255, 369, 428, 464

designer brands, 406

designer clothes, 231

Desmond Morris, 93, 332

desolation of defeat, 175

despair, 397

desperation, 182

despondency, 37, 397

destiny, 64, 95, 330, 352

detachment, 295, 466

Devil's Island, 169

devious, 171

devotional life, 175, 414

diabetes, 3, 26, 258, 268, 309, 319, 425, 427, 439, 461

E

F

H

J

jet-lagged, 415

Jewish, 27, 97, 141, 142, 149, 233, 236, 411, 470, 471

Jewish immortality, 141

Jews, 138, 142, 305, 338

Jim Fixx, 287

job strain, 533

Johari Window, The, 209

John F. Kennedy, 58, 257

Johnson, Samuel, 102, 534

joie de vivre, 22, 138

Jostein Gaarder, 487

Journey, The 487

joy, 16, 22, 37, 109, 212, 214, 215, 231, 259, 294, 311, 349, 354, 392, 408, 410, 469, 486

Judaism, 233, 411

Judeo-Christianity, 358

judgement, 156, 356

justice, 156

justification, 218, 381

juvenile mind, 197

K

Kahneman, Daniel, 4, 188

Kennedy, John F., 58, 257

Kennedy, Robert, 395

Kenny Nicholls, 108, 406

KGB, 162

kidney disease, 439

kindliness, 232, 410

kinins, 318

Kirk, Charlie, 297

knight's move thinking, 275

knighthood, 173

knowledge, 143, 365

knowledge and communication, 392

known self, 209

kudos, 173, 453

L

labelling, 273, 455

M

nature and nurture, 370

naval officer cadets, 351, 352

navigate other people, 179

Neanderthalensis, Homo, 178

nebula thinking, 57

need, 201

need for speed, 311

need to be included, 205

need to give, 206

need to impress, 133

need(s) (various), 2, 9, 26, 42, 43, 49, 59, 65, 67, 73, 100, 112, 113, 124, 139, 141, 164, 166, 170, 174, 194, 195, 199, 201, 202, 204, 205, 206, 207, 209, 213, 214, 215, 228, 231, 237, 241, 252, 261, 263, 273, 277, 280, 307, 326, 331, 341, 344, 345, 348, 355, 360, 366, 368, 369, 389, 392, 399, 408, 419, 435, 441, 452, 454, 461, 481, 490, 491, 495

needy, 129, 202, 335, 366

negative situations, 34

neighbour(s), 240, 344, 363, 368, 370, 385, 403, 407

nerds, 186, 198, 390

nerve endings, 184, 318

net gain, 233, 411

Netanyahu, B, 46

Q

T

U

vocation, 61, 62, 440, 458, 506, 507

vulnerability, 113, 250, 354

vulnerable, 53, 198, 225, 233, 472

W

Wabi Sabi, 50

waiting lists, 364, 418

wakefulness, 84, 103, 104, 261, 339, 430, 431, 482

Wall Street crash, 284

war, 174

warrior virtues, 156

warriors, 160, 407

wartime, 261, 289, 480

waste of time', 312

wasting time, 109, 296

wasting time, 227

Watergate, 47, 271

wax and wane, 103

way of life, 453

Wayne, John, 95, 340, 468

Y

Z

www.ingramcontent.com/pod-product-compliance
Lightning Source LLC
Chambersburg PA
CBHW050212270326
41914CB00003BA/380